OXFORD STATISTICAL SCIENCE SERIES

OXFORD STATISTICAL SCIENCE SERIES

1. A. C. Atkinson: *Plots, transformations, and regression*
2. M. Stone: *Coordinate-free multivariable statistics*
3. W. J. Krzanowski: *Principles of multivariate analysis: a user's perspective*
4. M. Aitkin, D. Anderson, B. Francis, and J. Hinde: *Statistical modelling in GLIM*
5. Peter J. Diggle: *Time series: a biostatistical introduction*
6. Howell Tong: *Non-linear time series: a dynamical system approach*
7. V. P. Godambe: *Estimating functions*
8. A. C. Atkinson and A. N. Donev: *Optimum and related models*
9. U. N. Bhat and I. V. Basawa: *Queuing and related models*
10. J. K. Lindsey: *Models for repeated measurements*
11. N. T. Longford: *Random coefficient models*
12. P. J. Brown: *Measurement, regression, and calibration*
13. Peter J. Diggle, Kung-Yee Liang, and Scott L. Zeger: *Analysis of longitudinal data*
14. J. I. Ansell and M. J. Phillips: *Practical methods for reliability data analysis*
15. J. K. Lindsey: *Modelling frequency and count data*
16. J. L. Jensen: *Saddlepoint approximations*
17. Steffen L. Lauritzen: *Graphical models*
18. A. W. Bowman and A. Azzalini: *Applied smoothing methods for data analysis*
19. J. K. Lindsey: *Models for repeated measurements* Second edition
20. Michael Evans and Tim Swartz: *Approximating integrals via Monte Carlo and deterministic methods*
21. D. F. Andrews and J. E. Stafford: *Symbolic computation for statistical inference*
22. T. A. Severini: *Likelihood methods in statistics*
23. W. J. Krzanowski: *Principles of multivariate analysis: a user's perspective* Updated edition
24. J. Durbin and S. J. Koopman: *Time series analysis by state space models*
25. Peter J. Diggle, Patrick J. Heagerty, Kung-Yee Liang, Scott L. Zeger: *Analysis of Longitudinal Data* Second edition
26. J. K. Lindsey: *Nonlinear models in medical statistics*
27. Peter J. Green, Nils L. Hjort, and Sylvia Richardson: *Highly structured stochastic systems*
28. Margaret S. Pepe: *Statistical evaluation of medical tests*

Analysis of Longitudinal Data

SECOND EDITION

PETER J. DIGGLE

Director, Medical Statistics Unit
Lancaster University

PATRICK J. HEAGERTY

Biostatistics Department
University of Washington

KUNG-YEE LIANG

and

SCOTT L. ZEGER

School of Hygiene & Public Health
Johns Hopkins University, Maryland

OXFORD
UNIVERSITY PRESS

OXFORD
UNIVERSITY PRESS

Great Clarendon Street, Oxford OX2 6DP

Oxford University Press is a department of the University of Oxford.
It furthers the University's objective of excellence in research, scholarship,
and education by publishing worldwide in

Oxford New York

Auckland Cape Town Dar es Salaam Hong Kong Karachi
Kuala Lumpur Madrid Melbourne Mexico City Nairobi
New Delhi Taipei Toronto Shanghai

With offices in

Argentina Austria Brazil Chile Czech Republic France Greece
Guatemala Hungary Italy Japan South Korea Poland Portugal
Singapore Switzerland Thailand Turkey Ukraine Vietnam

Published in the United States
by Oxford University Press Inc., New York

First edition 1994
Second edition 2002
Reprinted 2003, 2004

A catalogue record for this book is available from the British Library

Library of Congress Cataloging in Publication Data

(Data available)

ISBN 0 19 852484 6

10 9 8 7 6 5 4

Printed in Great Britain
on acid-free paper by
Biddles Ltd., King's Lynn, Norfolk

To Mandy, Claudia, Yung-Kuang, Joanne,
Jono, Hannah, Amelia, Margaret, Chao-Kang,
Chao-Wei, Max, and David

Preface

This book describes statistical models and methods for the analysis of longitudinal data, with a strong emphasis on applications in the biological and health sciences. The technical level of the book is roughly that of a first year postgraduate course in statistics. However, we have tried to write in such a way that readers with a lower level of technical knowledge, but experience of dealing with longitudinal data from an applied point of view, will be able to appreciate and evaluate the main ideas. Also, we hope that readers with interests across a wide spectrum of application areas will find the ideas relevant and interesting.

In classical univariate statistics, a basic assumption is that each of a number of subjects, or experimental units, gives rise to a single measurement on some relevant variable, termed the *response*. In multivariate statistics, the single measurement on each subject is replaced by a vector of measurements. For example, in a univariate medical study we might measure the blood pressure of each subject, whereas in a multivariate study we might measure blood pressure, heart-rate, temperature, and so on. In longitudinal studies, each subject again gives rise to a vector of measurements, but these now represent the same physical quantity measured at a sequence of observation times. Thus, for example, we might measure a subject's blood pressure on each of five successive days.

Longitudinal data therefore combine elements of multivariate and time series data. However, they differ from classical multivariate data in that the time series aspect of the data typically imparts a much more highly structured pattern of interdependence among measurements than for standard multivariate data sets; and they differ from classical time series data in consisting of a large number of short series, one from each subject, rather than a single, long series.

The book is organized as follows. The first three chapters provide an introduction to the subject, and cover basic issues of design and exploratory analysis. Chapters 4, 5, and 6 develop linear models and associated statistical methods for data sets in which the response variable is a continuous measurement. Chapters 7, 8, 9, 10, and 11 are concerned with generalized linear models for discrete response variables. Chapter 12 discusses the issues which arise when a variable which we wish to use as an explanatory variable in a longitudinal regression model is, in fact, a stochastic process which may interact with the response process in complex ways. Chapter 13 considers how to deal with missing values in longitudinal studies, with a focus on attrition or dropout, that is the premature permination of the intended sequences of measurements on some subjects. Chapter 14 gives a brief account of a number of additional topics. Appendix A is a short review of the statistical background assumed in the main body of the book.

We have chosen not to discuss software explicitly in the book. Many commercially available packages, for example Splus, MLn, SAS, Mplus or GENSTAT, include some facilities for longitudinal data analysis. However, none of the currently available packages contains enough facilities to cope with the full range of longitudinal data analysis problems which we cover in the book. For our own analyses, we have used the S system (Becker *et al.*, 1988; Chambers and Hastie, 1992) with additional user-defined functions for longitudinal data analysis and, more recently, the R system which is a publically available software environment not unlike Splus (see `www.r-project.org`).

We have also made a number of more substantial changes to the text. In particular, the chapter on missing values is now about three times the length of its counterpart in the first edition, and we have added three new chapters which reflect recent methodological developments.

Most of the data sets used in the book are in the public domain, and can be down-loaded from the first author's web-site, `http://www.maths.lancs.ac.uk/~diggle/` or from the second author's web-site, `http://faculty.washington.edu/heagerty/`.

The book remains incomplete, in the sense that it reflects our own knowledge and experience of longitudinal data problems as they have arisen in our work as biostatisticians. We are aware of other relevant work in econometrics, and in the social sciences more generally, but whilst we have included some references to this related work in the second edition, we have not attempted to cover it in detail.

Many friends and colleagues have helped us with this project. Patty Hubbard typed much of the book. Mary Joy Argo facilitated its production. Larry Magder, Daniel Tsou, Bev Mellen-Harrison, Beth Melton, John Hanfelt, Stirling Hilton, Larry Moulton, Nick Lange, Joanne Katz, Howard Mackey, Jon Wakefield, and Thomas Lumley gave assistance with computing, preparation of diagrams, and reading the draft. We gratefully acknowledge support from a Merck Development Grant to Johns Hopkins

University. In this second edition, we have corrected a number of typographical errors in the first edition and have tried to clarify some of our explanations. We thank those readers of the first edition who pointed out faults of both kinds, and accept responsibility for any remaining errors and obscurities.

Lancaster	P. J. D.
Seattle	P. J. H.
Baltimore	K. Y. L.
November 2001	S. L. Z.

Contents

1 Introduction 1
1.1 Longitudinal studies 1
1.2 Examples 3
1.3 Notation 15
1.4 Merits of longitudinal studies 16
1.5 Approaches to longitudinal data analysis 17
1.6 Organization of subsequent chapters 20

2 Design considerations 22
2.1 Introduction 22
2.2 Bias 22
2.3 Efficiency 24
2.4 Sample size calculations 26
2.4.1 Continuous responses 28
2.4.2 Binary responses 30
2.5 Further reading 31

3 Exploring longitudinal data 33
3.1 Introduction 33
3.2 Graphical presentation of longitudinal data 34
3.3 Fitting smooth curves to longitudinal data 41
3.4 Exploring correlation structure 46
3.5 Exploring association amongst categorical responses 52
3.6 Further reading 53

4 General linear models for longitudinal data 54
4.1 Motivation 54
4.2 The general linear model with correlated errors 55
4.2.1 The uniform correlation model 55
4.2.2 The exponential correlation model 56
4.2.3 Two-stage least-squares estimation and random effects models 57
4.3 Weighted least-squares estimation 59
4.4 Maximum likelihood estimation under Gaussian assumptions 64
4.5 Restricted maximum likelihood estimation 66
4.6 Robust estimation of standard errors 70

5 Parametric models for covariance structure 81
5.1 Introduction 81
5.2 Models 82
5.2.1 Pure serial correlation 84
5.2.2 Serial correlation plus measurement error 89
5.2.3 Random intercept plus serial correlation plus measurement error 90
5.2.4 Random effects plus measurement error 91
5.3 Model-fitting 93
5.3.1 Formulation 94
5.3.2 Estimation 95
5.3.3 Inference 97
5.3.4 Diagnostics 98
5.4 Examples 99
5.5 Estimation of individual trajectories 110
5.6 Further reading 113

6 Analysis of variance methods 114
6.1 Preliminaries 114
6.2 Time-by-time ANOVA 115
6.3 Derived variables 116
6.4 Repeated measures 123
6.5 Conclusions 125

7 Generalized linear models for longitudinal data 126
7.1 Marginal models 126
7.2 Random effects models 128
7.3 Transition (Markov) models 130
7.4 Contrasting approaches 131
7.5 Inferences 137

8 Marginal models 141
8.1 Introduction 141
8.2 Binary responses 142
8.2.1 The log-linear model 142
8.2.2 Log-linear models for marginal means 143
8.2.3 Generalized estimating equations 146
8.3 Examples 148
8.4 Counted responses 160
8.4.1 Parametric modelling for count data 160
8.4.2 Generalized estimating equation approach 162
8.5 Sample size calculations revisited 165
8.6 Further reading 167

9 Random effects models 169
9.1 Introduction 169
9.2 Estimation for generalized linear mixed models 171
9.2.1 Conditional likelihood 171
9.2.2 Maximum likelihood estimation 172
9.3 Logistic regression for binary responses 175
9.3.1 Conditional likelihood approach 175
9.3.2 Random effects models for binary data 178
9.3.3 Examples of logistic models with Gaussian random effects 180
9.4 Counted responses 184
9.4.1 Conditional likelihood method 184
9.4.2 Random effects models for counts 186
9.4.3 Poisson–Gaussian random effects models 188
9.5 Further reading 189

10 Transition models 190
10.1 General 190
10.2 Fitting transition models 192
10.3 Transition models for categorical data 194
10.3.1 Indonesian children's study example 197
10.3.2 Ordered categorical data 201
10.4 Log-linear transition models for count data 204
10.5 Further reading 206

11 Likelihood-based methods for categorical data 208
11.1 Introduction 208
11.1.1 Notation and definitions 209
11.2 Generalized linear mixed models 209
11.2.1 Maximum likelihood algorithms 212
11.2.2 Bayesian methods 214
11.3 Marginalized models 216
11.3.1 An example using the Gaussian linear model 218
11.3.2 Marginalized log-linear models 220
11.3.3 Marginalized latent variable models 222
11.3.4 Marginalized transition models 225
11.3.5 Summary 231
11.4 Examples 231
11.4.1 Crossover data 231
11.4.2 Madras schizophrenia data 234
11.5 Summary and further reading 243

12 Time-dependent covariates 245
12.1 Introduction 245
12.2 An example: the MSCM study 247

12.3 Stochastic covariates 253
12.3.1 Estimation issues with cross-sectional models 254
12.3.2 A simulation illustration 256
12.3.3 MSCM data and cross-sectional analysis 257
12.3.4 Summary 258
12.4 Lagged covariates 259
12.4.1 A single lagged covariate 259
12.4.2 Multiple lagged covariates 260
12.4.3 MSCM data and lagged covariates 261
12.4.4 Summary 265
12.5 Time-dependent confounders 265
12.5.1 Feedback: response is an intermediate and a confounder 266
12.5.2 MSCM data and endogeneity 268
12.5.3 Targets of inference 269
12.5.4 Estimation using *g*-computation 273
12.5.5 MSCM data and *g*-computation 275
12.5.6 Estimation using inverse probability of treatment weights (IPTW) 276
12.5.7 MSCM data and marginal structural models using IPTW 279
12.5.8 Summary 280
12.6 Summary and further reading 280

13 Missing values in longitudinal data 282
13.1 Introduction 282
13.2 Classification of missing value mechanisms 283
13.3 Intermittent missing values and dropouts 284
13.4 Simple solutions and their limitations 287
13.4.1 Last observation carried forward 287
13.4.2 Complete case analysis 288
13.5 Testing for completely random dropouts 288
13.6 Generalized estimating equations under a random missingness mechanism 293
13.7 Modelling the dropout process 295
13.7.1 Selection models 295
13.7.2 Pattern mixture models 299
13.7.3 Random effect models 301
13.7.4 Contrasting assumptions: a graphical representation 303
13.8 A longitudinal trial of drug therapies for schizophrenia 305
13.9 Discussion 316

14 Additional topics 319
14.1 Non-parametric modelling of the mean response 319
14.1.1 Further reading 326
14.2 Non-linear regression modelling 326
14.2.1 Correlated errors 328
14.2.2 Non-linear random effects 329
14.3 Joint modelling of longitudinal measurements and recurrent events 329
14.4 Multivariate longitudinal data 332

Appendix Statistical background 337
A.1 Introduction 337
A.2 The linear model and the method of least squares 337
A.3 Multivariate Gaussian theory 339
A.4 Likelihood inference 340
A.5 Generalized linear models 343
A.5.1 Logistic regression 343
A.5.2 Poisson regression 344
A.5.3 The general class 345
A.6 Quasi-likelihood 346

Bibliography 349

Index 369

1
Introduction

1.1 Longitudinal studies

The defining characteristic of a longitudinal study is that individuals are measured repeatedly through time. Longitudinal studies are in contrast to cross-sectional studies, in which a single outcome is measured for each individual. While it is often possible to address the same scientific questions with a longitudinal or cross-sectional study, the major advantage of the former is its capacity to separate what in the context of population studies are called *cohort* and *age* effects. The idea is illustrated in Fig. 1.1. In Fig. 1.1(a), reading ability is plotted against age for a hypothetical cross-sectional study of children. Reading ability appears to be poorer among older children; little else can be said. In Fig. 1.1(b), we suppose the same data were obtained in a longitudinal study in which each individual was measured twice. Now it is clear that while younger children began at a higher reading level, everyone improved with time. Such a pattern might have resulted from introducing elementary education into a poor rural community beginning with the younger children. If the data set were as in Fig. 1.1(c), a different explanation would be required. The cross-sectional and longitudinal patterns now tell the same unusual story – that reading ability deteriorates with age.

The point of this example is that longitudinal studies (Fig. 1.1(b) and (c)) can distinguish changes over time within individuals (ageing effects) from differences among people in their baseline levels (cohort effects). Cross-sectional studies cannot. This concept is developed in more detail in Section 1.4.

In some studies, a third timescale the *period*, or calendar date of a measurement, is also important. Any two of age, period, and cohort determine the third. For example, an individual's age and birth cohort at a given measurement determine the date. Analyses which must consider all three scales require external assumptions which unfortunately are difficult to validate. See Mason and Feinberg (1985) for details.

Longitudinal data can be collected either prospectively, following subjects forward in time, or retrospectively, by extracting multiple

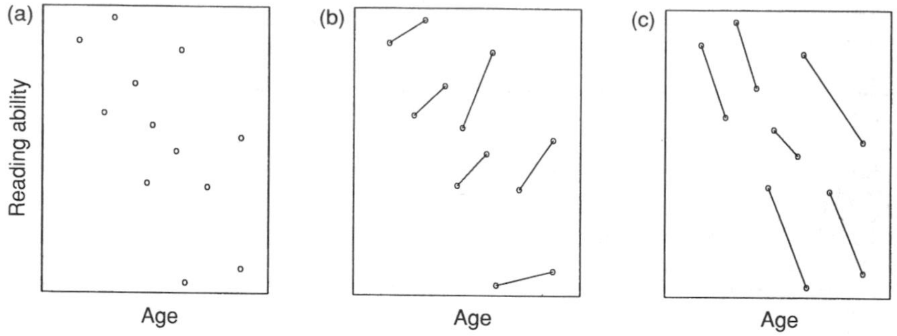

Fig. 1.1. Hypothetical data on the relationship between reading ability and age.

measurements on each person from historical records. The statistical methods discussed in this book apply to both situations. Longitudinal data are more commonly collected prospectively since the quality of repeated measurements collected from past records or from a person's recollection may be inferior (Goldfarb, 1960).

Clinical trials are prospective studies which often have time to a clinical outcome as the principal response. The dependence of this univariate measure on treatment and other factors is the subject of *survival analysis* (Cox, 1972). This book does not discuss survival problems. The interested reader is referred to Cox and Oakes (1984) or Kalbfleisch and Prentice (1980).

The defining feature of a longitudinal data set is repeated observations on individuals enabling direct study of change. Longitudinal data require special statistical methods because the set of observations on one subject tends to be intercorrelated. This correlation must be taken into account to draw valid scientific inferences.

The issue of accounting for correlation also arises when analysing a single long *time series* of measurements. Diggle (1990) discusses time series analysis in the biological sciences. Analysis of longitudinal data tends to be simpler because subjects can usually be assumed independent. Valid inferences can be made by borrowing strength across people. That is, the consistency of a pattern across subjects is the basis for substantive conclusions. For this reason, inferences from longitudinal studies can be made more robust to model assumptions than those from time series data, particularly to assumptions about the nature of the correlation.

Sociologists and economists often refer to longitudinal studies as *panel studies*. Although many of the statistical methods which we discuss in this book will be applicable to the analysis of data from the social sciences, our emphasis is firmly motivated by our experience of longitudinal data problems arising in the biological health sciences. A somewhat different emphasis would have been appropriate for many social science applications, and is reflected in books written with such applications in mind. See, for example, Goldstein (1979), Plewis (1985), or Heckman and Singer (1985).

1.2 Examples

We now introduce seven longitudinal data sets to illustrate the kinds of scientific and statistical issues which arise with longitudinal studies. These and other data sets will be used throughout the book for illustration of the relevant methodology. The examples have been chosen from the biological and health sciences to represent a range of challenges for analysis. After presenting each data set, common and distinguishing features are discussed.

Example 1.1. CD4+ cell numbers

The human immune deficiency virus (HIV) causes AIDS by reducing a person's ability to fight infection. HIV attacks an immune cell called the CD4+ cell which orchestrates the body's immunoresponse to infectious agents. An uninfected individual has around 1100 cells per millilitre of blood. CD4+ cells decrease in number with time from infection so that an infected person's CD4+ cell number can be used to monitor disease progression. Figure 1.2 displays 2376 values of CD4+ cell number plotted against time since seroconversion (time when HIV becomes detectable) for 369 infected men enrolled in the Multicenter AIDS Cohort Study or MACS (Kaslow *et al.*, 1987).

In Fig. 1.2, repeated measurements for some individuals are connected to accentuate the longitudinal nature of the study. An important objective

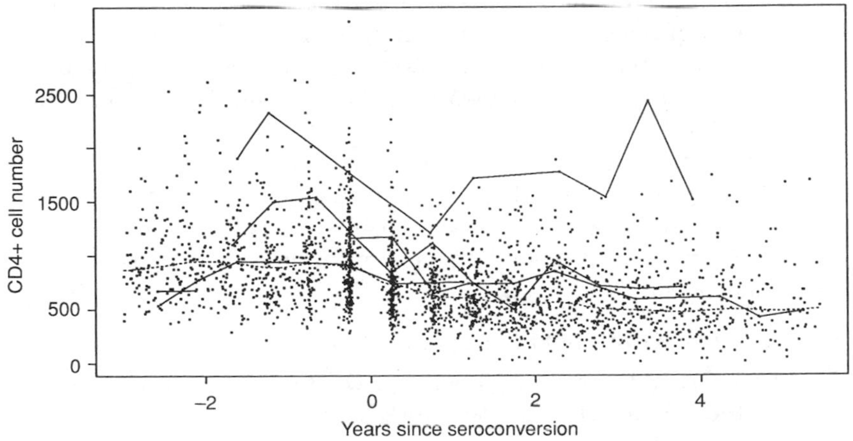

Fig. 1.2. Relationship between CD4+ cell numbers and time since seroconversion due to infection with the HIV virus. · : individual counts; ——: sequences of measurements for randomly selected subjects; ....: lowess curve.

of MACS is to characterize the typical time course of CD4+ cell depletion. This helps to clarify the interaction of HIV with the immune system and can assist when counselling infected men. A non-parametric smooth curve (Zeger and Diggle, 1994) has been added to the figure to highlight the average trend. Note that the average CD4+ cell number is constant until the time of seroconversion and then decreases, more quickly at first.

Objectives of a longitudinal analysis of these data are to

(1) estimate the average time course of CD4+ cell depletion;

(2) estimate the time course for individual men taking account of the measurement error in CD4+ cell determinations;

(3) characterize the degree of heterogeneity across men in the rate of progression;

(4) identify factors which predict CD4+ cell changes.

Example 1.2. Indonesian children's health study

Alfred Sommer and colleagues conducted a study (which we will refer to as the Indonesian Children's Health Study or ICHS) in the Aceh province of Indonesia to determine the causes and effects of vitamin A deficiency in pre-school children (Sommer, 1982). Over 3000 children were medically examined quarterly for up to six visits to assess whether they suffered from respiratory or diarrhoeal infection and xerophthalmia, an ocular manifestation of vitamin A deficiency. Weight and height were also measured. We will focus on the question of whether vitamin A deficient children are at increased risk of respiratory infection, one of the leading causes of morbidity and mortality in children from the developing world. Such a relationship is plausible because vitamin A is required for the integrity of epithelial cells, the first line of defence against infection in the respiratory tract. It has public health significance because vitamin A deficiency can be eliminated by diet modification or if necessary by food fortification for only a few pence per child per year.

The data on 275 children are summarized in Table 1.1. The objectives of analysis are to estimate the increase in risk of respiratory infection for children who are vitamin A deficient while controlling for other demographic factors, and to estimate the degree of heterogeneity in the risk of disease among children.

Example 1.3. Growth of Sitka spruce

Dr Peter Lucas of the Biological Sciences Division at Lancaster University provided these data on the growth of Sitka spruce trees. The study objective is to assess the effect of ozone pollution on tree growth. As ozone pollution is common in urban areas, the impact of increased ozone concentrations on tree growth is of considerable interest. The response variable is log tree size, where size is conventionally measured by the product of tree height

Table 1.1. Summary of 1200 observations of respiratory infection (RI), xerophthalmia and age on 275 children from the ICHS (Sommer, 1982).

		Age						
Xerophthalmia	RI	1	2	3	4	5	6	7
No	No	90	236	330	176	143	65	5
	Yes	8	36	39	9	7	1	0
Yes	No	0	2	18	15	8	4	1
	Yes	0	0	7	0	0	0	0

and diameter squared. The data for 79 trees over two growing seasons are listed in Table 1.2, and displayed graphically in Fig. 1.3. A total of 54 trees were grown with ozone exposure at 70 ppb; 25 were grown under control conditions. The objective is to compare the growth patterns of trees under the two conditions.

In Fig. 1.3, two features are immediately obvious. Firstly, the trees are indeed growing over the duration of the experiment – the mean size is an increasing function of time. The one or two exceptions to this general rule could reflect random variation about the mean or, less interestingly from a scientific point of view, errors of measurement. Secondly, the trees tend to preserve their rank order throughout the study – trees which are relatively large at the start tend to be relatively large always. This phenomenon, a by-product of a component of random variation between experimental units, is very common in longitudinal data and should feature in the formulation of any general class of models.

Example 1.4. Protein content of milk

In this example, milk was collected weekly from 79 Australian cows and analysed for its protein content. The cows were maintained on one of three diets: barley, a mixture of barley and lupins, or lupins alone. The data were provided by Ms Alison Frensham, and are listed in Table 1.3. Figure 1.4 displays the three subsets of the data corresponding to each of the three diets. The repeated measurements on each animal are joined to accentuate the longitudinal nature of the data set. The objective of the study is to determine how diet affects the protein in milk. It appears from the figure that barley gives higher values than the mixture, which in turn gives higher values than lupins alone. A plot of the average traces for each group (Diggle, 1990) confirms this pattern. One problem with simple inferences, however, is that in this example, time is measured in weeks since calving, and

Table 1.2. Measurements of log-size for Sitka spruce trees grown in normal or ozone-enriched environments. Within each year, the data are organized in four blocks, corresponding to four controlled environment chambers. The first two chambers, containing 27 trees each, have an ozone-enriched atmosphere, the remaining two, containing 12 and 13 trees respectively, have a normal (control) atmosphere. Data below are from the first chamber only.

Time in days since 1 January 1988												
152	174	201	227	258	469	496	528	556	579	613	639	674
4.51	4.98	5.41	5.9	6.15	6.16	6.18	6.48	6.65	6.87	6.95	6.99	7.04
4.24	4.2	4.68	4.92	4.96	5.2	5.22	5.39	5.65	5.71	5.78	5.82	5.85
3.98	4.36	4.79	4.99	5.03	5.87	5.88	6.04	6.34	6.49	6.58	6.65	6.61
4.36	4.77	5.1	5.3	5.36	5.53	5.56	5.68	5.93	6.21	6.26	6.2	6.19
4.34	4.95	5.42	5.97	6.28	6.5	6.5	6.79	6.83	7.1	7.17	7.21	7.16
4.59	5.08	5.36	5.76	6	6.33	6.34	6.39	6.78	6.91	6.99	7.01	7.05
4.41	4.56	4.95	5.23	5.33	6.13	6.14	6.36	6.57	6.78	6.82	6.81	6.86
4.24	4.64	4.95	5.38	5.48	5.61	5.63	5.82	6.18	6.42	6.48	6.47	6.46
4.82	5.17	5.76	6.12	6.24	6.48	6.5	6.77	7.14	7.26	7.3	6.91	7.28
3.84	4.17	4.67	4.67	4.8	4.94	4.94	5.05	5.33	5.53	5.56	5.57	5.6
4.07	4.31	4.9	5.1	5.1	5.26	5.26	5.38	5.66	5.81	5.84	5.93	5.89
4.28	4.8	5.27	5.55	5.65	5.76	5.77	5.98	6.18	6.39	6.43	6.44	6.41
4.47	4.89	5.23	5.55	5.74	5.99	6.01	6.08	6.39	6.45	6.57	6.57	6.58
4.46	4.84	5.11	5.34	5.46	5.47	5.49	5.7	5.93	6.06	6.15	6.12	6.12
4.6	4.08	4.17	4.35	4.59	4.65	4.69	5.01	5.21	5.38	5.58	5.46	5.5
3.73	4.15	4.61	4.87	4.93	5.24	5.25	5.25	5.45	5.65	5.65	5.76	5.83
4.67	4.88	5.18	5.34	5.49	6.44	6.44	6.61	6.74	7.06	7.11	7.04	7.11
2.96	3.47	3.76	3.89	4.3	4.15	4.15	4.41	4.72	4.76	4.93	4.98	5.07
3.24	3.93	4.76	4.62	4.64	4.63	4.64	4.77	5.08	5.27	5.3	5.43	5.2
4.36	4.77	5.02	5.26	5.45	5.44	5.44	5.49	5.73	5.77	6.01	5.96	5.96
4.04	4.64	4.86	5.09	5.25	5.25	5.27	5.5	5.65	5.69	5.97	5.97	5.89
3.53	4.25	4.68	4.97	5.18	5.64	5.64	5.53	5.74	5.78	5.94	6.18	5.99
4.22	4.69	5.07	5.37	5.58	5.76	5.8	6.11	6.37	6.35	6.58	6.55	6.55
2.79	3.1	3.3	3.38	3.55	3.61	3.65	3.93	4.18	4.13	4.36	4.43	4.39
3.3	3.9	4.34	4.96	5.4	5.46	5.49	5.77	6.03	6.07	6.2	6.26	6.28
3.34	3.81	4.21	4.54	4.86	4.93	4.96	5.15	5.48	5.49	5.7	5.74	5.74
3.76	4.36	4.7	5.44	5.32	5.65	5.67	5.63	6.04	6.02	6.05	6.03	5.91

the experiment was terminated 19 weeks after the earliest calving. Thus, about half of the 79 sequences of milk protein measurements are incomplete. Calving date may well be associated, directly or indirectly, with the physiological processes that also determine protein content. If this is the case, the missing observations should not be ignored in inference. This issue is taken up in Chapter 11.

Note how the multitude of lines in Fig. 1.4 confuses the group comparison. On the other hand, the lines are useful to show the variability across

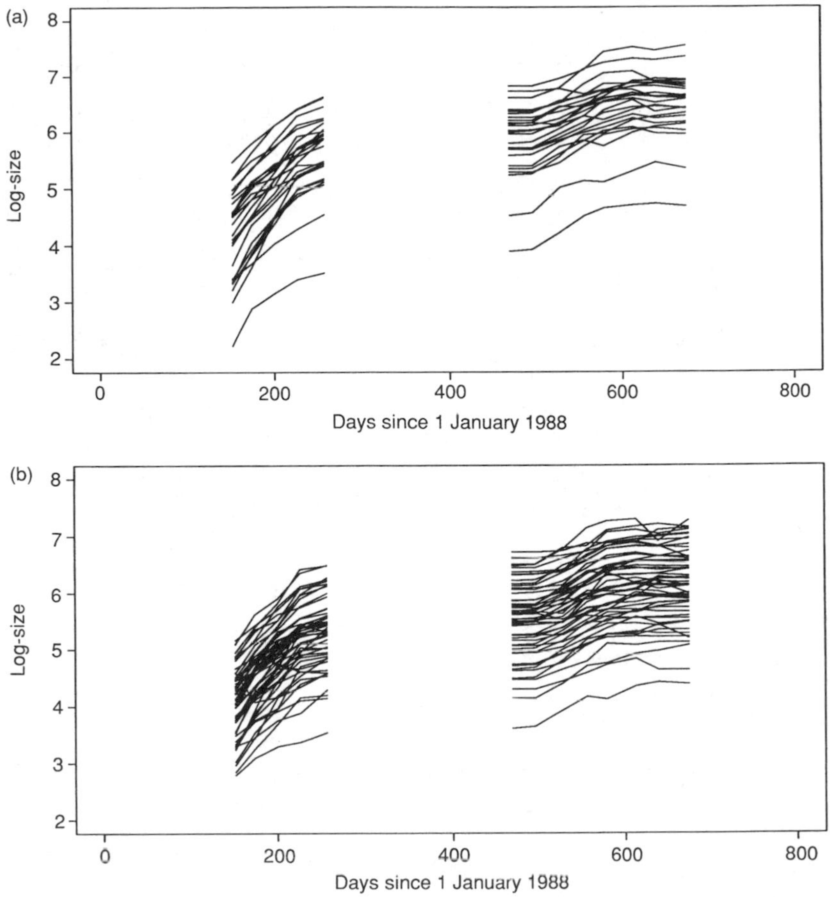

Fig. 1.3. Log-size of 79 Sitka spruce over two growing seasons: (a) control; (b) ozone-treated.

time and among individuals. Chapter 3 discusses compromise displays which more effectively capture patterns in longitudinal data.

Example 1.5. Crossover trial

Jones and Kenward (1987) report a data set from a three-period crossover trial of an analgesic drug for relieving pain from primary dysmenorrhoea (menstrual cramps). Three levels of the analgesic (control, low and high) were given to each of 86 women. Women were randomized to one of the six possible orders for administering the three treatment levels so that the effect of the prior treatment on the current response or *carry-over effect* could be assessed. Table 1.4 is a cross-tabulation of the eight possible outcome categories with the six orderings. Ignoring for now the

Table 1.3. Percentage protein content of milk samples taken at weekly intervals. In the original experiment, 79 cows were allocated at random amongst three diets. cows 1–25, barley; cows 26–52, barley + lupins; cows 53–79, lupins. Data below are from the barley diet only. 9.99 signifies missing.

3.63	3.57	3.47	3.65	3.89	3.73	3.77	3.90	3.78	3.82	3.83	3.71	4.10	4.02	4.13	4.08	4.22	4.44	4.30
3.24	3.25	3.29	3.09	3.38	3.33	3.00	3.16	3.34	3.32	3.31	3.27	3.41	3.45	3.12	3.42	3.40	3.17	3.00
3.98	3.60	3.43	3.30	3.29	3.25	2.93	3.20	3.27	3.22	2.93	2.92	2.82	2.64	9.99	9.99	9.99	9.99	9.99
3.66	3.50	3.05	2.90	2.72	3.11	3.05	2.80	3.20	3.18	3.14	3.18	3.24	3.37	3.30	3.40	3.35	3.28	9.99
4.34	3.76	3.68	3.51	3.45	3.53	3.60	3.77	3.90	3.87	3.61	3.85	3.94	3.87	3.60	3.06	3.47	3.50	3.42
4.36	3.71	3.42	3.95	4.06	3.73	3.92	3.99	3.70	3.88	3.71	3.62	3.74	3.42	9.99	9.99	9.99	9.99	9.99
4.17	3.60	3.52	3.10	3.78	3.42	3.66	3.64	3.83	3.73	3.72	3.65	3.50	3.32	2.95	3.34	3.51	3.17	9.99
4.40	3.86	3.56	3.32	3.64	3.57	3.47	3.97	9.99	3.78	3.98	3.90	4.05	4.06	4.05	3.92	3.65	3.60	3.74
3.40	3.42	3.51	3.39	3.35	3.13	3.21	3.50	3.55	3.28	3.75	3.55	3.53	3.52	3.77	3.77	3.74	4.00	3.87
3.75	3.89	3.65	3.42	3.32	3.27	3.34	3.35	3.09	3.65	3.53	3.50	3.63	3.91	3.73	3.71	4.18	3.97	4.06
4.20	3.59	3.55	3.27	3.19	3.60	3.50	3.55	3.60	3.75	3.75	3.75	3.89	3.87	3.60	3.68	3.68	3.56	3.34
4.02	3.76	3.60	3.53	3.95	3.26	3.73	3.96	9.99	3.70	9.99	3.45	3.50	3.13	9.99	9.99	9.99	9.99	9.99
4.02	3.90	3.73	3.55	3.71	3.40	3.49	3.74	3.61	3.42	3.46	3.40	3.38	3.13	9.99	9.99	9.99	9.99	9.99
3.90	3.33	3.25	3.22	3.35	3.24	3.16	3.33	3.12	2.93	2.84	3.07	3.02	2.75	9.99	9.99	9.99	9.99	9.99
3.81	4.00	3.57	3.47	3.52	3.63	3.45	3.50	3.71	3.55	3.13	3.04	3.31	3.22	2.92	9.99	9.99	9.99	9.99
3.62	3.22	3.62	3.02	3.28	3.15	3.52	3.22	3.45	3.51	3.38	3.00	2.94	3.52	3.48	3.02	9.99	9.99	9.99
3.66	3.66	3.28	3.10	2.66	3.00	3.15	3.01	3.50	3.29	3.16	3.33	3.50	3.46	3.48	3.98	3.70	3.36	3.55
4.44	3.85	3.55	3.22	3.40	3.28	3.42	3.35	3.01	3.55	3.70	3.73	3.65	3.78	3.82	3.75	3.95	3.85	3.72
4.23	3.75	3.82	3.60	4.09	3.84	3.62	3.36	3.65	3.41	3.15	3.68	3.54	3.75	3.72	4.05	3.60	3.88	3.98
3.82	9.99	3.27	3.33	3.25	2.97	3.57	3.43	3.50	3.58	3.70	3.55	3.58	3.70	3.60	3.42	3.33	3.53	3.40
3.53	3.10	3.90	3.48	3.35	3.35	3.65	3.56	3.27	3.61	3.66	3.47	3.34	3.32	3.22	3.18	9.99	9.99	9.99
4.47	3.86	3.34	3.49	3.74	3.24	3.71	3.46	3.88	3.60	4.00	3.83	3.80	4.12	3.98	3.77	3.52	3.50	3.42
3.93	3.79	3.68	3.58	3.76	3.66	3.57	3.85	3.75	3.37	3.00	3.24	3.44	3.23	9.99	9.99	9.99	9.99	9.99
3.27	3.84	3.46	3.44	3.40	3.50	3.63	3.47	3.32	3.47	3.40	3.27	3.74	3.76	3.68	3.68	3.93	3.80	3.52
3.32	3.61	3.25	3.48	3.58	3.47	3.60	3.51	3.74	3.50	3.08	2.77	3.22	3.35	3.14	9.99	9.99	9.99	9.99

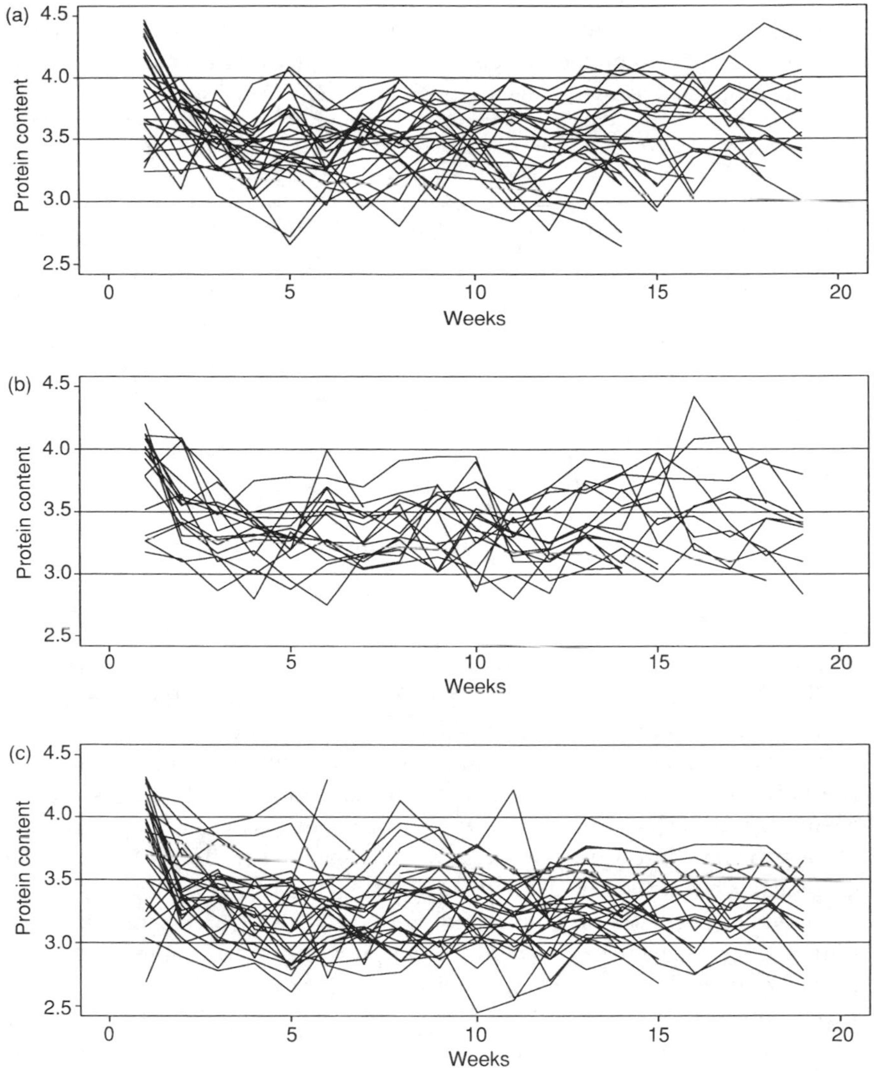

Fig. 1.4. Protein content of milk samples from 79 cows: (a) barley diet (25 cows); (b) mixed diet (27 cows); (c) lupins diet (27 cows).

order of treatment, pain was relieved for 22 women (26%) on placebo, 61 (71%) on low analgesic, and 69 (80%) on high analgesic. This pattern is consistent with the treatment being beneficial. However, there may be carry-over or other treatment by period interactions which can also explain the observed pattern. This must be determined in a longitudinal data analysis.

Table 1.4. Number of patients for each treatment and response sequence in three-period crossover trial of analgesic treatment for pain from primary dysmenorrhoea (Jones and Kenward, 1987).

Treatment sequence*	Response sequence in periods 1, 2, 3 (0 = no relief; 1 = relief)								
	000	100	010	001	110	101	011	111	Total
012	0	0	2	2	1	0	9	1	15
021	2	1	0	0	0	0	9	4	16
102	0	1	1	1	0	8	3	1	15
120	0	1	1	1	8	0	0	1	12
201	3	0	0	0	1	7	2	1	14
210	1	5	0	0	4	3	1	0	14
Total	6	8	4	4	14	18	24	8	86

*Treatment: 0 = placebo; 1 = low; 2 = high analgesic.

Example 1.6. Epileptic seizures

This example comprises data from a clinical trial of 59 epileptics, analysed by Thall and Vail (1990) and by Breslow and Clayton (1993). For each patient, the number of epileptic seizures was recorded during a baseline period of eight weeks. Patients were then randomized to treatment with the anti-epileptic drug progabide, or to placebo in addition to standard chemotherapy. The number of seizures was then recorded in four consecutive two-week intervals. These data are reprinted in Table 1.5, and are graphically displayed using boxplots (Tukey, 1977) in Fig. 1.5. The medical question is whether the progabide reduces the rate of epileptic seizures. Figure 1.5 is suggestive of a small reduction in the average number except, possibly, at week two. Inferences must take into account the very strong variation among people in the baseline level of seizures, which appears to persist across time. In this case, the natural heterogeneity in rates will facilitate the detection of a treatment effect as will be discussed in later chapters.

Example 1.7. A clinical trial of drug therapies for schizophrenia

Our final example considers data from a randomized clinical trial comparing different drug regimes in the treatment of chronic schizophrenia. The data were provided by Dr Peter Ouyang, Janssen Research Foundation.

We have data from 523 patients, randomly allocated amongst the following six treatments: placebo, haloperidol 20 mg and risperidone at dose levels 2, 6, 10, and 16 mg. Haloperidol is regarded as a standard therapy. Risperidone is described as ‘a novel chemical compound with useful

Table 1.5. Four successive two-week seizure counts for each of 59 epileptics. Covariates are adjuvant treatment (0 = placebo, 1 = progabide), eight-week baseline seizure counts, and age (in years).

Y_1	Y_2	Y_3	Y_4	Trt.	Base	Age	Y_1	Y_2	Y_3	Y_4	Trt.	Base	Age
5	3	3	3	0	11	31	0	4	3	0	1	19	20
3	5	3	3	0	11	30	3	6	1	3	1	10	20
2	4	0	5	0	6	25	2	6	7	4	1	19	18
4	4	1	4	0	8	36	4	3	1	3	1	24	24
7	18	9	21	0	66	22	22	17	19	16	1	31	30
5	2	8	7	0	27	29	5	4	7	4	1	14	35
6	4	0	2	0	12	31	2	4	0	4	1	11	57
40	20	23	12	0	52	42	3	7	7	7	1	67	20
5	6	6	5	0	23	37	4	18	2	5	1	41	22
14	13	6	0	0	10	28	2	1	1	0	1	7	28
26	12	6	22	0	52	36	0	2	4	0	1	22	23
12	6	8	5	0	33	24	5	4	0	3	1	13	40
4	4	6	2	0	18	23	11	14	25	15	1	46	43
7	9	12	14	0	42	36	10	5	3	8	1	36	21
16	24	10	9	0	87	26	19	7	6	7	1	38	35
11	0	0	5	0	50	26	1	1	2	4	1	7	25
0	0	3	3	0	18	28	6	10	8	8	1	36	26
37	29	28	29	0	111	31	2	1	0	0	1	11	25
3	5	2	5	0	18	32	102	65	72	63	1	151	22
3	0	6	7	0	20	21	4	3	2	4	1	22	32
3	4	3	4	0	12	29	8	6	5	7	1	42	25
3	4	3	4	0	9	21	1	3	1	5	1	32	35
2	3	3	5	0	17	32	18	11	28	13	1	56	21
8	12	2	8	0	28	25	6	3	4	0	1	24	41
18	24	76	25	0	55	30	3	5	4	3	1	16	32
2	1	2	1	0	9	40	1	23	19	8	1	22	26
3	1	4	2	0	10	19	2	3	0	1	1	25	21
13	15	13	12	0	47	22	0	0	0	0	1	13	36
11	14	9	8	1	76	18	1	4	3	2	1	12	37
8	7	9	4	1	38	32							

pharmacological characteristics, as has been demonstrated in *in vitro* and *in vivo* experiments.' The primary response variable was the total score obtained on the Positive and Negative Symptom Rating Scale (PANSS), a measure of psychiatric disorder. The study design specified that this score should be taken at weeks −1, 0, 1, 2, 4, 6, and 8, where −1 refers to selection into the trial and 0 refers to baseline. The week between selection and baseline was used to establish a stable regime of medication for each patient. Eligibility criteria included: age between 18 and 65; good general health; total score at selection between 60 and 120. A reduction of 20 in the mean score was regarded as demonstrating a clinical improvement.

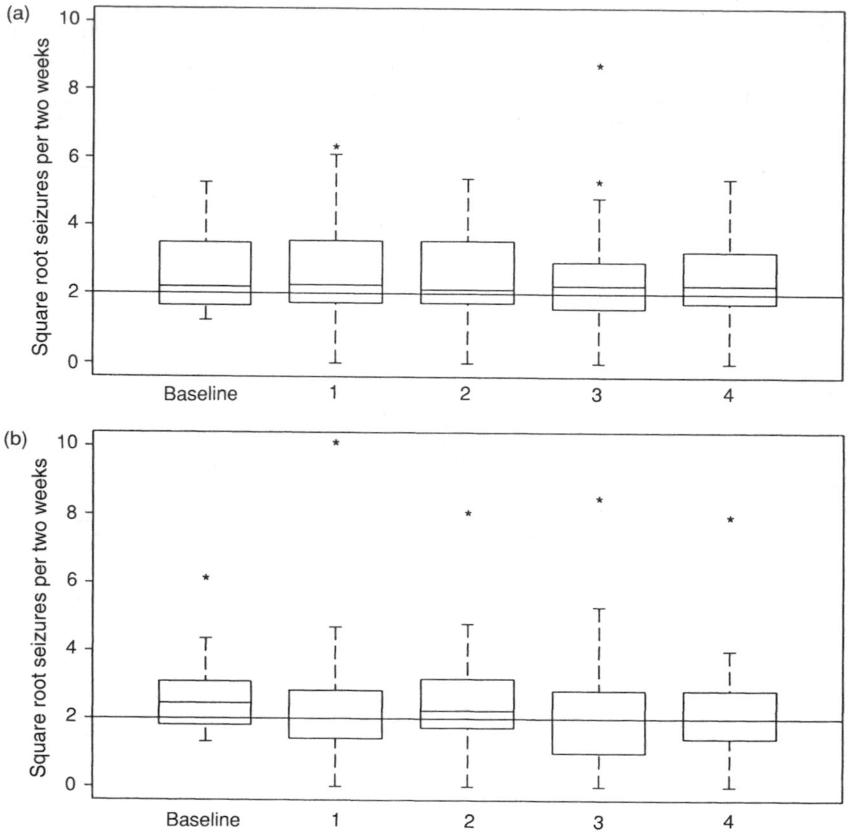

Fig. 1.5. Boxplots of square-root-transformed seizure rates for epileptics at baseline and for four subsequent two-week periods: (a) placebo; (b) progabide-treated.

Of the 523 patients, only 253 are listed as completing the study, although a further 16 provided a complete sequence of PANSS scores as the criterion for completion included a follow-up interview. Table 1.6 gives the distribution of the stated reasons for dropout. Table 1.7 gives the numbers of dropouts and completers in each of the six treatment groups. The most common reason for dropout is 'inadequate response', which accounts for 183 out of the 270 dropouts. The highest dropout rate occurs in the placebo group, followed by the haloperidol group and the lowest dose risperidone group. One patient provided no data at all after the selection visit, and was not considered further in the analysis.

Figure 1.6 shows the observed mean response as a function of time within each treatment group, that is each average is over those patients who have not yet dropped out. All six groups show a mean response profile with

Table 1.6. Frequency distribution of reasons for dropout in the clinical trial of drug therapies for schizophrenia.

Abnormal lab result	4
Adverse experience	26
Inadequate response	183
Inter-current illness	3
Lost to follow-up	3
Other reason	7
Uncooperative	25
Withdrew consent	19

Table 1.7. Numbers of dropouts and completers by treatment group in the schizophrenia trial. The treatment codes are: p = placebo, h = haloperidol 20 mg, r2 = risperidone 2 mg, r6 = risperidone 6 mg, r10 = risperidone 10 mg, r16 = risperidone 16 mg.

	p	h	r2	r6	r10	r16	Total
Dropouts	61	51	51	34	39	34	270
Completers	27	36	36	52	48	54	253
Total	88	87	87	86	87	88	523

the following features: increasing between selection and baseline; decreasing post-baseline; slower rate of decrease towards the end of the study. The mean response in the placebo group shows a much smaller overall decrease than any of the five active treatment groups. The risperidone treatments all show a faster rate of decrease than haloperidol initially, but the final mean responses for all five active treatment groups are similar. The overall reduction in mean response within each active treatment group is very roughly from 90 to 70, which appears to meet the criterion for clinical improvement. However, at each time-point these observed means are, necessarily, calculated only from those subjects who have not yet dropped out of the study, and should therefore be interpreted as conditional means. As we shall see in Chapter 13, these conditional means may be substantially different from the means which are estimated in an analysis of the data which ignores the dropout problem.

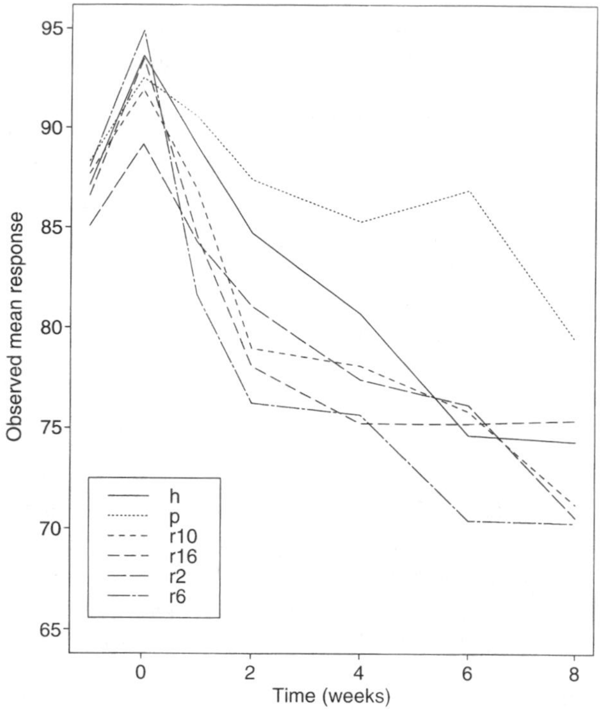

Fig. 1.6. Observed mean response profiles for the schizophrenia trial data. The treatment codes are: p = placebo, h = haloperidol 20 mg, r2 = risperidone 2 mg, r6 = risperidone 6 mg, r10 = risperidone 10 mg, r16 = risperidone 16 mg.

In all seven examples, there are repeated observations on each experimental unit. The units can reasonably be assumed independent of one another, but the multiple responses within each unit are likely to be correlated. The scientific objectives of each study can be formulated as regression problems whose purpose is to describe the dependence of the response on explanatory variables.

There are important differences among the examples as well. The responses in Examples 1.1 (CD4+ cells), 1.3 (tree size), 1.4 (protein content), and 1.7 (schizophrenia trial) are continuous variables which, perhaps after transformation, can be adequately described by linear statistical models. However, the response is binary in Examples 1.2 (respiratory disease) and 1.5 (presence of pain); and is a count in Example 1.6 (number of seizures). Linear models will not suffice here. The choice of statistical model must depend on the type of outcome variable. Second, the relative magnitudes of the number of experimental units and number of observations per unit vary across the six examples. For example, the ICHS had over 3000 participants with at most seven observations per person. The Sitka spruce data set includes only 79 trees, each with 23 measurements. Finally, the objectives of the studies differ. For example, in the CD4+ data set, inferences are to be made about the individual subject so that counselling can be provided, whereas in the crossover trial, the average response in the population for each of the two treatments is the focus. These differences influence the specific approach to analysis as discussed in detail throughout the book.

1.3 Notation

To the extent possible, the book will describe in words the major ideas underlying longitudinal data analysis. However, details and precise statements often require a mathematical formulation. This section presents the notation to be followed.

In general, we will use capital letters to represent random variables or matrices, relying on the context to distinguish the two, and small letters for specific observations. Scalars and matrices will be in normal type, vectors will be in bold type.

Turning to specific points of notation, we let Y_{ij} represent a response variable and $\boldsymbol{x}_{ij}$ a vector of length p (p-vector) of explanatory variables observed at time t_{ij}, for observation $j = 1, \dots, n_i$ on subject $i = 1, \dots, m$. The mean and variance of Y_{ij} are represented by $\mathrm{E}(Y_{ij}) = \mu_{ij}$ and $\mathrm{Var}(Y_{ij}) = v_{ij}$. The set of repeated outcomes for subject i are collected into an n_i-vector, $\boldsymbol{Y_i} = (Y_{i1}, \dots, Y_{in_i})$, with mean $\mathrm{E}(\boldsymbol{Y_i}) = \boldsymbol{\mu_i}$ and $n_i \times n_i$ covariance matrix $\mathrm{Var}(\boldsymbol{Y_i}) = V_i$, where the jk element of V_i is the covariance between Y_{ij} and Y_{ik}, denoted by $\mathrm{Cov}(Y_{ij}, Y_{ik}) = v_{ijk}$. We use R_i for the $n_i \times n_i$ correlation matrix of $\boldsymbol{Y_i}$. The responses for all units are referred to as $\boldsymbol{Y} = (\boldsymbol{Y}_1, \dots, \boldsymbol{Y}_m)$, which is an N-vector with $N = \sum_{i=1}^{m} n_i$.

Most longitudinal analyses are based on a regression model such as the linear model,

$$\begin{aligned} Y_{ij} &= \beta_1 x_{ij1} + \beta_2 x_{ij2} + \cdots + \beta_p x_{ijp} + \epsilon_{ij} \\ &= \boldsymbol{x_{ij}}'\boldsymbol{\beta} + \epsilon_{ij}, \end{aligned}$$

where $\boldsymbol{\beta} = (\beta_1, \dots, \beta_p)$ is a p-vector of unknown regression coefficients and ϵ_{ij} is a zero-mean random variable representing the deviation of the response from the model prediction, $\boldsymbol{x_{ij}}'\boldsymbol{\beta}$. Typically, $x_{ij1} = 1$ for all i and all j, and β_1 is then the intercept term in the linear model.

In matrix notation, the regression equation for the ith subject takes the form

$$\boldsymbol{Y_i} = X_i \boldsymbol{\beta} + \boldsymbol{\epsilon_i},$$

where X_i is a $n_i \times p$ matrix with $\boldsymbol{x_{ij}}$ in the jth row and $\boldsymbol{\epsilon_i} = (\epsilon_{i1}, \dots, \epsilon_{in_i})$.

Note that in longitudinal studies, the natural experimental unit is not the individual measurement Y_{ij}, but the sequence, $\boldsymbol{Y_i}$, of measurements on an individual subject. For example, when we talk about replication we refer to the number of subjects, not the number of individual measurements. We shall use the following terms interchangeably, according to context: subject, experimental unit, person, animal, individual.

1.4 Merits of longitudinal studies

As mentioned above, the prime advantage of a longitudinal study is its effectiveness for studying change. The artificial reading example of Fig. 1.1 can easily be generalized to the class of linear regression models using the new notation. The distinction between cross-sectional and longitudinal inference is made clearer by consideration of the simple linear regression without intercept. The general case follows naturally by thinking of the explanatory variable as a vector rather than a scalar.

In a cross-sectional study ($n_i = 1$) we are restricted to the model

$$Y_{i1} = \beta_{\mathrm{C}} x_{i1} + \epsilon_{i1}, \quad i = 1, \ldots, m, \tag{1.4.1}$$

where β_{C} represents the difference in average Y across two sub-populations which differ by one unit in x. With repeated observations, the linear model can be extended to the form

$$Y_{ij} = \beta_{\mathrm{C}} x_{i1} + \beta_{\mathrm{L}}(x_{ij} - x_{i1}) + \epsilon_{ij}, \quad j = 1, \ldots, n_i; \; i = 1, \ldots, m, \tag{1.4.2}$$

(Ware *et al.*, 1990). Note that when $j = 1$, (1.4.2) reduces to (1.4.1) so β_{C} has the same cross-sectional interpretation. However, we can now also estimate β_{L} whose interpretation is made clear by subtracting (1.4.1) from (1.4.2) to obtain

$$(Y_{ij} - Y_{i1}) = \beta_{\mathrm{L}}(x_{ij} - x_{i1}) + \epsilon_{ij} - \epsilon_{i1}.$$

That is, β_{L} represents the expected change in Y over time per unit change in x for a given subject.

In Fig. 1.1(b), β_{C} and β_{L} have opposite signs; in Fig. 1.1(c), they have the same sign. To estimate how individuals change with time from a cross-sectional study, we must assume $\beta_{\mathrm{C}} = \beta_{\mathrm{L}}$. With a longitudinal study, this strong assumption is unnecessary since both can be estimated.

Even when $\beta_{\mathrm{C}} = \beta_{\mathrm{L}}$, longitudinal studies tend to be more powerful than cross-sectional studies. The basis of inference about β_{C} is a comparison of individuals with a particular value of x to others with a different value. In contrast, the parameter β_{L} is estimated by comparing a person's response at two times, assuming x changes with time. In a longitudinal study, each person can be thought of as serving as his or her own control. For most vectr vs scalar-definition?

outcomes, there is considerable variability across individuals due to the influence of unmeasured characteristics such as genetic make-up, environmental exposures, personal habits, and so on. These tend to persist over time. Their influence is cancelled in the estimation of β_L; they obscure the estimation of β_C.

Another merit of the longitudinal study is its ability to distinguish the degree of variation in Y across time for one person from the variation in Y among people. This partitioning of the variation in Y is important for the following reason. Much of statistical analysis can be viewed as estimating unobserved quantities. For example, in the CD4+ problem we want to estimate a man's immune status as reflected in his CD4+ level. With cross-sectional data, one man's estimate must draw upon data from others to overcome measurement error. But averaging across people ignores the natural differences in CD4+ level among persons. With repeated values, we can borrow strength across time for the person of interest as well as across people. If there is little variability among people, one man's estimate can rely on data for others as in the cross-sectional case. However, if the variation across people is large, we might prefer to use only data for the individual. Given longitudinal data, we can acknowledge the naturally occurring differences among subjects when estimating a person's current value or predicting his future one.

1.5 Approaches to longitudinal data analysis

With one observation on each experimental unit, we are confined to modelling the population average of Y, called the *marginal* mean response; there is no other choice. With repeated measurements, there are several different approaches that can be adopted. A simple and often effective strategy is to

(1) reduce the repeated values into one or two summaries;

(2) analyse each summary variable as a function of covariates, $\boldsymbol{x}_i$.

For example, with the Sitka spruce data of Example 1.3, the linear growth rate of each tree can be estimated and the rates compared across the ozone groups. This so-called *two-stage* or *derived variable* analysis, which dates at least from Wishart (1938), works when $\boldsymbol{x}_{ij} = \boldsymbol{x}_i$ for all i and j since the summary value which results from stage (1) can only be regressed on $\boldsymbol{x}_i$ in stage (2). This approach is less useful if important explanatory variables change over time.

In lieu of reducing the repeated responses to summary statistics, we can model the individual Y_{ij} in terms of $\boldsymbol{x}_{ij}$. This book will discuss three distinct strategies.

The first is to model the marginal mean as in a cross-sectional study. For example, in the ICHS, the frequency of respiratory disease in children who are and are not vitamin A deficient would be compared. Or in the CD4+ example, the average CD4+ level would be characterized as a function of time. Since repeated values are not likely to be independent, this *marginal analysis* must also include assumptions about the form of the correlation. For example, in the linear model we can assume $\mathrm{E}(\boldsymbol{Y_i}) = X_i\boldsymbol{\beta}$, and $\mathrm{Var}(\boldsymbol{Y_i}) = V_i(\boldsymbol{\alpha})$ where $\boldsymbol{\beta}$ and $\boldsymbol{\alpha}$ must be estimated. The marginal model approach has the advantage of separately modelling the mean and covariance. As will be discussed below, valid inferences about $\boldsymbol{\beta}$ can sometimes be made even when an incorrect form for $V(\boldsymbol{\alpha})$ is assumed.

A second approach, the random effects model, assumes that correlation arises among repeated responses because the regression coefficients vary across individuals. Here, we model the conditional expectation of Y_{ij} given the person-specific coefficients, $\boldsymbol{\beta_i}$, by

$$\mathrm{E}(Y_{ij} \mid \boldsymbol{\beta_i}) = \boldsymbol{x}'_{\boldsymbol{ij}}\boldsymbol{\beta_i}. \tag{1.5.1}$$

Because there is too little data on a single person to estimate $\boldsymbol{\beta_i}$ from $(\boldsymbol{Y_i}, X_i)$ alone, we further assume that the $\boldsymbol{\beta_i}$'s are independent realizations from some distribution with mean $\boldsymbol{\beta}$. If we write $\boldsymbol{\beta_i} = \boldsymbol{\beta} + \boldsymbol{U_i}$ where $\boldsymbol{\beta}$ is fixed and $\boldsymbol{U_i}$ is a zero-mean random variable, then the basic heterogeneity assumption can be restated in terms of the latent variables, $\boldsymbol{U_i}$. That is, there are unobserved factors represented by the $\boldsymbol{U_i}$'s that are common to all responses for a given person but which vary across people, thus inducing the correlation. In the ICHS, it is reasonable to assume that the propensity of respiratory infection naturally varies across children irrespective of their vitamain A status, due to genetic and environmental factors which cannot be easily measured. Random effects models are particularly useful when inferences are to be made about individuals as in the CD4+ example.

The final approach, which we will refer to as a *transition model* (Ware *et al.*, 1988) focuses on the conditional expectation of Y_{ij} given past outcomes, $Y_{ij-1}, \ldots, Y_{i1}$. Here the data-analyst specifies a regression model for the conditional expectation, $\mathrm{E}(Y_{ij} \mid Y_{ij-1}, \ldots, Y_{i1}, \boldsymbol{x_{ij}})$, as an explicit function of $\boldsymbol{x_{ij}}$ and of the past responses. An example for equally spaced binary data is the logistic regression

$$\log \frac{\Pr(Y_{ij} = 1 \mid Y_{ij-1}, \ldots, Y_{i1}, \boldsymbol{x_{ij}})}{1 - \Pr(Y_{ij} = 1 \mid Y_{ij-1}, \ldots, Y_{i1}, \boldsymbol{x_{ij}})} = \boldsymbol{x_{ij}}'\boldsymbol{\beta} + \alpha Y_{ij-1}. \tag{1.5.2}$$

Transition models like (1.5.2) combine the assumptions about the dependence of Y on x and the correlation among repeated Y's into a single equation. As an example, the chance of respiratory infection for a child in the ICHS might depend on whether she was vitamin A deficient but also on whether she had an infection at the prior visit.

In each of the three approaches, we model both the dependence of the response on the explanatory variables and the autocorrelation among the responses. With cross-sectional data, only the dependence of Y on $\boldsymbol{x}$ need be specified; there is no correlation. There are at least three consequences of ignoring the correlation when it exists in longitudinal data:

(1) incorrect inferences about regression coefficients, $\boldsymbol{\beta}$;

(2) estimates of $\boldsymbol{\beta}$ which are inefficient, that is, less precise than possible;

(3) sub-optimal protection against biases causes by missing data.

To illustrate the first two, suppose $Y_{ij} = \beta_0 + \beta_1 t_j + \epsilon_{ij}$, $t_j = -3, -2, \ldots, 2, 3$ where the errors, ϵ_{ij}, follow the first-order autoregressive model, $\epsilon_{ij} = \alpha\epsilon_{ij-1} + Z_{ij}$ and the Z_{ij}'s are independent, mean zero, Gaussian variates. Suppose further that we ignore the correlation and use ordinary least squares (OLS) to obtain a slope estimate, $\hat{\boldsymbol{\beta}}_{\text{OLS}}$, and an estimate of its variance, $\hat{V}_{\text{OLS}}$. Let $\hat{\boldsymbol{\beta}}$ be the optimal estimator of $\boldsymbol{\beta}$ obtained by taking the correlation into account. Figure 1.7 shows the true variances of $\hat{\boldsymbol{\beta}}_{\text{OLS}}$ and $\hat{\boldsymbol{\beta}}$ as well as the stated variance from OLS, $\hat{V}_{\text{OLS}}$, as a function of the correlation, α, between observations one time unit apart. Note first that $\hat{V}_{\text{OLS}}$ can be grossly incorrect when the correlation is substantial. Ignoring correlation leads to invalid assessment of the evidence about trend. Second, $\hat{\boldsymbol{\beta}}$ is less variable than $\hat{\boldsymbol{\beta}}_{\text{OLS}}$. That is, better use is made of the available information about the trend by accounting for correlation. The two costs listed above are true for most regression problems and correlation patterns encountered in practice.

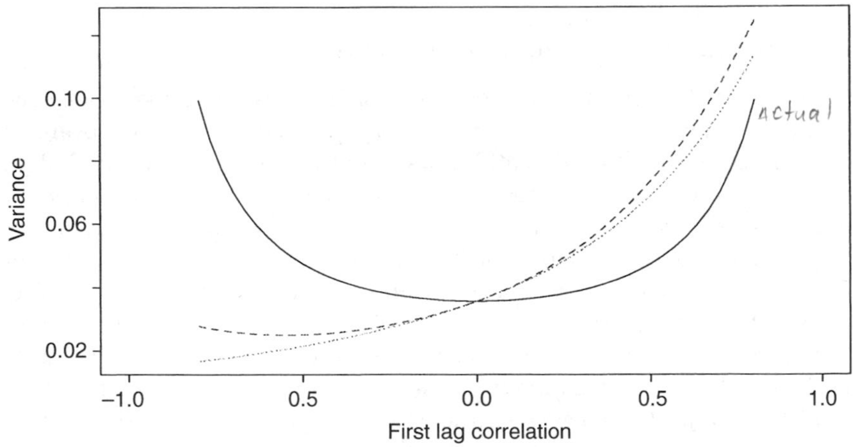

Fig. 1.7. Actual and estimated variances of OLS estimates, and actual variance of optimally weighted least-squares estimates, as functions of the correlation between successive measurements: ——: reported by OLS – – –: actual for OLS ....: best possible.

Longitudinal data analysis problems can be partitioned into two groups:

(1) those where the regression of Y on $\boldsymbol{x}$ is the scientific focus and the number of experimental units (m) is much greater than the number of observations per unit (n);

(2) problems where the correlation is of prime interest or where m is small.

Using the MACS data in Example 1.1 to estimate the average number of CD4+ cells as a function of time since seroconversion falls into group 1. The nature of the correlation among repeated observations is immaterial to this purpose and m is large relative to n. Estimation of one individual's CD4+ curve is of type 2 since the correlation structure must be correctly modelled. Drawing correct inferences about the effect of ozone on Sitka spruce growth (Example 1.3) is also of type 2 since m and n are of similar size.

The classification scheme above is imprecise, but is nevertheless useful as a rough guide to strategies for analysis. With objectives of type 1, the data analyst must invest the majority of time in correctly modelling the mean, that is, including all necessary explanatory variables and their interactions and identifying the best functional form for each predictor. Less time need be spent in modelling the correlation. As we will show in Chapter 4, if m is large relative to n a robust variance estimate can be used to draw valid inferences about regression parameters even when the correlation is misspecified. In group 2, however, both the mean and covariance models must be approximately correct to obtain valid inferences.

1.6 Organization of subsequent chapters

This chapter has given a brief overview of the ideas underlying longitudinal data analysis. Chapter 2 discusses design issues such as choosing the number of persons (experimental units) and the number of repeated observations to attain a given power. Analytic methods begin in Chapter 3, which focuses on exploratory tools for displaying the data and summarizing the mean and correlation patterns. The linear model for longitudinal data is treated in Chapters 4–6. In Chapter 4, the emphasis is on problems of type 1, where relatively less effort will be devoted to careful modelling of the covariance structure. Details necessary for modelling covariances are given in Chapter 5. Chapter 6 discusses traditional analysis of variance models for repeated measures, a special case of the linear model. Chapters 7–11 treat extensions to the longitudinal data setting of generalized linear models (GLMs) for discrete and/or continuous responses. The three approaches based upon marginal, random effects and transitional models are contrasted in Chapter 7. Each approach is then discussed in detail, with the focus on the analysis of two important special cases, in which the response variable is either a binary outcome or a count, whilst Chapter 11 describes recent methodological developments which integrate the different approaches. Chapter 12 describes the problems which can arise when a time-varying explanatory variable is derived from a stochastic process which may interact with the response process in a complex manner; in particular, this requires careful consideration of what form of conditioning is appropriate. Chapter 13 discusses the problems raised by missing values, which frequently arise in longitudinal studies. Chapter 14 gives short introductions to several additional topics which have been the focus of recent research: non-parametric and non-linear modelling; multivariate extensions, including joint modelling of longitudinal measurements and recurrent events. Appendix A is a brief review of the statistical theory of linear and GLMs for regression analysis with independent observations, which provides the foundation for the longitudinal methodology developed in the rest of the book.

2
Design considerations

2.1 Introduction

In this chapter we contrast cross-sectional and longitudinal studies from the design perspective. As discussed in Chapter 1, the major advantage of a longitudinal study is its ability to distinguish the cross-sectional and longitudinal relationships between the explanatory variables and the response. The price associated with this advantage is the potential higher cost incurred by repeated sampling of individuals. At the design stage, we can benefit from guestimates of the potential size of bias from a cross-sectional study and the increase in precision of inferences from a longitudinal study. This information can then be weighed either formally or informally against the additional cost of repeated sampling. Then if a longitudinal study is selected, we must choose the number of persons and number of measurements on each.

In Sections 2.2 and 2.3 we quantify the potential bias of a cross-sectional study as well as its efficiency relative to a longitudinal study. Section 2.4 presents sample size calculations when the response variables are either continuous or dichotomous.

2.2 Bias

As the discussion of the reading example in Section 1.4 demonstrates, it is possible for the association between an explanatory variable, x, and response, Y, determined from a cross-sectional study to be very different from the association measured in a longitudinal study.

We begin our study of bias by formalizing this idea using the model from Section 1.4. Consider a response variable that both changes over time and varies among subjects. Examples include age, blood pressure, or weight. Adopting the notation given in Section 1.3, we begin with a model of the form

$$Y_{ij} = \beta_0 + \beta x_{ij} + \epsilon_{ij}, \quad j = 1, \ldots, n; \; i = 1, \ldots, m. \qquad (2.2.1)$$

Re-expressing (2.2.1) as

$$Y_{ij} = \beta_0 + \underline{\beta x_{i1}} + \beta(x_{ij} - x_{i1}) + \epsilon_{ij}, \tag{2.2.2}$$

we note that this model assumes implicitly that the cross-sectional effect due to x_{i1} is the same as the longitudinal effect represented by $x_{ij} - x_{i1}$ on the right-hand side. This assumption is rather a strong one and doomed to fail in many studies. The model can be modified by allowing each person to have their own intercept, β_{0i}, that is, by replacing $\beta_0 + \beta x_{i1}$ with β_{0i} so that

$$Y_{ij} = \beta_{0i} + \beta(x_{ij} - x_{i1}) + \epsilon_{ij}. \tag{2.2.3}$$

Both (2.2.1) and (2.2.3) represent extreme cases for modelling the cross-sectional variation in the response variable at baseline. In the former case, one assumes that the cross-sectional association with x_{i1} is the same as the longitudinal effect; in the latter case, the baseline level is allowed to be different for every person. An intermediate and often more effective way to modify (2.2.1) is to assume a model of the form

$$Y_{ij} = \beta_0 + \beta_{\mathrm{C}} x_{i1} + \beta_{\mathrm{L}}(x_{ij} - x_{i1}) + \epsilon_{ij}, \tag{2.2.4}$$

as suggested in Section 1.4. The inclusion of x_{i1} in the model with separate coefficient β_{C} allows both cross-sectional and longitudinal effects to be examined separately. We can also use this form to test whether the cross-sectional and longitudinal effects of particular explanatory variables are the same, that is, whether $\beta_{\mathrm{C}} = \beta_{\mathrm{L}}$. From a second perspective, one may simply view x_{i1} as a confounding variable whose absence may bias our estimate of the true longitudinal effect.

We now examine the bias of the least-squares estimate of β derived from the model (2.2.1). The estimate is

$$\hat{\beta} = \sum_{i=1}^{m}\sum_{j=1}^{n}(x_{ij} - \bar{x})(y_{ij} - \bar{y}) \Big/ \sum_{i=1}^{m}\sum_{j=1}^{n}(x_{ij} - \bar{x})^2,$$

where $\bar{x} = \sum_{ij} x_{ij}/(nm)$ and $\bar{y} = \sum_{ij} y_{ij}/(nm)$. When the true model is (2.2.4), simple algebra leads to

$$\mathrm{E}(\hat{\beta}) = \beta_{\mathrm{L}} + \frac{\sum_{i=1}^{m} n(x_{i1} - \bar{x}_1)(\bar{x}_i - \bar{x})}{\sum_{i=1}^{m}\sum_{j=1}^{n}(x_{ij} - \bar{x})^2}(\beta_{\mathrm{C}} - \beta_{\mathrm{L}}),$$

where $\bar{x}_i = \sum_j x_{ij}/n$ and $\bar{x}_1 = \sum_i x_{i1}/m$. Thus the cross-sectional estimate $\hat{\beta}$, which assumes $\beta_{\mathrm{L}} = \beta_{\mathrm{C}}$, is a biased estimate of β_{L} and is unbiased only if either $\beta_{\mathrm{L}} = \beta_{\mathrm{C}}$ or the variables $\{x_{i1}\}$ and $\{\bar{x}_i\}$ are orthogonal to each other. The latter result is of no surprise if one re-expresses (2.2.4) as

$$Y_{ij} = \beta_0 + \beta_L x_{ij} + x_{i1}(\beta_C - \beta_L) + \epsilon_{ij}. \qquad (2.2.5)$$

In this re-expression, (2.2.1) is seen as a special case of (2.2.4) where the variable x_{i1} has been omitted from the model.

The direction of the bias in $\hat{\beta}$ as an estimate for the longitudinal effect, β_L, depends upon the correlation between x_{i1} and $\bar{x}_i$, as is clear from the expression for $E(\hat{\beta})$ above. The main message to be conveyed here is that when dealing with covariates which change over time and vary across subjects at the baseline, it is good practice to use model (2.2.4) instead of (2.2.1). The former model allows one to separate the longitudinal effect, which describes individual change, from the cross-sectional effect where comparison on Y is made between individuals with different x's.

2.3 Efficiency

The previous section addressed the issue of bias in cross-sectional studies of change. Even when $\beta_C = \beta_L$, longitudinal studies tend to be more powerful, as we now examine in detail. Assuming the model specified in (2.2.1), the variance of $\hat{\beta}_C$, which uses the data from the first visit only, is

$$\mathrm{Var}(\hat{\beta}_C) = \sigma^2 \Big/ \sum_{i=1}^{m} (x_{i1} - \bar{x}_1)^2,$$

where $\sigma^2 = \mathrm{Var}(\epsilon_{ij})$. On the other hand, the variance of $\hat{\beta}_L$, which uses all the data, is the lower right entry of

$$\sigma^2 \left\{ \sum_{i=1}^{m} (X_i' R_i^{-1} X_i) \right\}^{-1},$$

where R_i is the $n_i \times n_i$ correlation matrix for $\boldsymbol{Y_i} = (Y_{i1}, \ldots, Y_{in_i})$ and

$$X_i' = \begin{pmatrix} 1 & 1 & \cdots & 1 \\ x_{i1} & x_{i2} & \cdots & x_{in_i} \end{pmatrix}.$$

We can address the question of how much more can be learned by taking repeated measurements on each person by comparing the variances of $\hat{\beta}_L$ and $\hat{\beta}_C$ in (2.2.5) when $\beta_C = \beta_L$. We use $e = \mathrm{Var}(\hat{\beta}_L)/\mathrm{Var}(\hat{\beta}_C)$ as the specific measure of efficiency. The smaller the value of e the greater is the information gained by taking additional measurements on each person.

As expected, the value of e depends on the true structure of the correlation matrix. We consider two correlation matrices commonly occurring in longitudinal studies. For simplicity, we continue to assume $n_i = n$ for all i.

In case 1, we assume the uniform correlation matrix, $R_{jk} = 1$ if $j = k$ and $R_{jk} = \rho$ for any $j \neq k$. The e function defined above then reduces to

$$e = \frac{\{1 + (n-1)\rho\}(1-\rho)}{n(1+\delta)\{1 - p + n\rho\delta/(1+\delta)\}},$$

where

$$\delta = \frac{\text{the averaged within-subject variation in } x}{\text{the between-subjects variation in } x \text{ at visit 1}}$$
$$= \frac{\sum_{i,j}(x_{ij} - \bar{x}_i)^2/\{m(n-1)\}}{\sum_i(\bar{x}_i - \bar{x})^2/(m-1)}.$$

Figure 2.1 gives plots of e against δ for some selected values of ρ and n. Except when δ is small and the common correlation ρ is high, there is much to be gained by conducting longitudinal studies even when the number of repeated observations is as small as two.

In case 2, we consider the situation when the true correlation matrix has the form $R_{jk} = \rho^{|j-k|}$. This is the correlation structure of a first order autoregressive process discussed in Chapter 5. In this case

$$e = \frac{1-\rho^2}{(1-\rho)\{n - (n-2)\rho\} + \delta\gamma/(n+1)},$$

where $\gamma = n(n+1) - 2(n-3)(n+1)\rho + (n-3)(n-2)\rho^2$. The message regarding efficiency gain is similar as can be seen in Fig. 2.2.

We note that in either case, e is a decreasing function of δ. One implication for design is that we may obtain a more efficient (less variable) estimate of β by increasing the within-subject variation in x when possible. Suppose x_{ij} is the age of person i at visit j so that β represents the time rate of change of the response variable. With three observations for each person, it is better, all other factors being equal, to arrange the visits at years 0, 1, and 3 rather than 0, 1, and 2. In the former design, the within-subject variation in x is $\{(0-4/3)^2 + (1-4/3)^2 + (3-4/3)^2\}/3 = 1.45$ as opposed to $\{(0-1)^2 + (1-1)^2 + (2-1)^2\}/3 = 0.67$ in the latter case. The efficiency for the former design depends on the type of correlation structure, the magnitude of ρ, and the between-subject variation in x at visit 1 (the denominator of δ). For example, with exchangeable correlation structure with $\rho = 0.5$ and the between-subject variation at visit one equal to 10, the variance of $\hat{\beta}$ for the (0, 1, 3) design is only 78% of that for the (0, 1, 2) design. In other words, delaying the last visit from year two to year three is equivalent to increasing the number of persons in the study by a factor of $0.78^{-1} = 1.28$.

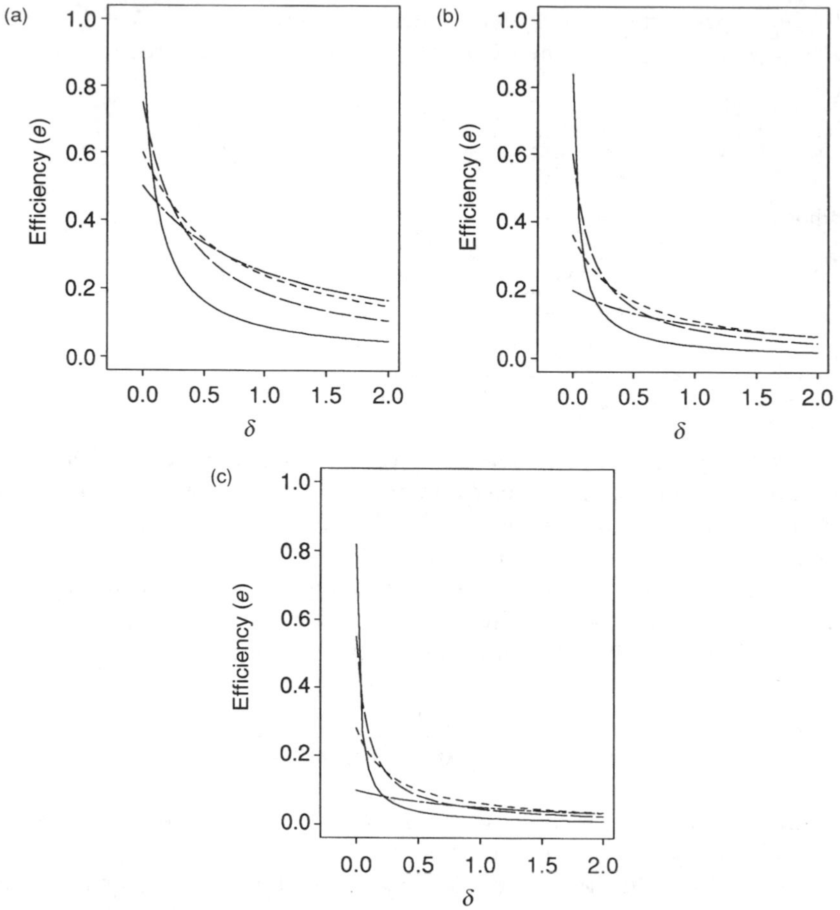

Fig. 2.1. Relationship between relative efficiency of cross-sectional and longitudinal estimation and nature of variation in x, with uniform correlation structure and n observations per subject: (a) $n = 2$; (b) $n = 5$; (c) $n = 10$. ——: $\rho = 0.8$; – – –: $\rho = 0.5$; - - - -: $\rho = 0.2$; – · – · –: $\rho = 0.0$.

2.4 Sample size calculations

As with cross-sectional studies, investigators conducting longitudinal studies need to know in advance the number of subjects approximately required to achieve a specified statistical power. In any study, investigators must provide the following quantities to determine the required sample sizes.

1. **Type I error rate** (α): This quantity, denoted α, is the probability that the study will reject the null hypothesis when it is correct;

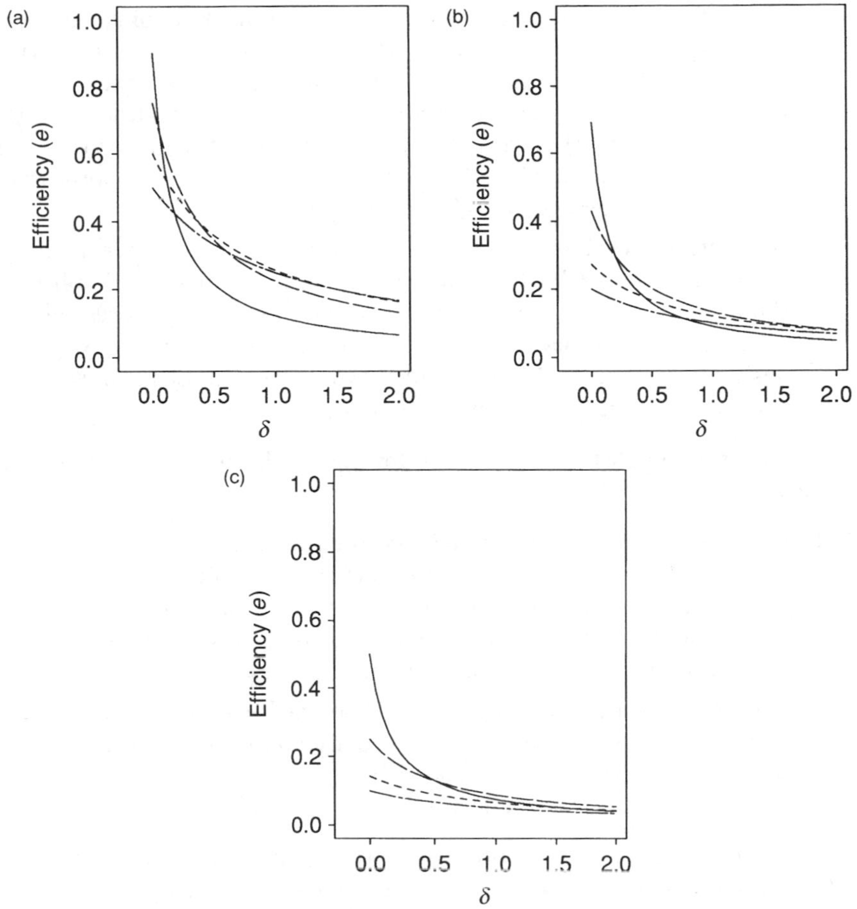

Fig. 2.2. Relationship between relative efficiency of cross-sectional and longitudinal estimation and nature of variation in x, with exponential correlation structure and n observations per subject: (a) $n = 2$; (b) $n = 5$; (c) $n = 10$. ——: $\rho = 0.8$; – – –: $\rho = 0.5$; - - - -: $\rho = 0.2$; — · — · —: $\rho = 0.0$.

for example, it would correspond to the probability of declaring a significant difference between treatment and control groups when the treatment is useless. A typical choice of α is 0.05.

2. **Smallest meaningful difference to be detected** (d): The investigators typically want their study to reject the null hypothesis with high probability when the parameter of interest deviates from its value under the null hypothesis by an amount d or more, where the value of d is chosen to be of practical significance. We call this value the smallest meaningful difference.

3. **Power** (P): The power, P, of a statistical test is the probability that the study rejects the null hypothesis when it is incorrect. Of course, this must depend on *how* incorrect is the null hypothesis, as the power must approach the type I error rate, α, as the deviation from the null hypothesis approaches zero. A typical requirement might be that the power is at least 0.9 when the deviation from the null hypothesis is at least d, the smallest meaningful difference.
4. **Measurement variation** (σ^2): For a continuous response variable, Y_{ij}, the quantity $\sigma^2 = \text{Var}(Y_{ij})$ measures the unexplained variability in the response. The value of σ^2 is sometimes available to a reasonable approximation through either pilot studies or similar studies previously reported in the literature. Otherwise, the statistician must elicit from the investigator a plausible guess at its value.

In longitudinal studies, the following additional quantities are needed:

5. **Number of repeated observations per person** (n): The number, n, of observations per person may be constrained by practical considerations, or may need to be balanced against the sample size. For a given total cost, the investigator may be free to choose between a small value of n and a large sample size, or vice versa.
6. **Correlation among the repeated observations**: As with the measurement variance, the pattern of correlation among repeated observations can sometimes be estimated from previous studies. When this is not possible, a reasonable guess must be made.

In the remainder of this section, we give sample size formulas separately for continuous and binary responses. For simplicity, we present only formulas for two-group comparisons. However, the principles apply to general study designs, the formulas for which will be developed and presented in Chapter 8.

2.4.1 *Continuous responses*

We consider the simple problem of comparing two groups, A and B. We assume that in group A, the response depends on a single explanatory variable as follows:

$$Y_{ij} = \beta_{0\text{A}} + \beta_{1\text{A}} x_{ij} + \epsilon_{ij}, \quad j = 1, \ldots, n; \ i = 1, \ldots, m.$$

In group B, the same equation holds but with different coefficients, $\beta_{0\text{B}}$ and $\beta_{1\text{B}}$. Both groups have the same number of subjects, m; each person has n repeated observations. We assume that $\text{Var}(\epsilon_{ij}) = \sigma^2$ and $\text{Corr}(Y_{ij}, Y_{ik}) = \rho$ for all $j \neq k$. In addition, we assume that each person has the same set of explanatory variables so that $x_{ij} = x_j$. A typical example of such x_j is the duration between the first and the jth visit, in which case $\beta_{1\mathrm{A}}$ and $\beta_{1\mathrm{B}}$ are the rates of change in Y for groups A and B respectively.

Let z_p denote the pth quantile of a standard Gaussian distribution and $d = \beta_{1\mathrm{B}} - \beta_{1\mathrm{A}}$ be the meaningful difference of interest. With n fixed and known, the number of subjects per group that are needed to achieve type I error rate α and power P, is

$$m = \frac{2(z_\alpha + z_Q)^2\sigma^2(1-\rho)}{ns_x^2d^2}, \tag{2.4.1}$$

where $Q = 1 - P$ and $s_x^2 = \sum_j (x_j - \bar{x})^2/n$, the within-subject variance of the x_j.

To illustrate, consider a hypothetical clinical trial on the effect of a new treatment in reducing blood pressure. Three visits, including the baseline visit, are planned at years 0, 2, and 5. Thus, $n = 3$ and $s_x^2 = 4.22$. For type I error rate $\alpha = 0.05$, power $P = 0.8$ and smallest meaningful difference $d = 0.5\,\mathrm{mmHg/year}$, the table below gives the number of subjects needed for both treated and control groups for some selected values of ρ and σ^2.

	σ^2		
ρ	100	200	300
0.2	313	625	937
0.5	195	391	586
0.8	79	157	235

Note that for each value of σ^2, the required sample size decreases as the correlation, ρ, increases.

Finally, the sample size formula presented above can be extended easily to correlation structures other than the exchangeable one. Let R, a $n \times n$ matrix be the common correlation matrix for each subject. In this case, one simply replaces $\sigma^2(1-\rho)/(ns_x^2)$ in (2.4.1) by the lower right entry of the following 2×2 matrix

$$\begin{pmatrix} 1 & \cdots & 1 \\ x_1 & \cdots & x_n \end{pmatrix} R^{-1} \begin{pmatrix} 1 & x_1 \\ \vdots & \vdots \\ 1 & x_n \end{pmatrix}.$$

A second important type of problem is to estimate the time-averaged difference in a response between two groups. The appropriate statistical model is written as

$$Y_{ij} = \beta_0 + \beta_1 x_i + \epsilon_{ij}, \quad j = 1, \ldots, n; \;\; i = 1, \ldots, 2m,$$

where x_i is the treatment assignment indicator variable for the ith subject. Let d be the meaningful difference between the average response for groups A and B. The number of subjects needed per group is

$$\begin{aligned} m &= 2(z_\alpha + z_Q)^2 \sigma^2 \{1 + (n-1)\rho\}/nd^2 \\ &= 2(z_\alpha + z_Q)^2 \{1 + (n-1)\rho\}/(n\Delta^2), \end{aligned} \tag{2.4.2}$$

where $\Delta = d/\sigma$ is the smallest meaningful difference in standard deviation units. For $\alpha = 0.05, P = 0.8$, and $n = 3$, the table below gives the sample size needed per group for some selected values of ρ and Δ.

	Δ (%)			
ρ	20	30	40	50
0.2	146	65	37	24
0.5	208	93	52	34
0.8	270	120	68	44

Note that in this case, for each value of σ^2, the required sample size increases with the correlation, ρ.

It may seem counter-intuitive at first glance that the sample size formula is decreasing in ρ in the first case, but increasing in the second case. The explanation is that in the first case, the parameter of interest, β, is the rate of the change in Y. As a result, the contribution from each subject to the estimation of β is a linear contrast of the Y's whose variance is decreasing in ρ. However, in the second case, the parameter of interest is the expected average of the Y's for individuals in a group and the variance of the corresponding estimate is increasing in ρ.

For an arbitrary correlation matrix, R, the number of subjects needed per group is readily modified by replacing $\{1 + (n-1)\rho\}/n$ in (2.4.2) by $(\mathbf{1}'R^{-1}\mathbf{1})^{-1}$, where $\mathbf{1}$ is a $n \times 1$ vector of ones.

2.4.2 *Binary responses*

For a binary response variable, we consider the situation similar to the last case in Section 2.4.1. That is, we assume

$$\Pr(Y_{ij} = 1) = \begin{cases} p_{\mathrm{A}} & \text{in group A} \\ p_{\mathrm{B}} & \text{in group B} \end{cases} \quad j = 1, \ldots, n; \;\; i = 1, \ldots, m.$$

Assuming also that $\text{Corr}(Y_{ij}, Y_{ik}) = \rho$ for all $j \neq k$ and that d is the smallest meaningful difference between the response probabilities for groups A and B, the number of subjects needed per group is

$$m = \frac{\left\{z_\alpha(2\bar{p}\bar{q})^{1/2} + z_Q(p_A q_A + p_B q_B)^{1/2}\right\}^2 (1 + (n-1)\rho)}{nd^2},$$

where $\bar{p} = (p_A + p_B)/2$ and $\bar{q} = 1 - \bar{p}$. For $\alpha = 0.05$, $P = 0.8$, $n = 3$, and $p_A = 0.5$, the table below gives the sample size needed per group for some selected ρ and $d = p_B - p_A$. As in the analogous problem with a continuous

	d		
ρ	0.3	0.2	0.1
0.2	15	35	143
0.5	21	49	204
0.8	27	64	265

response variable, the required sample size increases with the correlation, ρ. Furthermore, the same modification of the sample size formula can be used for general correlation structures as described above.

In summary, this section has shown that correlation between repeated observations can affect required sample sizes differently, depending on the problem. A simple rule of thumb is that positive correlation increases the variance, and hence the required sample size for a given power, when estimating group averages or differences between averages for more than one group. In contrast, positive correlation decreases the required sample size when estimating a change over time within individuals, or differences between groups in the average change.

2.5 Further reading

In this chapter, we have discussed some of the most basic design considerations which arise with longitudinal studies. In particular, we have assumed that each subject is allocated to a single treatment group for the duration of the study.

There is an extensive literature on the more sophisticated design issues which arise in the related area of crossover trials, in which each subject receives a sequence of different treatments, with the order of presentation of the treatments varying between subjects. Much of this work emphasizes the construction of designs which enable valid inferences to be made in the presence of carry-over effects, whereby the response to a given treatment may include a residual dependence on the previous treatment.

Two of the earliest references to crossover designs are Williams (1949) and Patterson (1951). Later developments are discussed in Hedayat and Afsarinejad (1975, 1978), Afsarinejad (1983), and Bishop and Jones (1984). The books by Jones and Kenward (1989) and by Senn (1992) give general introductions to the design and analysis of crossover trials. The work by Liu and Liang (1997) on sample size calculations for correlated data will be utilized and presented in Chapter 8.

3
Exploring longitudinal data

3.1 Introduction

Longitudinal data analysis, like other statistical methods, has two components which operate side by side: exploratory and confirmatory analysis. Exploratory data analysis (EDA) is detective work. It comprises techniques to visualize patterns in data. Confirmatory analysis is judicial work, weighing evidence in data for, or against hypotheses. This chapter discusses methods for exploring longitudinal data.

John W. Tukey, the father of EDA, said, 'EDA can never be the whole story, but nothing else can serve as the foundation stone – as the first step' (Tukey, 1977). Data analysis must begin by making displays that expose the patterns relevant to the scientific question. The best methods are capable of uncovering patterns which are unexpected. Like a good detective, the data analyst must keep an open mind ready to discover new clues.

There is no single prescription for making effective graphical displays of longitudinal data, but the following are a few simple guidelines:

(1) show as much of the relevant raw data as possible rather than only data summaries;

(2) highlight aggregate patterns of potential scientific interest;

(3) identify both cross-sectional and longitudinal patterns as distinguished in Section 1.1;

(4) make easy the identification of unusual individuals or unusual observations.

Most longitudinal analyses address the relationship of a response with explanatory variables, often including time. Hence, a scatterplot of the response against an explanatory variable is a basic display. Section 3.2 discusses scatterplots designed to follow the guidelines above. Special attention is given to large data sets where care is required to avoid graphs that are excessively busy. Section 3.3 discusses smoothing techniques that highlight the typical response as a function of an explanatory variable without reliance on specific parametric models. Smoothing splines, kernel estimators, and a robust method, *lowess*, are reviewed. Section 3.4 discusses methods to explore the association among repeated observations for an individual. When observations are made at equally spaced times, association is conveniently measured in terms of correlation. With unequally spaced observations, the variogram is often more effective. In this chapter, the main focus is on continuous responses, although in Section 3.5 we also describe the lorelogram (Heagerty and Zeger, 1998), a graphical method for exploring association structure in longitudinal categorical data. Other data displays for discrete data are illustrated in later chapters.

3.2 Graphical presentation of longitudinal data

With longitudinal data, an obvious first graph is the scatterplot of the response variable against time.

Example 3.1. Weights of pigs

Table 3.1 lists some data provided by Dr Philip McCloud (Monash University, Melbourne) on the weights of 48 pigs measured in nine successive weeks. Figure 3.1 displays the data graphically. Lines connect

Table 3.1. Bodyweights of pigs in nine successive weeks of follow-up. The full data-set consists of measurements on 48 pigs. Data below are for 16 pigs only.

Week								
1	2	3	4	5	6	7	8	9
24.0	32.0	39.0	42.5	48.0	54.5	61.0	65.0	72.0
22.5	30.5	40.5	45.0	51.0	58.5	64.0	72.0	78.0
22.5	28.0	36.5	41.0	47.5	55.0	61.0	68.0	76.0
24.0	31.5	39.5	44.5	51.0	56.0	59.5	64.0	67.0
24.5	31.5	37.0	42.5	48.0	54.0	58.0	63.0	65.5
23.0	30.0	35.5	41.0	48.0	51.5	56.5	63.5	69.5
22.5	28.5	36.0	43.5	47.0	53.5	59.5	67.5	73.5
23.5	30.5	38.0	41.0	48.5	55.0	59.5	66.5	73.0
20.0	27.5	33.0	39.0	43.5	49.0	54.5	59.5	65.0
25.5	32.5	39.5	47.0	53.0	58.5	63.0	69.5	76.0
24.5	31.0	40.5	46.0	51.5	57.0	62.5	69.5	76.0
24.0	29.0	39.0	44.0	50.5	57.0	61.5	68.0	73.5
23.5	30.5	36.5	42.0	47.0	55.0	59.0	65.5	73.0
21.5	30.5	37.0	42.5	48.0	52.5	58.5	63.0	69.5
25.0	32.0	38.5	44.0	51.0	59.0	66.0	75.5	86.0
21.5	28.5	34.0	39.5	45.0	51.0	58.0	64.5	72.5

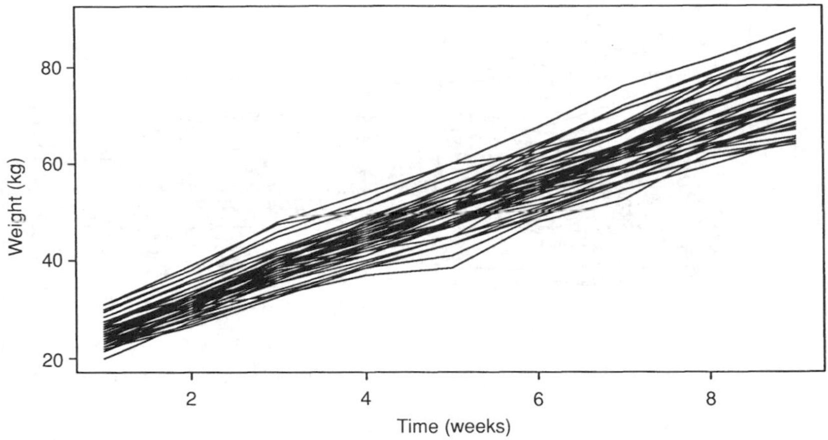

Fig. 3.1. Data on the weights of 48 pigs over a nine-week period.

the repeated observations for each animal. This simple graph makes apparent a number of important patterns. First, all animals are gaining weight. Second, the pigs which are largest at the beginning of the observation period tend to be largest throughout. This phenomenon is called 'tracking'. Third, the spread among the 48 animals is substantially smaller at the beginning of the study than at the end. This pattern of increasing variance over time could be explained in terms of variation in the growth rates of the individual animals.

Figure 3.1 is an adequate display for exploring these growth data, although it is hard to pick out individual response profiles. We can do slightly better by adding a second display obtained from the first by standardizing each observation. This is achieved by subtracting the mean, $\bar{y}_j$, and dividing by the standard deviation, s_j, of the 48 observations at time j, and replacing each y_{ij} by the standardized quantity $y^*_{ij} = (y_{ij} - \bar{y}_j)/s_j$. The resulting plot is shown in Fig. 3.2. Its effect is as if we were running a magnifying glass along the overall mean response profile, adjusting the magnification as we go so as to maintain a roughly constant amount of variation. As a result, the plot is able to highlight the degree of 'tracking', whereby animals tend to maintain their relative size over time. With large data sets, connected line graphs become unduly cluttered, and an alternative strategy for the basic time plot may be needed.

Example 3.2. CD4+ cell numbers

Figure 3.3 displays the CD4+ cell numbers for a subset of 100 seroconverters from the Multicenter AIDS Cohort Study (MACS) against the time variable, years since seroconversion. The plot includes only those men with

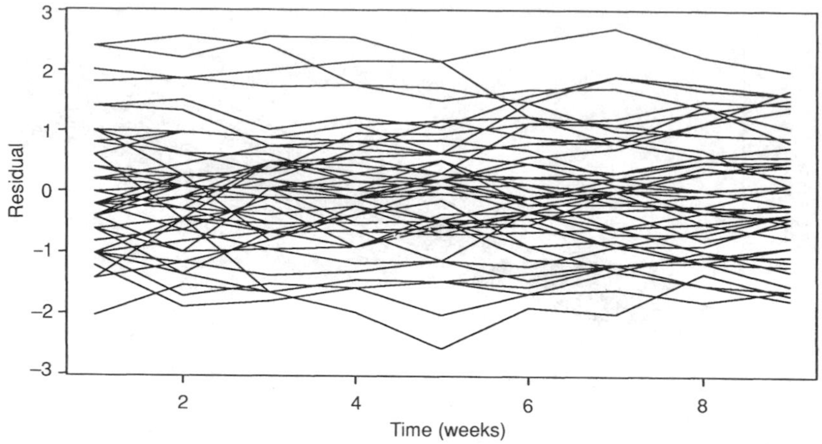

Fig. 3.2. Standardized residuals from data on the weights of pigs.

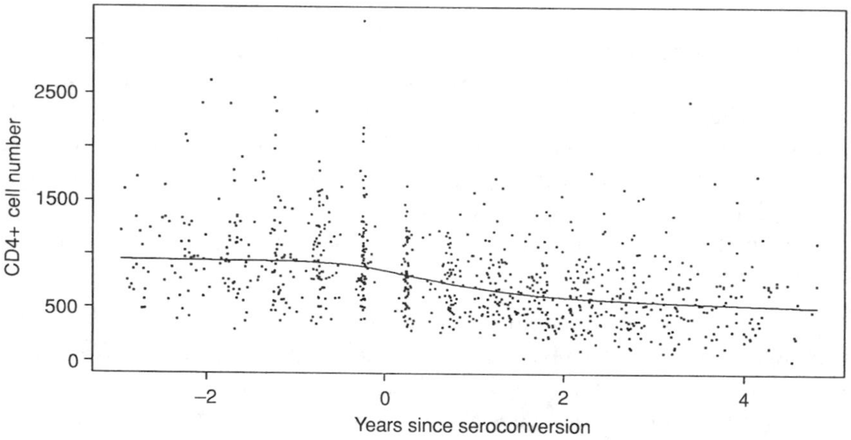

Fig. 3.3. CD4+ counts against time since seroconversion, with lowess smooth curve. · : data; ——: lowess curve.

at least seven observations that cover the date of seroconversion. We can see that the CD4+ cell numbers are relatively constant at about 1000 cells until the time of seroconversion and then decrease afterwards. This mean pattern is highlighted by the non-parametric curve also shown in Fig. 3.3. The curve was calculated using lowess (Cleveland, 1979); the degree of smoothness was chosen subjectively. The curve indicates that the rate of CD4+ cell loss may be more rapid immediately after seroconversion.

The repeated observations for an individual have not been connected in Fig. 3.3, so that it is not possible to discern whether the pattern of

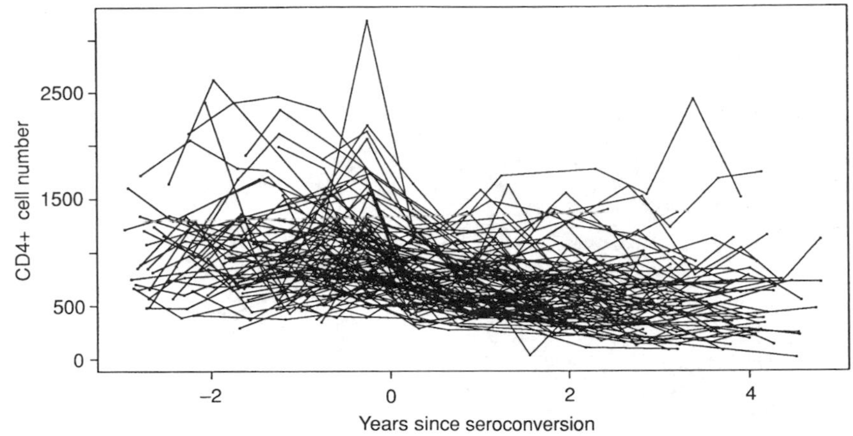

Fig. 3.4. CD4+ counts against time since seroconversion, with sequences of data on each subject shown as connected line segments.

decreasing cells is common to most individuals. That is, we cannot distinguish cross-sectional from longitudinal trends in the data. The reader is referred to Fig. 1.1 for a discussion of cross-sectional and longitudinal patterns.

Figure 3.4 displays the CD4+ cell data for all men, now with each person's repeated observations connected. Unfortunately, this plot is extremely busy, reducing its usefulness except perhaps from the perspective of an ink manufacturer.

The issue is clearly drawn by these two examples. On the one hand, we want to connect repeated measurements to display changes through time for individuals. On the other, presenting every person's curve creates little more than confusion in large data sets. The problem can be even more severe than in the CD4+ example. See Jones and Boadi-Boteng (1991) for a further illustration.

The ideal solution would be to display each individual's data with a very thin grey line and to use darker lines for the typical pattern as well as for a subset of persons. This is consistent with Tufte's (1990) 'micro/macro' design strategy whereby communication of statistical information is enhanced by adding detail in the background. Unfortunately, such a plot is difficult on the type of graphics devices which are available to many users. An alternative solution is to connect the repeated observations for only a judicious selection of individuals. Jones and Rice (1992) have proposed this idea for presenting a large number of curves. The simplest way to choose a subset is at random, as is done for seven people in Fig. 3.5.

There are two problems with random selection. First, it is possible to obtain a non-representative group by chance, especially when relatively

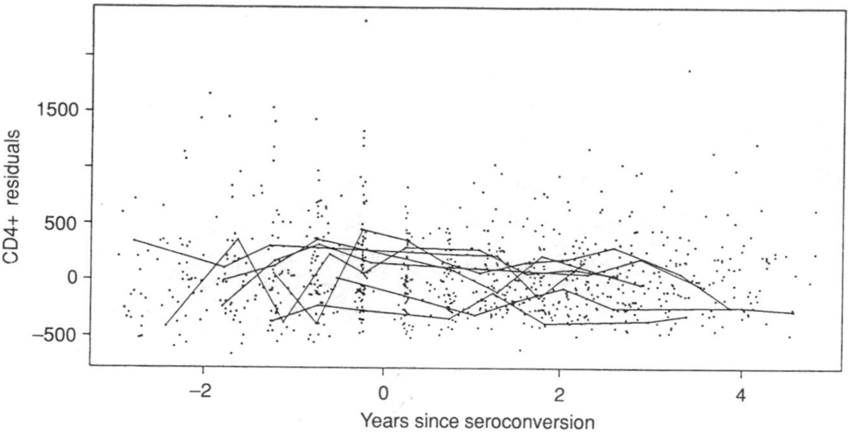

Fig. 3.5. CD4+ residuals against time since seroconversion, with sequences of data from randomly selected subjects shown as connected line segments.

few curves are to be highlighted. Second, this display is unlikely to uncover outlying individuals. We therefore prefer a second approach, in which individual curves are ordered with respect to some characteristic that is relevant to the model of interest. We then connect data for individuals with selected quantiles for this ordering statistic. Ordering statistics can be chosen to measure: the average level; variability within an individual; trend; or correlation between successive values. Resistant statistics are preferred for ordering, so that one or a few outlying observations do not determine an individual's summary score. The median, median absolute deviation, and biweight trend (Mosteller and Tukey, 1977) are examples.

When the data naturally divide into treatment groups, such as in Example 1.3, a separate plot can be made for each group, or one plot can be produced with a separate summary curve for each group and distinct plotting symbols for the data from each group.

For equally spaced observation times, Jones and Rice (1992) apply principal components analysis to identify ordering statistics. Principal components do not exploit the longitudinal nature of the data, nor do they adapt readily to situations with unequal numbers of observations or different sets of observation times across subjects.

Example 3.2. (continued)

Figure 3.3 displays the average number of CD4+ cells for the MACS seroconverters. Figure 3.6 shows the residuals from this average curve with the repeated values for nine individuals connected.

These persons had *median* residual value at the extrema or the 5th, 10th, 25th, 50th, 75th, 90th, or 95th percentile. We have used residuals rather than the raw data as this sometimes helps to uncover more subtle

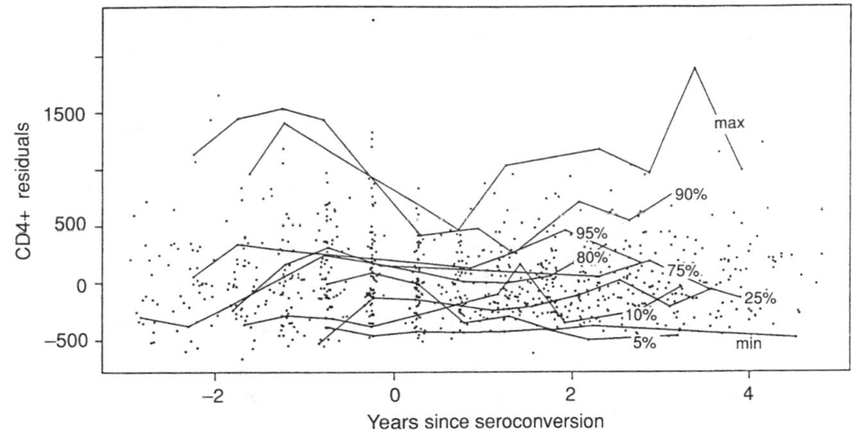

Fig. 3.6. CD4+ residuals against time since seroconversion, with sequences of data from systematically selected subjects shown as connected line segments.

patterns in individual curves. Note that the data for each individual tend to track at different levels of CD4+ cell numbers, but not nearly to the same extent as in Fig. 3.2. The CD4+ data have considerably more variation across time within a person.

Thus far, we have considered displays of the response against time. In many longitudinal problems, the primary focus is the relationship between the response and an explanatory variable other than time. For example, in the MACS data set, an interesting question is whether CD4+ cell number depends on the depressed mood of an individual. There is some prior belief that depressive symptoms are negatively correlated with the capacity for immune response. The MACS collected a measure of depressive symptoms called CESD; a higher score indicates greater depressive symptoms.

Example 3.3. Relationship between CD4+ cell numbers and CESD score

Figure 3.7 plots the residuals with time trends removed for CD4+ cell numbers against similar residuals for CESD scores. Also shown is a lowess curve, which is barely discernible from the horizontal line, $y = 0$. Thus, there is very little evidence for an association between depressive symptoms (CESD score) and immune response (CD4+ numbers), although such evidence as there is points to a negative association, a larger CESD score being associated with a lower CD4+ count.

An interesting question is whether the evidence for any such relationship would derive largely from differences across people, that is, from cross-sectional information, or from changes across time within a person. As previously discussed in Chapter 1, cross-sectional information is more likely biased by unobserved factors. In this example, 70 of the variation in

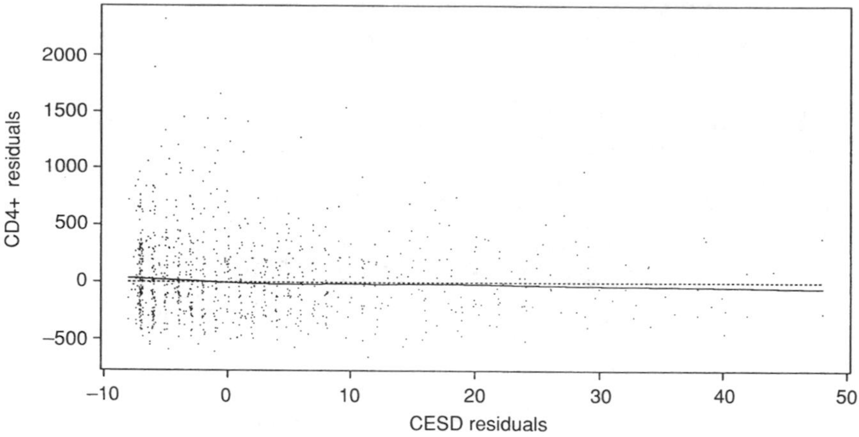

Fig. 3.7. CD4+ residuals against CESD residuals · : data; ——: lowess curve; - - -: $y = 0$.

CESD is within individuals, so that both cross-sectional and longitudinal information are present.

We would like to separate the cross-sectional and longitudinal evidence about the association between the response and explanatory variable in EDA. The model in equation (1.4.2)

$$Y_{ij} = \beta_C x_{i1} + \beta_L(x_{ij} - x_{i1}) + \epsilon_{ij}, \quad j = 1, \dots, n_i; \ \ i = 1, \dots, m,$$

expresses the outcomes in terms of the baseline value and the change in the explanatory variable. The model implies two facts:

(1) $Y_{i1} = \beta_C x_{i1} + \epsilon_{i1}$;

(2) $Y_{ij} - Y_{i1} = \beta_L(x_{ij} - x_{i1}) + \epsilon_{ij} - \epsilon_{i1}, \quad j = 2, \dots, n_i.$

This suggests making two scatterplots:

(1) y_{i1} against x_{i1}; and

(2) $y_{ij} - y_{i1}$ against $x_{ij} - x_{i1}$.

Example 3.3. (continued)

Figure 3.8 shows both scatterplots for the CD4+ and CESD data. There is no strong relationship between baseline CD4+ and CESD. That is, persons more depressed at baseline do not tend to have higher or lower CD4+ levels. Neither is there much relationship between the change in depression level with change in CD4+ members. Hence, there is little evidence of strong relationship in either the cross-sectional (a) or in the longitudinal (b) display. Nevertheless, such a graphical decomposition of the information into

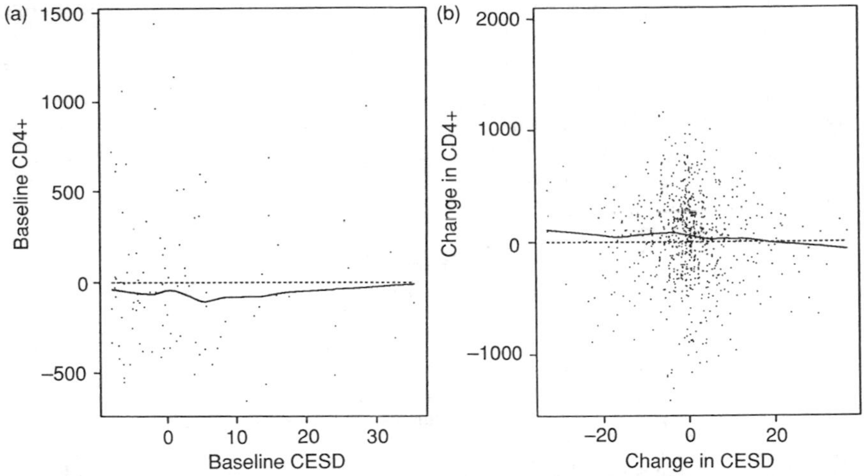

Fig. 3.8. Relationship between CD4+ residuals and CESD residuals. (a) cross-sectional (baseline residuals); (b) longitudinal (change in residuals); ·: data; ——: lowess curve; – –: $y = 0$.

the cross-sectional and longitudinal components can be useful, especially when the associations are different in direction or magnitudes.

3.3 Fitting smooth curves to longitudinal data

A curve-fitting method, lowess, was used in the previous section to highlight the average change in CD4+ cell numbers over time. Lowess is one of a number of non-parametric regression methods that can be used to estimate the mean response profile as a function of time. Other methods include kernel and spline estimation. Figure 3.9 is a scatterplot of CD4+ cell numbers against time using only a single observation, chosen at random, for each person. Smooth curves have been fitted by kernel estimation, smoothing splines, and lowess. All three methods give qualitatively similar results.

We now briefly review each of these smoothing techniques. Details can be found in Hastie and Tibshirani (1990) and the original references therein.

To simplify the discussion of smoothing, we assume there is a single observation on each individual, denoted y_i, observed at time t_i. The general problem is to estimate from data of the following form:

$$(t_i, y_i), \quad i = 1, \ldots, m,$$

an unknown mean response curve $\mu(t)$ in the underlying model

$$Y_i = \mu(t_i) + \epsilon_i, \tag{3.3.1}$$

where the ϵ_i are independent, mean-zero errors.

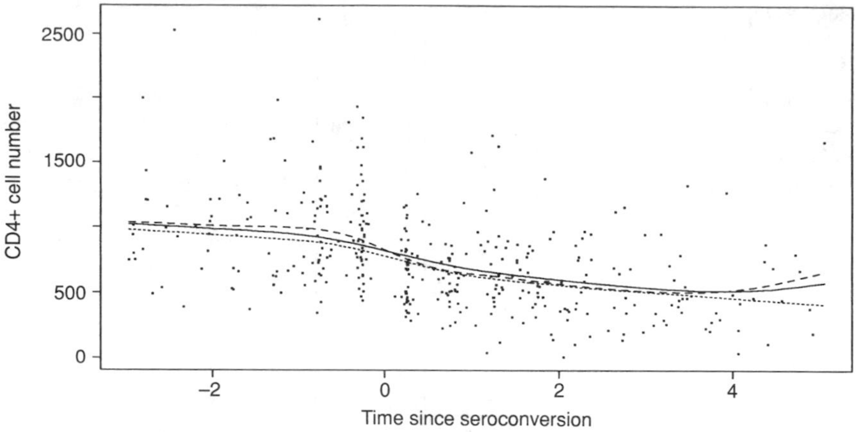

Fig. 3.9. Comparison between kernel, spline and lowess smooths of a subset of the CD4+ counts (one count per subject) · : data; ——: kernel; – – –: spline; ....: lowess.

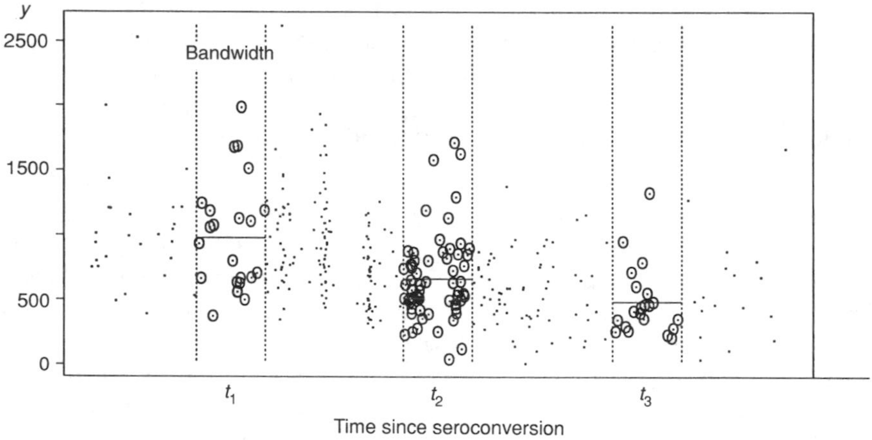

Fig. 3.10. Visualization of the kernel smoother (see text for detailed explanation).

The first method, kernel estimation, is visualized in Fig. 3.10. At the left side of the figure, a *window* is centred at t_1. Then $\hat{\mu}(t_1)$, the estimate of the mean response at time t_1, is just the average Y value of all points (highlighted by circles) which are visible in the window. Two other windows are shown in the centre and on the right of the plot for which we similarly obtain $\hat{\mu}(t_2)$ and $\hat{\mu}(t_3)$. To obtain an estimate of the smooth curve at every time, we simply slide a window from the extreme left across the data to the extreme right, calculating the average of the points within the window at every time.

If the window is so narrow as to contain only one observation at any time, the resulting estimate will interpolate the data. If it is so wide as to include all data at every time, the resulting estimate is a constant line equal to the average Y value. There is a continuum of curves, one for each possible window width. The wider the window, the smoother the resulting curve.

Taking a straight average of the points within each window is referred to as 'using a boxcar window' because $\hat{\mu}(t)$ is a weighted average of the y_i's with weights equal to zero or one. The weights form the shape of a boxcar (rail van) when plotted against time. An alternative, slightly better strategy is to use a weighting function that changes smoothly with time and gives more weight to the observations close to t. A common weight function is the Gaussian kernel, $K(u) = \exp(-0.5u^2)$. The kernel estimate is defined as

$$\hat{\mu}(t) = \sum_{i=1}^{m} w(t, t_i, h) y_i \Big/ \sum_{i=1}^{m} w(t, t_i, h), \qquad (3.3.2)$$

where $w(t, t_i, h) = K\{(t - t_i)/h\}$ and h is the *bandwidth* of the kernel. Larger values of h produce smoother curves.

Example 3.4. CD4+ cell numbers

Figure 3.11 shows the CD4+ data with kernel estimates of the conditional CD4+ mean as a function of time for two choices of the bandwidth. Note how the estimated curve is considerably smoother for the larger bandwidth.

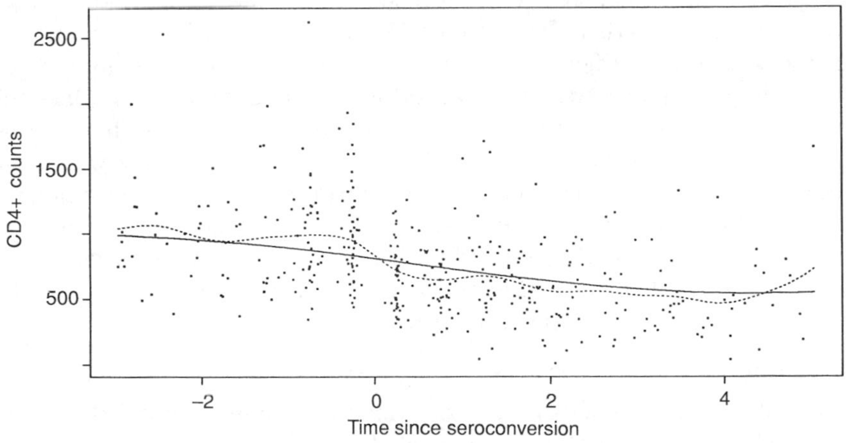

Fig. 3.11. Comparison between two kernel smoothers ——: large bandwidth ......: small bandwidth.

The second non-parametric curve in common use is the smoothing spline (Silverman, 1985). The name *spline* refers to a draftsman's tool which is a flexible rod used to interpolate smoothly, points in a design drawing. A cubic smoothing spline is the function, $s(t)$, which minimizes the criterion

$$J(\lambda) = \sum_{i=1}^{m} \{y_i - s(t_i)\}^2 + \lambda \int \{s''(t)\}^2 \, dt, \tag{3.3.3}$$

where $s''(t)$ is the second derivative of $s(t)$. The first term in (3.3.3) quantifies the fidelity of the function, $s(t)$, to the observations, y_i; the integral is a measure of curvature, or roughness of the function, sometimes called a *roughness penalty*. The constant λ determines the degree of smoothness of the spline. When λ is small, little weight is given to the roughness penalty and the spline will be less smooth.

The smoothing spline which minimizes the criterion above is a twice-differentiable piecewise cubic polynomial. It can be calculated from the observations $(t_i, y_i), i = 1, \ldots, m$ by solving relatively simple linear equations.

Silverman (1984) has shown that a cubic smoothing spline can be closely approximated by a kernel estimate with local bandwidth that is proportional to $g(t)^{-0.25}$ where $g(t)$ is the density of points in the vicinity of time t. While splines have adaptive bandwidths, the power -0.25 indicates that the effective bandwidths do not change very quickly with the density of observations.

The final method, lowess (Cleveland, 1979), is a natural extension of kernel methods made 'robust', that is less sensitive, to outlying Y values. The lowess curve estimate at time t_i starts by centring a window there as in Fig. 3.10. Rather than calculating a weighted mean of the points in the window, a weighted least-squares line is fitted. As before, more weight is given to observations close to the middle of the window. Once the line has been fitted, the residual (vertical) distance from the line to each point in the window is determined. The outliers, that is, points with large residuals, are then downweighted and the line is re-estimated. This process is iterated a few times. The net result is a fitted line that is insensitive to observations with outlying Y values. The value of the lowess curve at t_i is just the predicted value for the line. The entire lowess curve is obtained by repeating this process at the desired times.

Example 3.4. (continued)

Figure 3.12 shows kernel and lowess estimates of similar smoothness fitted to the CD4+ data where we have altered two of the points to create outliers. Note that the kernel estimator is affected more than lowess by the outliers. When exploring longitudinal data, it is good practice to use robust

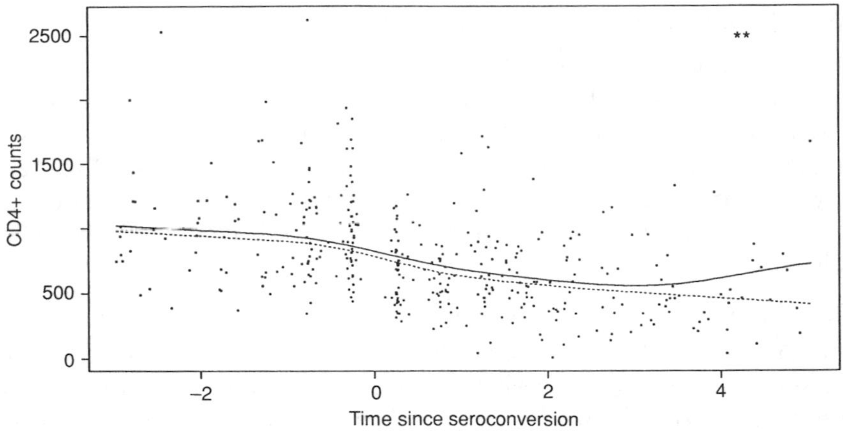

Fig. 3.12. Comparison between lowess and kernel smoothers, for data with two artificial outliers (shown as ⋆) ——: kernel ......: lowess.

smoothing methods as this avoids excessive dependence of results on a few observations.

With each of the non-parametric curve estimation techniques, there is a bandwidth parameter which controls the smoothness of the fitted curve. In choosing the bandwidth, there is a classic trade-off between bias and variance. The wider the bandwidth, the smaller the variance of the estimated curve at any fixed time since more observations have been averaged. But estimates which are smoother than the functions they are approximating are biased. The objective in curve estimation is to choose from the data a smoothness parameter that balances bias and variance.

A generally accepted aggregate measure that combines bias and variance is the *average predictive squared error* (PSE) defined by

$$\text{PSE}(\lambda) = \frac{1}{m}\sum_{i=1}^{m} \text{E}\{Y_i^* - \hat{\mu}(t_i;\lambda)\}^2, \tag{3.3.4}$$

where Y_i^* is a new observation at t_i. We cannot compare the observed y_i with the corresponding value, $\hat{\mu}(t_i)$, in the criterion above because the optimal curve would interpolate the points. PSE can be estimated by *cross-validation* where we compare the observed y_i to the predicted curve $\hat{\mu}^{-i}(t_i)$ obtained by leaving out the ith observation. The cross-validation criterion is given by

$$\text{CV}(\lambda) = \frac{1}{m}\sum_{i=1}^{m} \{y_i - \hat{\mu}^{-i}(t_i;\lambda)\}^2. \tag{3.3.5}$$

The expected value of CV(λ) is approximately equal to the average PSE. See Hastie and Tibshirani (1990) for further discussion.

3.4 Exploring correlation structure

In this section, graphical displays for exploring the degree of association in a longitudinal data set are considered. To remove the effects of explanatory variables, we first regress the response, y_{ij}, on the explanatory variables, $\boldsymbol{x}_{ij}$, to obtain residuals, $r_{ij} = y_{ij} - \boldsymbol{x}_{ij}'\hat{\beta}$. With data collected at a fixed number of equally spaced time points, correlation can be studied using a scatterplot matrix in which r_{ij} is plotted against r_{ik} for all $j < k = 1, \ldots, n$.

Example 3.5. CD4+ cell numbers

To illustrate the idea of a scatterplot matrix, we have rounded the CD4+ observation times to the nearest year, so that there are a maximum of seven observations between −2 and 4 for each individual. Figure 3.13 shows each of the 7 choose 2 scatterplots of responses from a person at different times.

Notice from the main diagonal of the scatterplot matrix that there is substantial positive correlation between repeated observations on the same individual that are one year apart. The degree of correlation decreases as the observations are moved farther from one another in time, which corresponds to moving farther from the diagonal. Notice also that the correlation is reasonably consistent along a diagonal in the matrix. This indicates that the correlation depends more strongly on the time between observations than on their absolute times.

If the residuals have constant mean and variance and if $\text{Corr}(y_{ij}, y_{ik})$ depends only on $|t_{ij} - t_{ik}|$, the process Y_{ij} is said to be *weakly stationary* (Box and Jenkins, 1970). This is a reasonable first approximation for the CD4+ data.

When each scatterplot in the matrix appears like a sample from the bivariate Gaussian (normal) distribution, we can summarize the association with a *correlation matrix*, comprised of a correlation coefficient for each plot.

Example 3.5. (continued)

The estimated correlation matrix for the CD4+ data is presented in Table 3.2. The correlations show some tendency to decrease with increasing time lag, but remain substantial at all lags. The estimated correlation of 0.89 at lag 6 is quite likely misleading, as it is calculated from only nine pairs of measurements.

Assuming stationarity, a single correlation estimate can be obtained for each distinct value of the time separation or *lag*, $|\, t_{ij} - t_{ik} \,|$. This corresponds to pooling observation pairs along the diagonals of the scatterplot matrix. This *autocorrelation function* for the CD4+ data takes the values presented in Table 3.3.

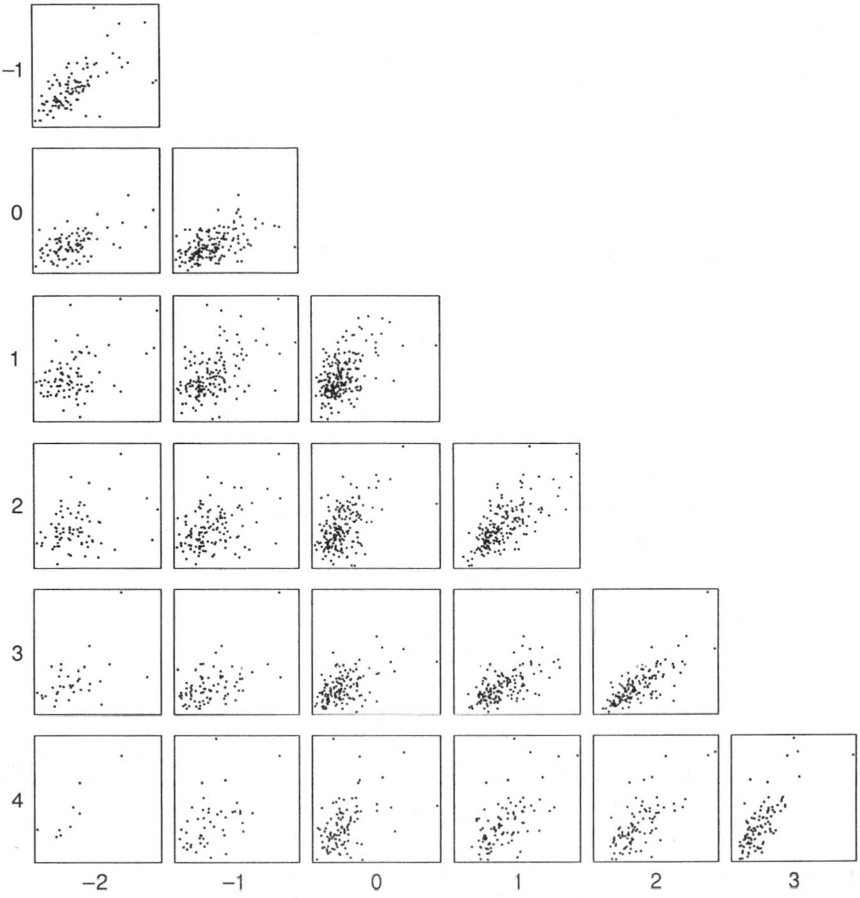

Fig. 3.13. Scatterplot matrix of CD4+ residuals. Axis labels are years relative to seroconversion.

It is obviously desirable to indicate the uncertainty in an estimated correlation coefficient when examining the correlation matrix or autocorrelation function. The simplest rule of thumb is that under the null condition of no correlation, a correlation coefficient has standard error which is roughly $1/\sqrt{N}$ where N is the number of independent pairs of observations in the calculation. Using this rule of thumb, a plot of the autocorrelation function can be enhanced with tolerance limits for a true autocorrelation of zero. These take the form of pairs of values $\pm 2/\sqrt{N_u}$, where N_u is the number of pairs of observations at lag u.

Example 3.5. (continued)

Figure 3.14 shows the estimated autocorrelation function for the CD4+ cell numbers, together with its associated tolerance limits for zero

Table 3.2. Estimated autocorrelation matrix for CD4+ residuals. Entries are $\mathrm{Corr}(Y_{ij}, Y_{ik})$, $1 = t_{ij} < t_{ik} \leq 7$ years.

	t_{ik}					
t_{ik}	1	2	3	4	5	6
2	0.66					
3	0.56	0.49				
4	0.41	0.47	0.51			
5	0.29	0.39	0.51	0.68		
6	0.48	0.52	0.51	0.65	0.75	
7	0.89	0.48	0.44	0.61	0.70	0.75

Table 3.3. Estimated autocorrelation function for CD4+ residuals. Entries are $\hat{\rho}(u) = \mathrm{Corr}(Y_{ij}, Y_{ij-u}), u = 1, \ldots, 6$.

u	1	2	3	4	5	6
$\hat{\rho}(u)$	0.60	0.54	0.46	0.42	0.47	0.89

autocorrelation. The size of the tolerance limit at lag 6 is an effective counter to spurious over-interpretation of the large estimated autocorrelation. All that can be said is that the autocorrelation at lag 6 is significantly greater than zero.

Calculating confidence intervals for non-zero autocorrelations is more complex. See Box and Jenkins (1970) for a detailed discussion.

In subsequent chapters, the autocorrelation function will be one tool for identifying sensible models for the correlation in a longitudinal data set. The empirical function described above will be contrasted with the theoretical correlations for a candidate model. Hence, the EDA displays are later useful for model criticism as well.

The autocorrelation function is most effective for studying equally spaced data that are roughly stationary. Autocorrelations are more difficult to estimate with irregularly spaced data unless we round observation times as was done above for the CD4+ data. An alternative function that describes the association among repeated values and is easily estimated with irregular observation times is the *variogram* (Diggle, 1990). For a stochastic process $Y(t)$, the variogram is defined as

$$\gamma(u) = \tfrac{1}{2}\mathrm{E}\left[\{Y(t) - Y(t-u)\}^2\right], \quad u \geq 0. \tag{3.4.1}$$

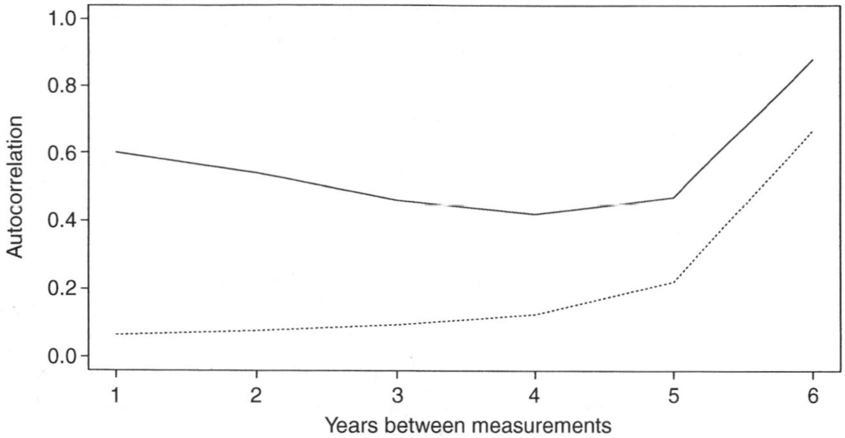

Fig. 3.14. Sample autocorrelation function of CD4+ residuals, and upper 95% tolerance limits assuming zero autocorrelation. ——: sample autocorrelation function ......: tolerance limits.

If $Y(t)$ is stationary, the variogram is directly related to the autocorrelation function, $\rho(u)$, by

$$\gamma(u) = \sigma^2 \{1 - \rho(u)\},$$

where σ^2 is the variance of $Y(t)$. However, the variogram is also well-defined for a limited class of non-stationary processes for which the *increments*, $Y(t) - Y(t-u)$, are stationary.

The origins of the variogram as a descriptive tool go back at least to Jowett (1952). It has since been used extensively in the body of methodology known as *geostatistics*, which is concerned primarily with the estimation of spatial variation (Journel and Huijbregts, 1978). In the longitudinal context, the empirical counterpart of the variogram, which we call the *sample variogram*, is calculated from observed half-squared-differences between pairs of residuals,

$$v_{ijk} = \tfrac{1}{2}(r_{ij} - r_{ik})^2,$$

and the corresponding time-differences

$$u_{ijk} = t_{ij} - t_{ik}.$$

If the times t_{ij} are not totally irregular, there will be more than one observation at each value of u. We then let $\hat{\gamma}(u)$ be the average of all of the v_{ijk} corresponding to that particular value of u. With highly irregular sampling times, the variogram can be estimated from the data (u_{ijk}, v_{ijk}),

$j < k = 1, \ldots, n_i$; $i = 1, \ldots, m$ by fitting a non-parametric curve. The process variance, σ^2, is estimated as the average of all half-squared-differences $\frac{1}{2}(y_{ij} - y_{lk})^2$ with $i \neq l$. The autocorrelation function at any lag u can then be estimated from the sample variogram by the formula

$$\hat{\rho}(u) = 1 - \hat{\gamma}(u)/\hat{\sigma}^2. \tag{3.4.2}$$

Example 3.6. CD4+ cell counts

An estimate of the variogram for the CD4+ data is pictured in Fig. 3.15. The diagram shows both the basic quantities (u_{ijk}, v_{ijk}) and a smooth estimate of $\gamma(u)$ which has been produced using lowess. Note that there are few data available for time differences of less than six months or beyond six years. Also, to accentuate the shape of the smooth estimate, we have truncated the vertical axis at 180 000. The variogram smoothly increases with lag corresponding to decreasing correlation as observations are separated in time, but appears almost to have levelled out by lag $u = 6$. This is in contrast to the apparent, albeit spurious, *rise* in the estimated autocorrelation at lag 6, as shown in Fig. 3.14. The explanation is that the non-parametric smoothing of the variogram recognizes the sparsity of data at lag $u = 6$, and incorporates information from the sample variogram at smaller values of u. This illustrates one advantage of the sample variogram for irregularly spaced data, by comparison with the sample autocorrelation function based on artificially rounded measurement times. The horizontal line on Fig. 3.15 is the variogram-based estimate of the process variance, which is substantially larger than the value of the sample variogram at lag $u = 6$. This suggests either that the autocorrelation has not decayed to zero within the range of the data or, if we accept the earlier observation that the variogram has almost levelled out, that positive correlation remains at arbitrarily large time separations. The latter is what we would expect if there is a component of variation between subjects, leading to a positive correlation between repeated measurements on the same subject, irrespective of their time separation.

Incidentally, the enormous random fluctuations in the basic quantities (u_{ijk}, v_{ijk}) are entirely typical. The marginal sampling distribution of each v_{ijk} is proportional to chi-squared on 1 degree of freedom.

Example 3.7. Milk protein measurements

We now construct an estimate of the variogram for the milk protein data. In a designed experiment such as this, we are able to use a *saturated* model for the mean response profiles. By this, we mean that we fit a separate parameter for the mean response at each of the 19 times in each of the three treatment groups. The ordinary least-squares (OLS) estimates of these 57 mean response parameters are just the corresponding observed means. The sample variogram of the resulting set of OLS residuals is shown

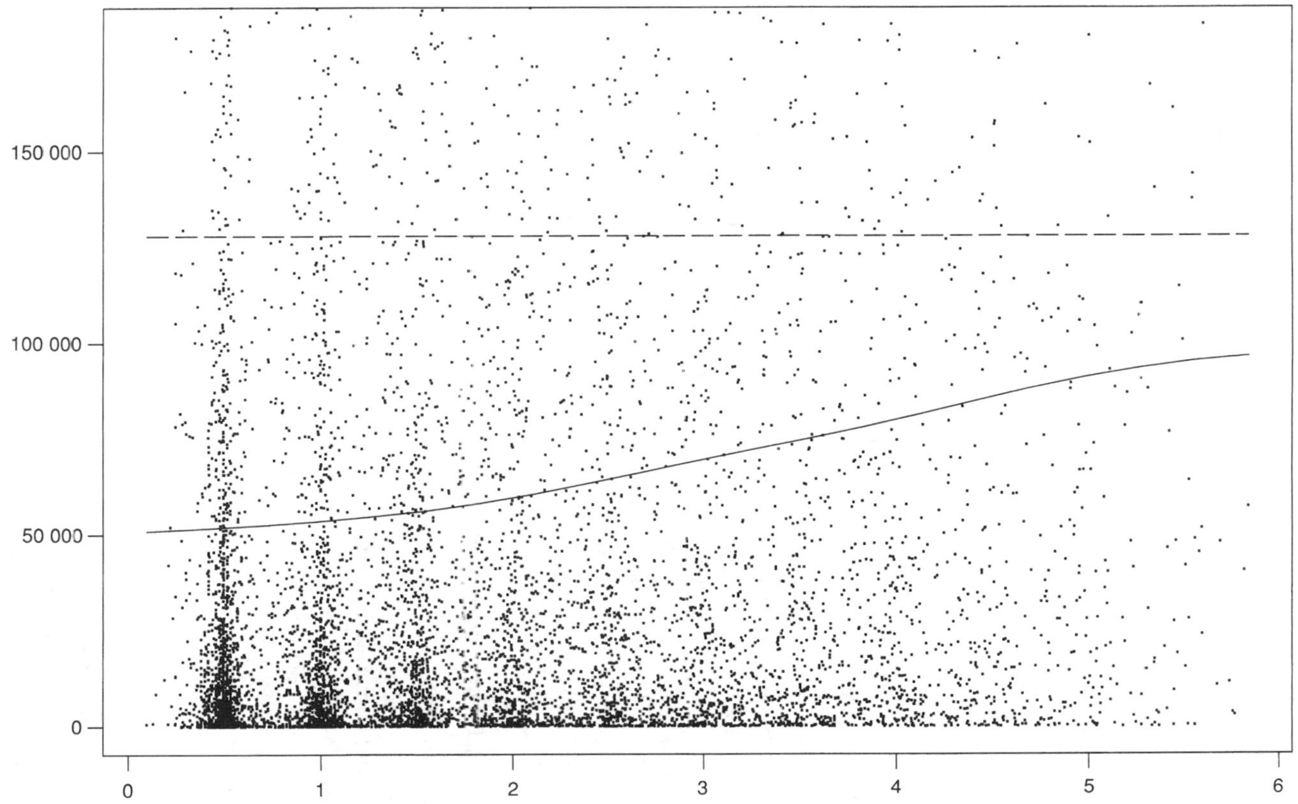

Fig. 3.15. Sample variogram of CD4+ residuals ·: individual points (u_{ijk}, v_{ijk}); ——: lowess smooth; – – –: residual variance.

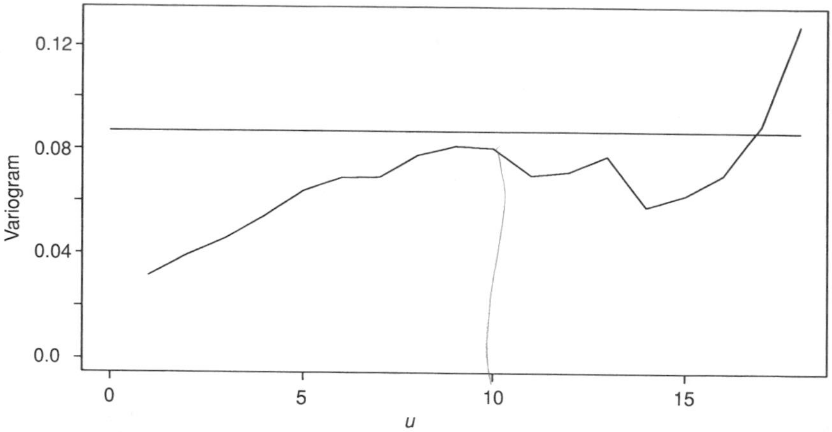

Fig. 3.16. Sample variogram of milk protein residuals. Horizontal line estimates process variance.

in Fig. 3.16. In contrast to the CD4+ example, the pattern is clear without further smoothing. The variogram rises steadily with increasing u, but levels off within the range spanned by the data. This levelling off suggests that the correlation has effectively decayed to zero by a time separation of about 10 weeks. The increase in $\hat{V}(u)$ at $u = 18$ is apparently inconsistent with this interpretation. However, this estimate is an average of rather few v_{ijk}, and is therefore unreliable. For a more detailed interpretation of this variogram estimate, see Example 5.1 of Section 5.4.

3.5 Exploring association amongst categorical responses

For a continuous-valued response variable, it is natural to seek initially to describe association in terms of the correlation structure between values of the response variable measured at different times. For a binary response, a correlation-based approach is less natural; for example, the permissible range of correlations between a pair of binary variables is constrained by their respective means. A more natural measure of association is the *log-odds ratio*. For a pair of binary variables, say Y_1 and Y_2, the odds ratio is

$$\gamma(Y_1, Y_2) = \frac{P(Y_1 = 1, Y_2 = 1)P(Y_1 = 0, Y_2 = 0)}{P(Y_1 = 1, Y_2 = 0)P(Y_1 = 0, Y_2 = 1)},$$

and the log-odds ratio is LOR $= \log \gamma$. For a longitudinal sequence $Y_1, \ldots, Y_n$ at measurement times $t_1, \ldots, t_n$, Heagerty and Zeger (1998) define the *lorelogram* to be the function

$$\text{LOR}(t_j, t_k) = \log \gamma(Y_j, Y_k).$$

In the special case that $\text{LOR}(t_j, t_k)$ depends only on $u_{jk} = |t_j - t_k|$ they call the resulting function the *isotropic* lorelogram. Note that this is analogous to the concept of second-order stationarity for a real-valued process $Y(t)$.

To estimate the lorelogram from replicated longitudinal data, y_{ij}, $j = 1, \ldots, n_i; i = 1, \ldots, m$, we use sample proportions across subjects in place of the theoretical probabilities which appear in the definition of γ. Section 11.4 gives a detailed example in which the *lorelogram* is used to study the association between repeated psychiatric symptoms on a cohort of schizophrenic patients.

3.6 Further reading

The modern rebirth of exploratory data analysis was led by John W. Tukey. The books by Tukey (1977) and by Mosteller and Tukey (1977) are the best original sources. A simpler introduction is provided by Velleman and Hoaglin (1981). Background information on graphical methods in statistics, as well as on lowess, can be found in Chambers *et al.* (1983). Two stimulating books on graphical displays of information are by Edward Tufte (1983, 1990). An excellent review of smoothing methods is available in the first three chapters of Hastie and Tibshirani (1990). Further reading, with an emphasis on the kernel method, is in Härdle (1990). Discussion of the estimation and interpretation of autocorrelation functions can be found in almost any book on time series analysis, but perhaps the most detailed account is in Box and Jenkins (1970). The variogram is described in more detail in Diggle (1990) whereas a more detailed treatment of the *lorelogram* is given in Heagerty and Zeger (1998).

4
General linear models for longitudinal data

4.1 Motivation

In this and the next chapter, our aim is to develop a general linear modelling framework for longitudinal data, in which the inferences we make about the regression parameters of primary interest recognize the likely correlation structure in the data. Two ways of achieving this are to build explicit parametric models of the covariance structure whose validity can be checked against the available data or, where possible, to use methods of inference which are robust to misspecification of the covariance structure. In this chapter, we first consider the general linear model for correlated data and discuss briefly some specific models for the covariance structure. We then consider general approaches to parameter estimation – general in the sense that they are not restricted to particular models for the covariance structure. We use weighted least-squares estimation for parameters which describe the mean response, and maximum likelihood or restricted maximum likelihood for covariance parameters. Finally, we develop and illustrate methods for robust estimaton of standard errors associated with weighted least-squares estimates of mean response parameters. In this context, the term 'robust' means that, whilst the estimates themselves may be derived by making a working assumption that the covariance structure is of a particular form, the associated standard errors are calculated in such a way that they remain valid whatever the true covariance structure.

In Chapter 5 we further develop explicit parametric models for the covariance structure and show how to fit these models to data. Models of this kind are particularly useful when the data consist of relatively long, irregularly spaced or incomplete sequences of observations. For data consisting of short, complete sequences and when the primary scientific objective involves inference about the mean response, the approach described in the present chapter, which avoids the need for a parametric specification of the covariance structure, should suffice.

4.2 The general linear model with correlated errors

Let y_{ij}, $j = 1, \ldots, n$ be the sequence of observed measurements on the ith of m subjects, and t_j, $j = 1, \ldots, n$ be the corresponding times at which the measurements are taken on each unit. We relax the assumption of a common set of times, t_j, later. Associated with each y_{ij} are the values, x_{ijk}, $k = 1, \ldots, p$, of p explanatory variables. We assume that the y_{ij} are realizations of random variables Y_{ij} which follow the regression model

$$Y_{ij} = \beta_1 x_{ij1} + \cdots + \beta_p x_{ijp} + \epsilon_{ij},$$

where the ϵ_{ij} are random sequences of length n associated with each of the m subjects. In the classical linear model, the ϵ_{ij} would be mutually independent $N(0, \sigma^2)$ random variables. In our context, the longitudinal structure of the data means that we expect the ϵ_{ij} to be correlated within subjects.

For a formal analysis of the linear model, a matrix formulation is preferable. Let $\boldsymbol{y}_i = (y_{i1}, \ldots, y_{in})$ be the observed sequence of measurements on the ith subject and $\boldsymbol{y} = (\boldsymbol{y}_1, \ldots, \boldsymbol{y}_m)$ the complete set of $N = nm$ measurements from m units. Let X be an $N \times p$ matrix of explanatory variables, with $\{n(i-1)+j\}$th row $(x_{ij1}, \ldots, x_{ijp})$. Let $\sigma^2 V$ be a block-diagonal matrix with non-zero $n \times n$ blocks $\sigma^2 V_0$, each representing the variance matrix for the vector of measurements on a single subject. Then, the general linear model (GLM) for longitudinal data treats $\boldsymbol{y}$ as a realization of a multivariate Gaussian random vector, $\boldsymbol{Y}$, with

$$\boldsymbol{Y} \sim MVN(X\boldsymbol{\beta}, \sigma^2 V). \qquad (4.2.1)$$

If we want to use the robust approach to analysing data generated by the model (4.2.1), the block-diagonal structure of $\sigma^2 V$ is crucial, because we will use the replication across units to estimate $\sigma^2 V$ without making any parametric assumptions about its form. Nevertheless, it is perhaps useful at this stage, in anticipation of the parametric modelling approach of Chapter 5, to consider what form the non-zero blocks $\sigma^2 V_0$ might take.

4.2.1 *The uniform correlation model*

In this model, we assume that there is a positive correlation, ρ, between any two measurements on the same subject. In matrix terms, this corresponds to

$$V_0 = (1-\rho)I + \rho J, \qquad (4.2.2)$$

where I denotes the $n \times n$ identity matrix and J the $n \times n$ matrix all of whose elements are 1.

A justification of this *uniform correlation* model is the following. Let the observed measurements, y_{ij}, be realizations of random variables, Y_{ij}, such that

$$Y_{ij} = \mu_{ij} + U_i + Z_{ij}, \quad i = 1, \ldots, m; \; j = 1, \ldots, n, \tag{4.2.3}$$

where $\mu_{ij} = \mathrm{E}(Y_{ij})$, the U_i are mutually independent $N(0, \nu^2)$ random variables, the Z_{ij} are mutually independent $N(0, \tau^2)$ random variables and the U_i and Z_{ij} are independent of one another. Then, the covariance structure of the data corresponds to (4.2.2) with $\rho = \nu^2/(\nu^2 + \tau^2)$ and $\sigma^2 = \nu^2 + \tau^2$. Note that (4.2.3) gives an interpretation of the uniform correlation model as one in which a linear model for the mean response incorporates a random intercept term with variance ν^2 between subjects. It therefore provides the foundation for a wider class of random coefficient models which we consider in Section 4.2.3 and, in more detail, in Chapter 9. Also, (4.2.3) provides a model-based justification for a so called *split-plot* analysis of variance approach to longitudinal data which we describe in Chapter 6.

4.2.2 *The exponential correlation model*

In this model, V_0 has jkth element, $v_{jk} = \mathrm{Cov}(Y_{ij}, Y_{ik})$, of the form

$$v_{jk} = \sigma^2 \exp(-\phi \, | \, t_j - t_k \, |). \tag{4.2.4}$$

In contrast to the uniform correlation model, the correlation between a pair of measurements on the same unit decays towards zero as the time separation between the measurements increases. The rate of decay is faster for larger values of ϕ. Figure 4.1 illustrates this with $\phi = 0.1$, 0.25, and 1.0. Note that if the observation times, t_j, are equally spaced, say $t_{j+1} - t_j = d$ for all j, then (4.2.4) is expressible as

$$v_{jk} = \sigma^2 \rho^{|j-k|}, \tag{4.2.5}$$

where $\rho = \exp(-\phi d)$ is the correlation between successive observations on the same subject.

A justification of (4.2.5) is to represent the random variables Y_{ij} as

$$Y_{ij} = \mu_{ij} + W_{ij}, \quad i = 1, \ldots, m; \; j = 1, \ldots, n, \tag{4.2.6}$$

where

$$W_{ij} = \rho W_{ij-1} + Z_{ij}, \tag{4.2.7}$$

and the Z_{ij} are mutually independent $N\{0, \sigma^2(1 - \rho^2)\}$ random variables, to give $\mathrm{Var}(Y_{ij}) = \mathrm{Var}(W_{ij}) = \sigma^2$ as required. In view of (4.2.6) and (4.2.7), the exponential correlation model is sometimes called the *first-order autoregressive model*, because (4.2.7) is the standard definition of

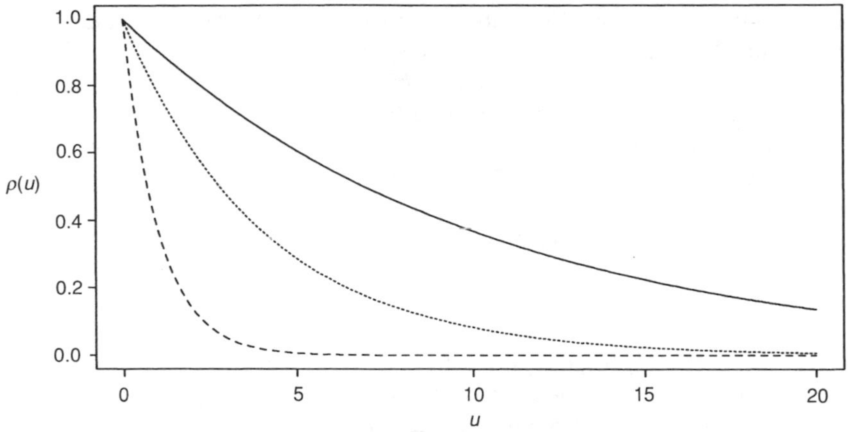

Fig. 4.1. The autocorrelation function for the exponential model. ——: $\phi = 0.1$; ....: $\phi = 0.25$; – – –: $\phi = 1.0$.

a discrete-time first-order autoregressive process (see, for example, Diggle, 1990, p. 34). This has led some authors to generalize the model by assuming the sequences, $W_{ij}, j = 1, \ldots, n$, in (4.2.6) to be mutually independent partial realizations of a general stationary autoregressive moving average process,

$$W_{ij} = \sum_{r=1}^{p} \rho_r W_{ij-r} + Z_{ij} + \sum_{s=1}^{q} \beta_s Z_{ij-s}. \tag{4.2.8}$$

Our view is that the discrete-time setting of (4.2.8) is often unnatural for longitudinal data and that a more natural generalization of (4.2.6) is to a model of the form

$$Y_{ij} = \mu_{ij} + W_i(t_j), \quad i = 1, \ldots, m; \; j = 1, \ldots, n, \tag{4.2.9}$$

where the sequences $W_i(t_j), j = 1, \ldots, n$ are realizations of mutually independent, continuous-time, stationary Gaussian processes $\{W_i(t), t \in R\}$ with a common covariance structure, $\gamma(u) = \text{Cov}\{W_i(t), W_i(t-u)\}$. Note that (4.2.9) automatically accomodates irregularly spaced times of measurement, t_j, and, incidentally, different times of measurement for different units, whereas either of the discrete-time models, (4.2.7) or (4.2.8), would be quite unnatural for irregularly spaced t_j.

4.2.3 *Two-stage least-squares estimation and random effects models*

Two-stage least squares provides a simple method of fitting a class of models in which the data-analyst recognises a partition of the random variation in a set of longitudinal data into two components, between and within subjects. A specific example motivates the general idea.

Imagine an investigation into the normal growth rate of children. The study involves the recruitment of a group of children, presumed to be a random sample from the population of interest, and the subsequent measurement of the weight of each child at a sequence of ages.

In the *first-stage* analysis of the results, we consider the growth trajectory of each child. A simple model is that the ith child's weight (possibly after appropriate transformation) varies randomly about a linear growth curve. Formally, we assume that

$$Y_{ij} = A_i + B_i x_{ij} + \epsilon_{ij}, \quad j = 1, \ldots, n_i; \; i = 1, \ldots, m, \tag{4.2.10}$$

in which Y_{ij} and x_{ij} respectively denote the (transformed) weight and age of the ith child on the jth measurement occasion, A_i and B_i determine the ith child's linear growth curve and the ϵ_{ij} are independent random deviations of the observed weight about this underlying growth curve, with mean zero and variance τ^2. We can fit the first-stage model (4.2.10) by ordinary least squares (OLS), to produce estimates $\hat{A}_i$, $\hat{B}_i$ and $\hat{\tau}^2$, each with an associated standard error. In particular, suppose that the estimated standard error of $\hat{B}_i$ is v_i, then a reasonable assumption is that

$$\hat{B}_i = B_i + Z_i, \quad i = 1, \ldots, m, \tag{4.2.11}$$

where the Z_i are mutually independent Gaussian random variables with respective variances v_i^2.

In the *second-stage* analysis of the results, we focus on the variation amongst the child-specific first-stage estimated regression coefficients. Children vary in their underlying growth rates. A reasonable assumption might therefore be that the B_i: $i = 1, \ldots, m$, are themselves an independent random sample from a Gaussian distribution with mean β and variance σ^2. Hence, the second-stage model is

$$B_i = \beta + \delta_i, \quad i = 1, \ldots, m, \tag{4.2.12}$$

in which the δ_i are an independent random sample from a Gaussian distribution with mean zero and variance σ^2.

If we now combine (4.2.11) and (4.2.12) we obtain

$$\hat{B}_i = \beta + \{\delta_i + Z_i\}, \tag{4.2.13}$$

in which each δ_i has the same variance σ^2, but the variances of the Z_i are different. Hence, the variances of the $\hat{B}_i$ are different, and an appropriate estimate of β would be a *weighted* mean of the $\hat{B}_i$.

We could apply a similar argument to the child-specific intercept parameters A_i, leading to a bivariate Gaussian second-stage model for the quantities (A_i, B_i): $i = 1, \ldots, m$. However, to simplify the presentation of what is intended only as a motivating example, suppose that $A_i = \alpha$, for all i. Then, we can combine the first-stage and second-stage models into a single equation for the entire set of data,

$$\begin{aligned} Y_{ij} &= \alpha + \{\beta + \delta_i\}x_{ij} + \epsilon_{ij} \\ &= \alpha + \beta x_{ij} + \{\delta_i x_{ij} + \epsilon_{ij}\} \\ &= \alpha + \beta x_{ij} + W_{ij}, \quad j = 1, \ldots, n_i; \ i = 1, \ldots, m. \end{aligned} \tag{4.2.14}$$

Now, the first two terms on the right-hand side of (4.2.14) define a linear regression model for the mean response, whilst the third identifies a set of random deviations W_{ij} which have different variances and are correlated within subjects. Specifically,

$$\text{Var}(W_{ij}) = \sigma^2 x_{ij}^2 + \tau^2,$$

and

$$\text{Cov}(W_{ij}, W_{ik}) = \sigma^2 x_{ij} x_{ik}.$$

This is a particular case of (4.2.1), in which the matrix V has diagonal elements $x_{ij}^2 + (\tau^2/\sigma^2)$ and off-diagonal elements $x_{ij}x_{ik}$. Thus, V involves a single unknown parameter, τ^2/σ^2. It follows that any method for fitting the GLM with correlated errors can be used to fit the present model in a single-stage calculation.

Models of this kind, in which the covariance structure of the data is induced by random variation amongst unobserved, subject-specific quantities, are called random effects models. We shall consider them in more detail in Section 5.2, and in Chapter 9.

4.3 Weighted least-squares estimation

We now return to the general formulation of (4.2.1), and consider the problem of estimating the regression parameter $\boldsymbol{\beta}$. The *weighted least-squares* estimator of $\boldsymbol{\beta}$, using a symmetric *weight matrix*, W, is the value, $\tilde{\boldsymbol{\beta}}_W$, which minimizes the quadratic form

$$(\boldsymbol{y} - X\boldsymbol{\beta})'W(\boldsymbol{y} - X\boldsymbol{\beta}). \tag{4.3.1}$$

Standard matrix manipulations give the explicit result

$$\tilde{\boldsymbol{\beta}}_W = (X'WX)^{-1}X'W\boldsymbol{y}. \tag{4.3.2}$$

Because $\boldsymbol{y}$ is a realization of a random vector $\boldsymbol{Y}$ with $E(\boldsymbol{Y}) = X\boldsymbol{\beta}$, the weighted least-squares estimator, $\tilde{\boldsymbol{\beta}}_W$, is unbiased, whatever the choice of W. Furthermore, since $\mathrm{Var}(\boldsymbol{Y}) = \sigma^2 V$, then

$$\mathrm{Var}(\tilde{\boldsymbol{\beta}}_W) = \sigma^2\{(X'WX)^{-1}X'W\}V\{WX(X'WX)^{-1}\}. \tag{4.3.3}$$

If $W = I$, the identity matrix, (4.3.2) reduces to the OLS estimator

$$\tilde{\boldsymbol{\beta}}_I = (X'X)^{-1}X'\boldsymbol{y}, \tag{4.3.4}$$

with

$$\mathrm{Var}(\tilde{\boldsymbol{\beta}}_I) = \sigma^2(X'X)^{-1}X'VX(X'X)^{-1}. \tag{4.3.5}$$

If $W = V^{-1}$, the estimator becomes

$$\hat{\boldsymbol{\beta}} = (X'V^{-1}X)^{-1}X'V^{-1}\boldsymbol{y}, \tag{4.3.6}$$

with

$$\mathrm{Var}(\hat{\boldsymbol{\beta}}) = \sigma^2(X'V^{-1}X)^{-1}. \tag{4.3.7}$$

The 'hat' notation anticipates that $\hat{\boldsymbol{\beta}}$ is the maximum likelihood estimator for $\boldsymbol{\beta}$ under the multivariate Gaussian assumption (4.2.1).

This last remark suggests, correctly, that the most efficient weighted least-squares estimator for $\boldsymbol{\beta}$ uses $W = V^{-1}$. However, to identify this optimal weighting matrix we need to know the complete correlation structure of the data – we do not need to know σ^2, because $\tilde{\boldsymbol{\beta}}_W$ is unchanged by proportional changes in all the elements of W. Because the correlation structure may be difficult to identify in practice, it is of interest to ask how much loss of efficiency might result from using a different W. Note that the relative efficiency of $\tilde{\boldsymbol{\beta}}_W$ and $\hat{\boldsymbol{\beta}}$ can be calculated from their respective variance matrices (4.3.3) and (4.3.7).

The relative efficiency of OLS depends on the precise interplay between the matrices X and V, as described by Bloomfield and Watson (1975). However, our experience has been that under the conditions encountered in a wide range of longitudinal data applications, the relative efficiency is often quite good. As a simple example, consider $m = 10$ units each observed at $n = 5$ time-points $t_j = -2, -1, 0, 1, 2$. Let the mean response at time t be $\mu(t) = \beta_0 + \beta_1 t$. We shall illustrate the relative efficiency of the OLS estimators for $\boldsymbol{\beta} = (\beta_0, \beta_1)$ under each of the covariance structures described in Section 4.2.

First, note that

$$(X'X)^{-1} = \begin{bmatrix} 50 & 0 \\ 0 & 100 \end{bmatrix}^{-1} = \begin{bmatrix} 0.02 & 0 \\ 0 & 0.01 \end{bmatrix}.$$

Now, suppose that V corresponds to the uniform correlation model (4.2.2) with

$$V_0 = (1-\rho)I + \rho J,$$

for some $0 \leq \rho < 1$. Then, straightforward matrix manipulations give

$$X'VX = \begin{bmatrix} 50(1+4\rho) & 0 \\ 0 & 100(1-\rho) \end{bmatrix},$$

and

$$\text{Var}(\tilde{\boldsymbol{\beta}}_I) = \sigma^2 \begin{bmatrix} 0.02(1+4\rho) & 0 \\ 0 & 0.01(1-\rho) \end{bmatrix}, \tag{4.3.8}$$

by substitution of $(X'X)^{-1}$ and $X'VX$ into (4.3.5). Similarly,

$$V_0^{-1} = (1-\rho)^{-1}I - \rho\{(1-\rho)(1+4\rho)\}^{-1}J,$$

$$X'V^{-1}X = \begin{bmatrix} 50(1+4\rho)^{-1} & 0 \\ 0 & 100(1-\rho)^{-1} \end{bmatrix},$$

and

$$\text{Var}(\hat{\boldsymbol{\beta}}) = \sigma^2 \begin{bmatrix} 0.02(1+4\rho) & 0 \\ 0 & 0.01(1-\rho) \end{bmatrix}, \tag{4.3.9}$$

from (4.3.7). Comparing (4.3.8) and (4.3.9), we see that they are identical, which implies that OLS is fully efficient in this case. An intuitive explanation is that with a common correlation between any two equally spaced measurements on the same unit, there is no reason to weight measurements differently. However, this is not always the case. For example, it would not be true if the number of measurements varied between units because, with $\rho > 0$, units with more measurements would then convey more information in total but *less* information per measurement, than units with fewer measurements.

Now suppose that V corresponds to the exponential correlation model (4.2.5), in which V_0 has jkth element

$$v_{jk} = \sigma^2 \rho^{|j-k|}.$$

Straightforward matrix manipulations now give $X'VX$ as

$$\begin{bmatrix} 10(5+8\rho+6\rho^2+4\rho^3+2\rho^4) & 0 \\ 0 & 20(5+4\rho-\rho^2-4\rho^3-4\rho^4) \end{bmatrix},$$

and $\text{Var}(\tilde{\boldsymbol{\beta}}_I)$ as

$$\sigma^2 \begin{bmatrix} 0.004(5+8\rho+6\rho^2+4\rho^3+2\rho^4) & 0 \\ 0 & 0.002(5+4\rho-\rho^2-4\rho^3-4\rho^4) \end{bmatrix}. \tag{4.3.10}$$

The matrix V_0^{-1} is tri-diagonal, with jkth element $(1-\rho^2)^{-1}w_{jk}$, and

$$\begin{aligned} w_{11} &= w_{55} = 1, \\ w_{22} &= w_{33} = w_{44} = 1+\rho^2, \\ w_{jj+1} &= w_{jj-1} = -\rho. \end{aligned}$$

Then,

$$X'V^{-1}X = (1-\rho^2)^{-1}\begin{bmatrix} 10(5-8\rho+3\rho^2) & 0 \\ 0 & 20(5-4\rho+\rho^2) \end{bmatrix},$$

and

$$\text{Var}(\hat{\boldsymbol{\beta}}) = \sigma^2(1-\rho^2)\begin{bmatrix} 0.1(5-8\rho+3\rho^2)^{-1} & 0 \\ 0 & 0.05(5-4\rho+\rho^2)^{-1} \end{bmatrix}. \tag{4.3.11}$$

The relative efficiencies, $e(\beta_k) = \text{Var}(\hat{\beta}_k)/\text{Var}(\tilde{\beta}_k)$, in this case are obtained from (4.3.10) and (4.3.11) as

$$e(\beta_0) = 25(1-\rho^2)\{(5-8\rho+3\rho^2)(5+8\rho+6\rho^2+4\rho^3+2\rho^4)\}^{-1},$$

and

$$e(\beta_1) = 25(1-\rho^2)\{(5-4\rho+\rho^2)(5+4\rho-\rho^2-4\rho^3-4\rho^4)\}^{-1}.$$

These are shown in Table 4.1 for a range of values of ρ. Note that all of the tabulated values are close to 1.

Comparisons of this kind suggest that in many circumstances where there is a balanced design, the OLS estimator, $\tilde{\boldsymbol{\beta}}$, is perfectly satisfactory for point estimation. However, this is not always the case. Consider, for

Table 4.1. Relative efficiency of OLS estimation in the linear regression example.

ρ	0.1	0.2	0.3	0.4	0.5
$e(\beta_0)$	0.998	0.992	0.983	0.973	0.963
$e(\beta_1)$	0.997	0.989	0.980	0.970	0.962
ρ	0.6	0.7	0.8	0.9	0.99
$e(\beta_0)$	0.955	0.952	0.956	0.970	0.996
$e(\beta_1)$	0.952	0.955	0.952	0.955	0.961

example, a two-treatment crossover design in which $n = 3$ measurements are taken, at unit time intervals, on each of $m = 8$ subjects. The sequences of treatments given to the eight subjects are AAA, AAB, ABA, ABB, BAA, BAB, BBA, and BBB (Fitzmaurice *et al.*, 1993). The model for the data is

$$Y_{ij} = \beta_0 + \beta_1 x_i + \epsilon_{ij},$$

where x_i is a binary indicator for treatment B and the ϵ_{ij} follow the exponential correlation model, as in the previous example, with autocorrelation ρ between successive measurements on any subject. The relative efficiencies $e(\beta_0)$ and $e(\beta_1)$ are given in Table 4.2. We see that OLS is tolerably efficient for β_0, but horribly inefficient for β_1 when ρ is large. In this example, efficient estimation of β_1 requires careful balancing of between-subject and within-subject comparisons of the two treatments, and the appropriate balance depends critically on the correlation structure.

Even when OLS is reasonably efficient, it is clear from the form of $\mathrm{Var}(\tilde{\boldsymbol{\beta}})$ given at (4.3.5) that interval estimation for $\boldsymbol{\beta}$ still requires information about $\sigma^2 V$, the variance matrix of the data. In particular, the usual formula for the variance of the least-squares estimator,

$$\mathrm{Var}(\tilde{\boldsymbol{\beta}}) = \sigma^2 (X'X)^{-1} \tag{4.3.12}$$

assumes that $V = I$, the identity matrix, and can be seriously misleading when this is not so.

A naive use of OLS would be to ignore the correlation structure in the data and to base interval estimation for $\boldsymbol{\beta}$ on the variance formula (4.3.12) with σ^2 replaced by its usual estimator, the residual mean square

$$\tilde{\boldsymbol{\sigma}}^2 = (nm - p)^{-1}(\boldsymbol{y} - X\tilde{\boldsymbol{\beta}})'(\boldsymbol{y} - X\tilde{\boldsymbol{\beta}}). \tag{4.3.13}$$

There are two sources of error in this naive approach when $V \neq I$. First, formula (4.3.12) is wrong for $\mathrm{Var}(\tilde{\boldsymbol{\beta}})$. Second, $\tilde{\sigma}^2$ is no longer an unbiased

Table 4.2. Relative efficiency of OLS estimation in the crossover example.

ρ	0.1	0.2	0.3	0.4	0.5
$e(\beta_0)$	0.993	0.974	0.946	0.914	0.880
$e(\beta_1)$	0.987	0.947	0.883	0.797	0.692
ρ	0.6	0.7	0.8	0.9	0.99
$e(\beta_0)$	0.846	0.815	0.788	0.766	0.751
$e(\beta_1)$	0.571	0.438	0.297	0.150	0.015

estimator for σ^2. To assess the combined effect of these two sources of error, we can compare the diagonal elements of $\text{Var}(\tilde{\boldsymbol{\beta}})$ as given by (4.3.5) with the corresponding diagonal elements of the matrix $\text{E}(\tilde{\sigma}^2)(X'X)^{-1}$. Some numerical examples are given in Chapter 1 and in Diggle (1990, Chapter 3), where the conclusion is that in the presence of positive autocorrelation, naive use of OLS can seriously over- or underestimate the variance of $\tilde{\boldsymbol{\beta}}$, depending on the design matrix.

4.4 Maximum likelihood estimation under Gaussian assumptions

One strategy for parameter estimation in the GLM is to consider simultaneous estimation of the parameters of interest, $\boldsymbol{\beta}$, and of the covariance parameters, σ^2 and V_0, using the likelihood function. Recall that V is a block-diagonal matrix with common non-zero blocks V_0. Under the Gaussian assumption (4.2.1), the log-likelihood for observed data $\boldsymbol{y}$ is

$$L(\boldsymbol{\beta}, \sigma^2, V_0) = -0.5\{nm \log(\sigma^2) + m \log(|\,V_0\,|) + \sigma^{-2}(\boldsymbol{y} - X\boldsymbol{\beta})'V^{-1}(\boldsymbol{y} - X\boldsymbol{\beta})\}. \tag{4.4.1}$$

For given V_0, the maximum likelihood estimator for $\boldsymbol{\beta}$ is the weighted least-squares estimator (4.3.6), namely

$$\hat{\boldsymbol{\beta}}(V_0) = (X'V^{-1}X)^{-1}X'V^{-1}\boldsymbol{y}. \tag{4.4.2}$$

Substitution into (4.4.1) gives

$$L\{\hat{\boldsymbol{\beta}}(V_0), \sigma^2, V_0\} = -0.5\{nm \log \sigma^2 + m \log(|\,V_0\,|) + \sigma^{-2}\text{RSS}(V_0)\}, \tag{4.4.3}$$

where

$$\text{RSS}(V_0) = \{\boldsymbol{y} - X\hat{\boldsymbol{\beta}}(V_0)\}'V^{-1}\{\boldsymbol{y} - X\hat{\boldsymbol{\beta}}(V_0)\}.$$

Now, differentiation of (4.4.3) with respect to σ^2 gives the maximum likelihood estimator for σ^2, again for fixed V_0, as

$$\hat{\sigma}^2(V_0) = \text{RSS}(V_0)/(nm). \tag{4.4.4}$$

Substitution of (4.4.2) and (4.4.4) into (4.4.1) now gives a reduced log-likelihood for V_0 which, apart from a constant term, is

$$L_r(V_0) = L\{\hat{\boldsymbol{\beta}}(V_0), \hat{\sigma}^2(V_0), V_0\} = -0.5m\{n \log \text{RSS}(V_0) + \log(|\,V_0\,|)\}. \tag{4.4.5}$$

Finally, maximization of $L_r(V_0)$ yields $\hat{V}_0$ and, by substitution into (4.4.2) and (4.4.4), the maximum likelihood estimators, $\hat{\boldsymbol{\beta}} \equiv \hat{\boldsymbol{\beta}}(\hat{V}_0)$ and $\hat{\sigma}^2 \equiv \hat{\sigma}^2(\hat{V}_0)$.

In general, maximization of (4.4.5) with respect to the distinct elements of V_0 requires numerical optimization techniques. The dimensionality of the optimization problem for V_0 is $\frac{1}{2}n(n-1)$ if we assume a common variance σ^2 at each of the n time-points, and $\frac{1}{2}n(n+1)-1$ otherwise. Also, the major computational work in evaluating $L(V_0)$ consists of calculating the determinant and inverse of a symmetric, positive-definite, $n \times n$ matrix.

Note that in using maximum likelihood for simultaneous estimation of $\boldsymbol{\beta}, \sigma^2$ and V_0, the form of the design matrix X is involved explicitly in the estimation of σ^2 and V_0. One consequence of this is that if we assume the wrong form for X, we may not even get consistent estimators for σ^2 and V_0. To combat this problem, a sensible strategy is to use an over-elaborate model for the mean response profiles in estimating the covariance structure of the data. When the data are from a designed experiment with no continuously varying explanatory variables, we recommend incorporating a separate parameter for the mean response at each time within each treatment, so defining a *saturated* model for the mean response profiles. This guarantees consistent estimates of the variance structure which we can then use in assessing whether a more economical parametrization of the mean structure can be justified.

In many observational studies this strategy is not feasible. In particular, whenever the data include one or more continuously varying covariates which are thought to affect the mean response, we need to decide whether to incorporate the covariate as a linear effect, using a single additional column in the X matrix, or as a quadratic or more general non-linear effect. In these circumstances, the concept of a saturated model breaks down.

Even when it is feasible, the saturated model strategy runs into another problem. For g treatments and n times of observation it requires $p = ng$ parameters to define the mean structure, and if this number is relatively large, the maximum likelihood estimates of σ^2 and V_0 may be seriously biased. For example, it is well known that when $V_0 = I$, an unbiased estimator for σ^2 requires a divisor $(nm - p)$ rather than nm in (4.4.4), and the problem is exacerbated by the autocorrelation structure in the data.

Maximum likelihood estimation therefore presents us with a conflict. We may need to use a design matrix with a large number of columns so as to obtain consistent estimates of the covariance structure, whereas approximately unbiased estimation requires a small number of columns. If we can be confident that a small number of columns will define an adequate model, the conflict is not a serious one. Otherwise, we need to consider other methods of estimation. One such is the method of restricted maximum likelihood (REML).

4.5 Restricted maximum likelihood estimation

The method of REML estimation, was introduced by Patterson and Thompson (1971) as a way of estimating variance components in a GLM. The objection to the standard maximum likelihood procedure is that it produces biased estimators of the covariance parameters. This is well known in the case of the GLM with independent errors,

$$\boldsymbol{Y} \sim MVN(X\boldsymbol{\beta}, \sigma^2 I). \tag{4.5.1}$$

In this case, the maximum likelihood estimator for σ^2 is $\hat{\sigma}^2 = \text{RSS}/(nm)$, where RSS denotes the residual sum of squares, whereas the usual unbiased estimator is $\tilde{\sigma}^2 = \text{RSS}/(nm - p)$, where p is the number of elements of $\boldsymbol{\beta}$. In fact, $\tilde{\sigma}^2$ is the REML estimator for σ^2 in the model (4.5.1).

In the case of the GLM with dependent errors,

$$\boldsymbol{Y} \sim MVN(X\boldsymbol{\beta}, \sigma^2 V), \tag{4.5.2}$$

the REML estimator is defined as a maximum likelihood estimator based on a linearly transformed set of data $\boldsymbol{Y}^* = A\boldsymbol{Y}$ such that the distribution of $\boldsymbol{Y}^*$ does not depend on $\boldsymbol{\beta}$. One way to achieve this is by taking A to be the matrix which converts $\boldsymbol{Y}$ to OLS residuals,

$$A = I - X(X'X)^{-1}X'. \tag{4.5.3}$$

Then, $\boldsymbol{Y}^*$ has a singular multivariate Gaussian distribution with mean zero, whatever the value of $\boldsymbol{\beta}$. To obtain a non-singular distribution, we could use only $nm - p$ rows of the matrix, A, defined at (4.5.3). It turns out that the resulting estimators for σ^2 and V do not depend on *which* rows we use, nor indeed on the particular choice of A: any full-rank matrix with the property that $\mathrm{E}(\boldsymbol{Y}^*) = \boldsymbol{0}$ for all $\boldsymbol{\beta}$ will give the same answer. Furthermore, from an operational viewpoint we do not need to make the transformation from $\boldsymbol{Y}$ to $\boldsymbol{Y}^*$ explicit. The algebraic details are as follows. Less mathematically inclined readers may wish to skim through the next few pages.

For the theoretical development it is convenient to re-absorb σ^2 into V, and write our model for the response vector $\boldsymbol{Y}$ as

$$\boldsymbol{Y} \sim MVN(X\boldsymbol{\beta}, H),$$

where $H \equiv H(\boldsymbol{\alpha})$, the variance matrix of $\boldsymbol{Y}$, is characterized by a vector of parameters $\boldsymbol{\alpha}$. Let A be the matrix defined in (4.5.3), and B the $nm \times (nm - p)$ matrix defined by the requirements that $BB' = A$ and $B'B = I$, where I denotes the $(nm - p) \times (nm - p)$ identity matrix. Finally, let $\boldsymbol{Z} = B'\boldsymbol{Y}$.

Now, for fixed $\boldsymbol{\alpha}$ the maximum likelihood estimator for $\boldsymbol{\beta}$ is the generalized least-squares estimator,

$$\hat{\boldsymbol{\beta}} = (X'H^{-1}X)^{-1}X'H^{-1}\boldsymbol{Y} = G\boldsymbol{Y},$$

say. Also, the respective pdf's of $\boldsymbol{Y}$ and $\hat{\boldsymbol{\beta}}$ are

$$f(\boldsymbol{y}) = (2\pi)^{-\frac{1}{2}nm} \mid H \mid^{-\frac{1}{2}} \exp\{-\tfrac{1}{2}(\boldsymbol{y} - X\boldsymbol{\beta})'H^{-1}(\boldsymbol{y} - X\boldsymbol{\beta})\},$$

and

$$g(\hat{\beta}) = (2\pi)^{-\frac{1}{2}p} \mid X'H^{-1}X \mid^{\frac{1}{2}} \exp\{-\tfrac{1}{2}(\hat{\boldsymbol{\beta}} - \boldsymbol{\beta})'(X'H^{-1}X)(\hat{\boldsymbol{\beta}} - \boldsymbol{\beta})\}.$$

Furthermore, $\mathrm{E}(\boldsymbol{Z}) = \boldsymbol{0}$ and $\boldsymbol{Z}$ and $\hat{\boldsymbol{\beta}}$ are independent, whatever the value of $\boldsymbol{\beta}$, as we now show.

First,

$$\mathrm{E}(\boldsymbol{Z}) = B'\mathrm{E}(\boldsymbol{Y}) = B'X\boldsymbol{\beta} = B'BB'X\boldsymbol{\beta},$$

since $B'B = I$. But since $BB' = A$, this gives

$$\mathrm{E}(\boldsymbol{Z}) = B'AX\boldsymbol{\beta},$$

and

$$AX = \{I - X(X'X)^{-1}X'\}X = X - X = 0,$$

hence $\mathrm{E}(\boldsymbol{Z}) = \boldsymbol{0}$ as required.

Secondly,

$$\begin{aligned}\mathrm{Cov}(\boldsymbol{Z}, \hat{\boldsymbol{\beta}}) &= \mathrm{E}\{\boldsymbol{Z}(\hat{\boldsymbol{\beta}} - \boldsymbol{\beta})'\} \\ &= \mathrm{E}\{B'\boldsymbol{Y}(\boldsymbol{Y}'G' - \boldsymbol{\beta}')\} \\ &= B'\mathrm{E}(\boldsymbol{Y}\boldsymbol{Y}')G' - B'\mathrm{E}(\boldsymbol{Y})\boldsymbol{\beta}' \\ &= B'\{\mathrm{Var}(\boldsymbol{Y}) + \mathrm{E}(\boldsymbol{Y})\mathrm{E}(\boldsymbol{Y})'\}G' - B'\mathrm{E}(\boldsymbol{Y})\boldsymbol{\beta}'.\end{aligned}$$

Now, substituting $\mathrm{E}(\boldsymbol{Y}) = X\boldsymbol{\beta}$ into this last expression gives

$$\mathrm{Cov}(\boldsymbol{Z}, \hat{\boldsymbol{\beta}}) = B'(H + X\boldsymbol{\beta}\boldsymbol{\beta}'X')G' - B'X\boldsymbol{\beta}\boldsymbol{\beta}'.$$

Also,

$$X'G' = X'H^{-1}X(X'H^{-1}X)^{-1} = I,$$

and

$$\begin{aligned}B'HG' &= B'HH^{-1}X(X'H^{-1}X)^{-1} \\ &= B'X(X'H^{-1}X)^{-1} = 0,\end{aligned}$$

because $B'X = B'AX = 0$ as in the proof that $\mathrm{E}(\boldsymbol{Z}) = 0$. It follows that $\mathrm{Cov}(\boldsymbol{Z}, \hat{\boldsymbol{\beta}}) = B'X\boldsymbol{\beta}\boldsymbol{\beta}' - B'X\boldsymbol{\beta}\boldsymbol{\beta}' = 0$. Finally, in the multivariate Gaussian setting, zero covariance is equivalent to independence. It follows that the algebraic form of the (singular) multivariate Gaussian pdf of $\boldsymbol{Z}$, expressed in terms of $\boldsymbol{Y}$, is proportional to the ratio $f(\boldsymbol{y})/g(\hat{\boldsymbol{\beta}})$. To obtain the explicit form of this ratio, we use the following standard result for the GLM,

$$(\boldsymbol{y} - X\boldsymbol{\beta})'H^{-1}(\boldsymbol{y} - X\boldsymbol{\beta}) = (\boldsymbol{y} - X\hat{\boldsymbol{\beta}})'H^{-1}(\boldsymbol{y} - X\hat{\boldsymbol{\beta}}) + (\hat{\boldsymbol{\beta}} - \boldsymbol{\beta})'(X'H^{-1}X)(\hat{\boldsymbol{\beta}} - \boldsymbol{\beta}).$$

Then, the pdf of $\boldsymbol{Z} = B'\boldsymbol{Y}$ is proportional to

$$\frac{f(\boldsymbol{y})}{g(\hat{\boldsymbol{\beta}})} = (2\pi)^{-\frac{1}{2}(nm-p)} \mid H \mid^{-\frac{1}{2}} \mid X'H^{-1}X \mid^{-\frac{1}{2}} \times \exp\left\{-\tfrac{1}{2}(\boldsymbol{y} - X\hat{\boldsymbol{\beta}})'H^{-1}(\boldsymbol{y} - X\hat{\boldsymbol{\beta}})\right\}, \qquad (4.5.4)$$

where the omitted constant of proportionality is the Jacobian of the transformation from $\boldsymbol{Y}$ to $(\boldsymbol{Z}, \hat{\boldsymbol{\beta}})$. Harville (1974) shows that the Jacobian reduces to $\mid X'X \mid^{-\frac{1}{2}}$, which does not depend on any of the parameters in the model and can therefore be ignored for making inferences about $\boldsymbol{\alpha}$ or $\boldsymbol{\beta}$. Note that the right-hand side of (4.5.4) is independent of A, and the same result would therefore hold for any $\boldsymbol{Z}$ such that $E(\boldsymbol{Z}) = 0$ and $\mathrm{Cov}(\boldsymbol{Z}, \hat{\boldsymbol{\beta}}) = 0$.

The practical implication of (4.5.4) is that the REML estimator, $\tilde{\boldsymbol{\alpha}}$, maximizes the log-likelihood

$$L^*(\boldsymbol{\alpha}) = -\tfrac{1}{2}\log \mid H \mid - \tfrac{1}{2}\log \mid X'H^{-1}X \mid - \tfrac{1}{2}(\boldsymbol{y} - X\hat{\boldsymbol{\beta}})'H^{-1}(\boldsymbol{y} - X\hat{\boldsymbol{\beta}}),$$

whereas the maximum likelihood estimator $\hat{\boldsymbol{\alpha}}$ maximizes

$$L(\boldsymbol{\alpha}) = -\tfrac{1}{2}\log \mid H \mid - \tfrac{1}{2}(\boldsymbol{y} - X\hat{\boldsymbol{\beta}})'H^{-1}(\boldsymbol{y} - X\hat{\boldsymbol{\beta}}).$$

It follows from this last result that the algorithm to implement REML estimation for the model (4.5.2) incorporates only a simple modification to the maximum likelihood algorithm derived in Section 4.4. Recall that we consider m units with n measurements per unit and that $\sigma^2 V$ is a block-diagonal matrix with non-zero $n \times n$ blocks $\sigma^2 V_0$ representing the variance matrix of the measurements on any one unit. Also, for given V_0 we write

$$\hat{\boldsymbol{\beta}}(V_0) = (X'V^{-1}X)^{-1}X'V^{-1}\boldsymbol{y}, \qquad (4.5.5)$$

and

$$\mathrm{RSS}(V_0) = \{\boldsymbol{y} - X\hat{\boldsymbol{\beta}}(V_0)\}'V^{-1}\{\boldsymbol{y} - X\hat{\boldsymbol{\beta}}(V_0)\}.$$

Then, the REML estimator for σ^2 is

$$\tilde{\sigma}^2(V_0) = \mathrm{RSS}(V_0)/(nm - p), \qquad (4.5.6)$$

where p is the number of elements of $\boldsymbol{\beta}$. The REML estimator for V_0 maximizes the reduced log-likelihood

$$L^*(V_0) = -\tfrac{1}{2}m\{n \log \text{RSS}(V_0) + \log(\,|\,V_0\,|\,)\} - \tfrac{1}{2}\log(\,|\,X'V^{-1}X\,|\,). \tag{4.5.7}$$

Finally, substitution of the resulting estimator $\tilde{V}_0$ into (4.5.5) and (4.5.6) gives the REML estimators $\tilde{\boldsymbol{\beta}} = \hat{\boldsymbol{\beta}}(\tilde{V}_0)$ and $\tilde{\sigma}^2 = \tilde{\sigma}^2(\tilde{V}_0)$.

It is instructive to compare the functions $L(V_0)$ and $L^*(V_0)$ defined at (4.4.5) and (4.5.7), respectively. The difference is the addition of the term $\frac{1}{2}\log(\,|\,X'V^{-1}X\,|\,)$ in (4.5.7). Note that $X'V^{-1}X$ is a $p \times p$ matrix, so this term is typically of order p, whereas $L(V_0)$ is of order nm suggesting, correctly, that the distinction between maximum likelihood and REML estimation is important only when p is relatively large. This is, of course, precisely the situation which can arise when we use a saturated or nearly saturated model for the mean response so as to obtain consistent estimation of the covariance structure, as we recommended in Section 4.4. Also, the order-of-magnitude argument breaks down when V is near-singular, that is, when there are strong correlations amongst the responses on an individual experimental unit, as is not uncommon in longitudinal studies.

Many authors have discussed the relative merits of maximum likelihood and REML estimators for covariance parameters. Early work, summarized by Patterson and Thompson (1971), concentrated on the estimation of variance components in designed experiments. Harville (1974) gives a Bayesian interpretation. More recently, Cullis and McGilchrist (1990) and Verbyla and Cullis (1990) apply REML in the longitudinal data setting, whilst Tunnicliffe-Wilson (1989) uses it for time series estimation under the name of marginal likelihood. One of Tunnicliffe-Wilson's examples shows very clearly how REML copes much more effectively with a near-singular variance matrix than does maximum likelihood estimation. General theoretical results are harder to find, because the two methods are asymptotically equivalent as either or both of m and n tend to infinity for fixed p. When p tends to infinity, comparisons unequivocally favour REML; for example, the usual procedure for a paired-sample t-test can be interpreted as a REML procedure with $n = 2$ observations on each pair, $p = m + 1$ parameters to define the m pair means and the single treatment effect, and a single unknown variance, σ^2, whereas a naive application of maximum likelihood estimation to this problem would give a seriously biased estimator for σ^2.

In summary, maximum likelihood and REML estimators will often give very similar results. However, when they do differ substantially, REML estimators should be less biased. Henceforth, we use the 'hat' notation to refer to maximum likelihood *or* REML estimators, except when the context does not make it clear which is intended.

4.6 Robust estimation of standard errors

The essential idea of the robust approach to inference for $\boldsymbol{\beta}$ is to use the generalized least-squares estimator $\tilde{\boldsymbol{\beta}}_W$ defined by (4.3.2),

$$\tilde{\beta}_W = (X'WX)^{-1}X'W\boldsymbol{y}, \tag{4.6.1}$$

in conjunction with an estimated variance matrix

$$\hat{R}_W = \{(X'WX)^{-1}X'W\}\hat{V}\{WX(X'WX)^{-1}\}, \tag{4.6.2}$$

where $\hat{V}$ is consistent for V whatever the true covariance structure. Note that in (4.6.2) we have re-absorbed the scale parameter σ^2 into V. For inference, we proceed as if

$$\tilde{\boldsymbol{\beta}}_W \sim MVN(\boldsymbol{\beta}, \hat{R}_W). \tag{4.6.3}$$

In this approach, we call W^{-1} the *working variance matrix*, to distinguish it from the true variance matrix, V. Typically, we use a relatively simple form for W^{-1} which we hope captures the qualitative structure of V. However, the crucial difference between this and a parametric modelling approach is that a poor choice of W will affect only the efficiency of our inferences for $\boldsymbol{\beta}$, not their validity. In particular, confidence intervals and tests of hypotheses derived from (4.6.3) will be asymptotically correct whatever the true form of V. This idea has a long history, dating back at least to Huber (1967). More recent references are White (1982), Liang and Zeger (1986) and Royall (1986).

The simplest possible implementation is to use the OLS estimator $\tilde{\boldsymbol{\beta}}$. This is equivalent to a working assumption that the measurements within a subject are uncorrelated, since we are then using $W^{-1} = I$ for the working variance matrix. Note, incidentally, that equations (4.3.2) and (4.3.3) do not change if the elements of W are multiplied by any constant, so that it would strictly be more correct to say that W^{-1} is *proportional* to the working variance matrix. For data with a smoothly decaying autocorrelation structure, a more efficient implementation might be obtained from a block-diagonal W^{-1}, with non-zero elements of the form $\exp\{-c\,|\,t_j - t_k\,|\,\}$, where c is a positive constant chosen roughly to match the rate of decay anticipated for the actual autocovariances of the data. In our experience, more elaborate choices for W^{-1} are often unnecessary.

For designed experiments in which we choose to fit the saturated model for the mean response, the explicit form of the robust estimator $\hat{V}$ required in (4.6.2) is obtained using the REML principle as follows. Suppose that measurements are made at each of n time-points t_j on m_h experimental units in the hth of g experimental treatment groups. Write the complete set of measurements as

$$y_{hij}, \quad h = 1, \ldots, g; \; i = 1, \ldots, m_h; \; j = 1, \ldots, n.$$

The saturated model for the mean response is

$$\mathrm{E}(Y_{hij}) = \mu_{hj}, \quad h = 1, \ldots, g; \; j = 1, \ldots, n,$$

and a saturated model for the covariance structure is that $V = \mathrm{Var}(\boldsymbol{Y})$ is block-diagonal, with all non-zero blocks equal to V_0, a positive definite but otherwise arbitrary $n \times n$ matrix.

This model falls within the general framework of Section 4.5, with a rather special form for the design matrix X. For example, with $g = 2$ treatments and replications $m_1 = 2$ and $m_2 = 3$ we have

$$X = \begin{bmatrix} I & O \\ I & O \\ O & I \\ O & I \\ O & I \end{bmatrix},$$

where I and O are, respectively, the $n \times n$ identity matrix and the $n \times n$ matrix of zeros. The extension to general g and $m_1, \ldots, m_g$ is obvious. It is then a straightforward exercise to deduce that the estimators for the μ_{hj} are the corresponding sample means,

$$\hat{\mu}_{hj} = m_h^{-1} \sum_{i=1}^{m_h} y_{hij},$$

and that the REML estimator for V_0 is

$$\hat{V}_0 = \left(\sum_{i=1}^{g} m_i - g \right)^{-1} \sum_{h=1}^{g} \sum_{i=1}^{m_h} (\boldsymbol{y}_{hi} - \hat{\boldsymbol{\mu}}_h)(\boldsymbol{y}_{hi} - \hat{\boldsymbol{\mu}}_h)', \tag{4.6.4}$$

where $\boldsymbol{y}_{hi} = (y_{hi1}, \ldots, y_{hin})'$ and $\hat{\boldsymbol{\mu}}_h = (\hat{\mu}_{h1}, \ldots, \hat{\mu}_{hn})'$. Then, the required estimate $\hat{V}$ is the block-diagonal matrix with non-zero blocks $\hat{V}_0$. Note that at this stage, we do not attempt to interpret the OLS fit. Its sole purpose is to provide a consistent estimate of V_0.

When the saturated model strategy is not feasible, typically when the data are from observational studies with continuously varying covariates, it is usually no longer possible to obtain an explicit expression for the REML estimate of V_0. However, the same basic idea applies. We make no assumption about the form of V_0, use an X matrix corresponding to the most elaborate model we are prepared to entertain for the mean response, and obtain the REML estimate, $\hat{V}_0$, by numerical maximization of (4.5.7).

To make robust inferences for $\boldsymbol{\beta}$, we now substitute $\hat{V}$ into (4.6.2), and use (4.6.3). Note that for these inferences about $\boldsymbol{\beta}$ we will typically use an X matrix with many fewer than the ng columns of the X matrix corresponding to the saturated model. Furthermore, if we want to test linear hypotheses about $\boldsymbol{\beta}$ within this model we can use the standard approach for the GLM. Suppose, for example, we wish to test the hypothesis $Q\boldsymbol{\beta} = \mathbf{0}$, where Q is a full-rank $q \times p$ matrix for some $q < p$. Then we deduce from (4.6.3) that

$$Q\hat{\boldsymbol{\beta}}_W \sim MVN(Q\boldsymbol{\beta}, Q\hat{R}_W Q').$$

An appropriate test statistic for the hypothesis that $Q\boldsymbol{\beta} = \mathbf{0}$ is

$$T = \hat{\boldsymbol{\beta}}_W' Q'(Q\hat{R}_W Q')^{-1} Q\hat{\boldsymbol{\beta}}_W, \tag{4.6.5}$$

and the approximate null sampling distribution of T is chi-squared on q degrees of freedom.

When measurement times are not common to all units, the robust approach can still be useful in the following, modified form. The required variance matrix V is still block-diagonal, but the non-zero blocks corresponding to the sets of measurements within units are no longer constant between units. Write V_{0i} for the $n_i \times n_i$ variance matrix of the set of measurements on the ith unit and $\boldsymbol{\mu}_i$ for the mean vector of these measurements. Estimate $\boldsymbol{\mu}_i$ by $\hat{\boldsymbol{\mu}}_i$, the OLS estimates from the most complicated model we are prepared to entertain for the mean response. Then, an estimate of V_{0i} is

$$\hat{V}_{0i} = (\boldsymbol{y}_i - \hat{\boldsymbol{\mu}}_i)(\boldsymbol{y}_i - \hat{\boldsymbol{\mu}}_i)'. \tag{4.6.6}$$

Our robust estimate of V is then $\hat{V}$, the block-diagonal matrix with non-zero blocks $\hat{V}_{0i}$ defined by (4.6.6).

A few comments on this procedure are in order. Firstly, the choice of a 'most complicated model' for the mean response is less clear-cut than in the case of a common set of measurement times for all units. At one extreme, if sets of measurement times are essentially unique for units as in the CD4+ data of Example 1.1, a saturated treatments by times model would result in $\hat{\boldsymbol{\mu}}_i = \boldsymbol{y}_i$ and $\hat{V}_{0i} = O$, a matrix of zeros. In this situation it is necessary, and sensible, to incorporate some smoothness into the assumed form for the variation in mean response over time. But it is not obvious precisely how to do this in practice. Fortunately, in many applications the replication of measurement times between units is sufficient to allow a sensible fit to a saturated treatments by times model provided, as always, that there are no important time-varying covariates.

A second comment is that $\hat{V}_{0i}$ defined by (4.6.6) is a *terrible* estimator for V_{0i}. For example, it is singular of rank 1, so the implied $\hat{\boldsymbol{V}}$ will be singular of rank m, the number of units. This is less serious than it sounds, because we only use $\hat{V}$ in (4.6.2) to evaluate the $p \times p$ matrix $\hat{R}_W$. The matrix multiplication in (4.6.2) achieves, in effect, the same ends as the explicit averaging over replicates in (4.6.4), to produce a useful estimate of R_W. Note that this argument breaks down unless p, the number of parameters defining the mean response for the most complicated model, is much less than m, the number of experimental units. It also breaks down when, in effect, any one regression parameter is estimated from only a small part of the data. For example, if (4.6.6) is used in conjunction with a saturated model for the mean response in a designed esperiment, it corresponds to using the within-treatment sample variance matrices to estimate the corresponding blocks of V_0. This is in contrast to (4.6.4), which pools the sample variance matrices from all g treatment groups to achieve a more precise estimate of V_0 under the declared assumption that V_0 is independent of treatment. For a further discussion, see White (1982), Zeger *et al.* (1985), Liang and Zeger (1986) and Zeger and Liang (1986).

Example 4.1. Growth of Sitka spruce with and without ozone

We now use the approach described above to analyse the data from Example 1.3. Recall that the data consist of measurements on 79 sitka spruce trees over two growing seasons. The trees were grown in four controlled environment chambers, of which the first two, containing 27 trees each, were treated with introduced ozone at 70 ppb whilst the remaining two, containing 12 and 13 trees, were controls. As the response variable we use a log-size measurement, $y = \log(hd^2)$ where h denotes height and d denotes stem diameter. The question of scientific interest concerns the effect of ozone on the growth pattern, rather than the growth pattern itself. Chamber effects were thought to be negligible and we shall see that this is borne out in the results.

Figure 4.2 shows the observed mean response in each of the four chambers. In the first year, the four curves are initially close but diverge progressively, with the control chambers showing a higher mean response than the treated chambers. In the second year, the curves are roughly parallel.

Turning to the covariance structure, we computed the REML estimates, $\hat{V}_0$, separately for each of the two years using a saturated model for the means in each case. That is, we used (4.6.4) with $g = 4$ in each case, and $n = 5$ and 8 for the 1988 and 1989 data, respectively. The resulting estimates are, for 1988,

$$\hat{V}_0 = \begin{pmatrix} 0.445 & 0.404 & 0.373 & 0.370 & 0.370 \\ & 0.397 & 0.372 & 0.375 & 0.376 \\ & & 0.370 & 0.372 & 0.371 \\ & & & 0.401 & 0.401 \\ & & & & 0.410 \end{pmatrix},$$

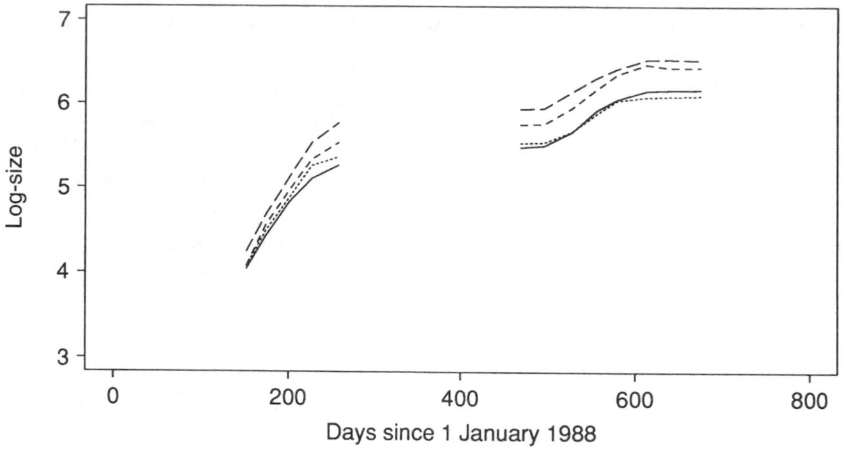

Fig. 4.2. Sitka spruce data: mean response profiles in each of the four growth chambers.

and, for 1989,

$$\hat{V}_0 = \begin{pmatrix} 0.457 & 0.454 & 0.427 & 0.417 & 0.433 & 0.422 & 0.408 & 0.418 \\ & 0.451 & 0.425 & 0.415 & 0.431 & 0.420 & 0.406 & 0.416 \\ & & 0.409 & 0.398 & 0.412 & 0.404 & 0.390 & 0.401 \\ & & & 0.396 & 0.410 & 0.402 & 0.388 & 0.400 \\ & & & & 0.434 & 0.422 & 0.405 & 0.418 \\ & & & & & 0.415 & 0.399 & 0.412 \\ & & & & & & 0.394 & 0.402 \\ & & & & & & & 0.416 \end{pmatrix}.$$

The most striking feature of each matrix $\hat{V}_0$ is its near-singularity. This arises because the dominant component of variation in the data is a random intercept between trees, as a result of which the variance structure approximates to that of the uniform correlation model 5.2.2 with ρ close to 1.

Using the estimated variance matrices $\hat{V}_0$, we can construct pointwise standard errors for the observed mean responses in the four chambers. These standard errors vary between about 0.1 and 0.2, suggesting that differences between chambers within experimental groups are negligible. We therefore proceed to model the data ignoring chambers.

Figure 4.3 shows the observed mean response in each of the two treatment groups. The two curves diverge progressively during 1988, the second year of the experiment, and are approximately parallel during 1989. The overall growth pattern is clearly non-linear, nor could it be well approximated by a low-order polynomial in time. For this reason, and because the

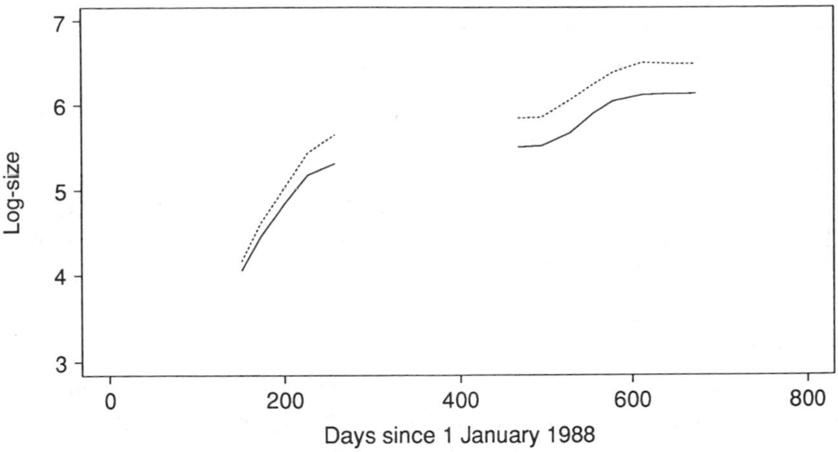

Fig. 4.3. Sitka spruce data: mean response profiles in control and ozone-treated groups. - - - -: control; ——: ozone-treated.

primary inferential focus is on the ozone effect, we make no attempt to model the overall growth pattern parametrically. Instead, we simply use a separate parameter, β_j say, for the treatment mean response at the jth time-point and concentrate our modelling efforts on the control versus treatment contrast.

For the 1988 data, we assume that this contrast is linear in time. Thus, if $\mu_1(t)$ and $\mu_2(t)$ represent the mean response at time t for treated and control trees, respectively, then

$$\mu_1(t_j) = \beta_j, \quad j = 1, \ldots, 5,$$

and

$$\mu_2(t_j) = \beta_j + \eta + \gamma t_j, \quad j = 1, \ldots, 5. \tag{4.6.7}$$

To estimate the parameters β_j, η and γ in (4.6.7) we use OLS, that is, $W = I$ in (4.6.1). To estimate the variance matrix of the parameter estimates, we use the estimated $\hat{V}_0$ in (4.6.2). The resulting estimates and standard errors are given in Table 4.3(a). The hypothesis of no treatment effect is that $\eta = \gamma = 0$. The test statistic for this hypothesis, derived from (4.6.5), is $T = 9.79$ on two degrees of freedom, corresponding to $p = 0.007$; this constitutes strong evidence of a negative treatment effect, that is, ozone suppresses growth. Note that for the linear model-fitting, we used a scaled time variable, $x = t/100$, where t is measured in days since 1 January 1988.

For the 1989 data, we assume that the control versus treatment contrast is constant in time. Thus,

$$\mu_1(t_j) = \beta_j, \quad j = 6, \ldots, 13.$$

Table 4.3. Ordinary least-squares estimates, and robust standard errors, for mean value parameters in the model fitted to the Sitka spruce data.

Parameter	β_1	β_2	β_3	β_4	β_5	η	γ
(a) 1988							
Estimate	4.060	4.470	4.483	5.179	5.316	−0.221	0.213
SE	0.090	0.086	0.083	0.086	0.087	0.220	0.077

	β_1	β_2	β_3	β_4	β_5	β_6	β_7	β_8	τ
(b) 1989									
Estimate	5.504	5.516	5.679	5.901	6.040	6.127	6.128	6.130	0.354
SE	0.091	0.090	0.087	0.086	0.089	0.088	0.086	0.088	0.156

and

$$\mu_2(t_j) = \beta_j + \eta, \quad j = 6, \ldots, 13. \tag{4.6.8}$$

To estimate the parameters in (4.6.8) and their standard errors, we again use $W = I$ and the estimated variance matrix $\hat{V}_0$ in (4.6.2). The resulting values are given in Table 4.3(b). The hypothesis of no treatment effect is that $\eta = 0$. The test statistic derived from (4.6.5) is $T = 5.15$ on one degree of freedom, corresponding to $p = 0.023$; alternatively, an approximate 95% confidence interval for η is 0.354 ± 0.306.

Figure 4.4 shows the estimated treatment mean response, $\hat{\mu}_1(t_j) = \hat{\beta}_j$, together with pointwise 95% confidence limits calculated as plus and minus two estimated standard errors; note that under the assumed model, both control and treated data contain information on the β_j. Figure 4.5 shows the observed mean differences between control and treated trees, with the estimated control versus treatment contrast. The model appears to fit the data well, and the analysis provides strong evidence that ozone suppresses early growth.

Incidentally, we obtained virtually identical results for the Sitka spruce data using an exponential working variance matrix, in which the (j,k)th element of W^{-1} is equal to $0.9^{|j-k|}$. This agrees with our general experience that the precise choice among reasonable working variance matrices is usually not critical.

Example 4.2. Weights of pigs

As a second example of the robust approach, we again consider the data on the weights of pigs, previously discussed in Example 3.1. There, we remarked that the overall growth curve was approximately linear, but that individual pigs appeared to vary both in their initial size and in their growth

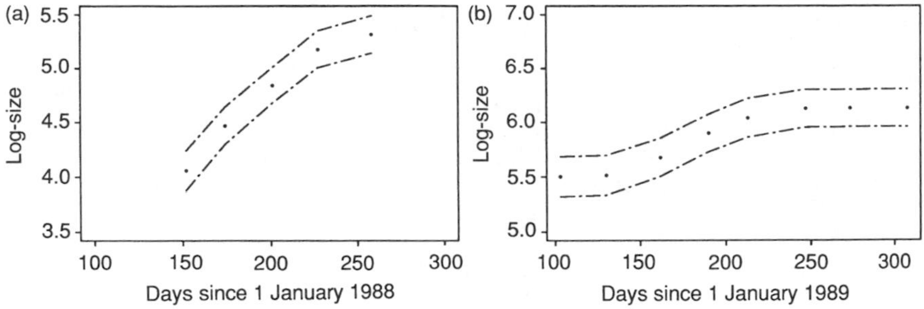

Fig. 4.4. Sitka spruce data: estimated response profiles, shown as solid dots, and 95% pointwise confidence limits for the ozone-treated group: (a) 1988 growing season; (b) 1989 growing season.

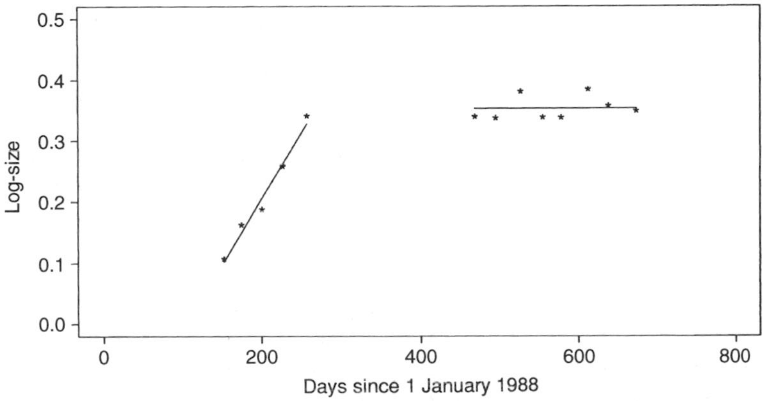

Fig. 4.5. Sitka spruce data: observed and fitted differences in mean response profiles between the control and ozone-treated groups. $\star$: observed; ——: fitted.

rates. Each pig was weighed in nine successive weeks. We therefore adopt the following as our working model for the weight, Y_{ij}, of the ith pig in the jth week:

$$Y_{ij} = \alpha + \beta x_j + U_i + W_i x_j + Z_{ij}, \quad j = 1, \ldots, 9; \; i = 1, \ldots, 48, \quad (4.6.9)$$

where $U_i \sim N(0, \sigma^2), W_i \sim N(0, \nu^2)$ and $Z_{ij} \sim N(0, \tau^2)$ are all mutually independent. In ((4.6.9)), the parameters α and β describe the mean growth curve, which we suppose to be the focus of scientific interest, and $x_j = j$ identifies weeks 1–9. The model implies that the variance matrix of

$\boldsymbol{Y}_i = (Y_{i1}, \ldots, Y_{i9})$ has jth diagonal element

$$v_{jj} = \sigma^2 + \tau^2 + \nu^2 x_j^2,$$

and jkth off-diagonal element

$$\sigma^2 + \nu^2 x_j x_k.$$

To convey the spirit of the robust approach, we now make some intentionally crude estimates of the parameters σ^2, ν^2 and τ^2 by simple visual inspection of Figs 3.1 and 3.2. First, from Fig. 3.1 we see that the range of initial weights is very roughly 10 kg. Taking this as, say, four standard deviations implies that

$$\sigma^2 + \tau^2 + \nu^2 \approx 6.25.$$

Treating the spread of final weights similarly implies a standard deviation of about 6 kg, hence

$$\sigma^2 + \tau^2 + \nu^2 \times 81 \approx 36.$$

These together imply that $\nu^2 \approx 0.4$ and $\sigma^2 + \tau^2 \approx 6$. Finally, from Fig. 3.2 the range of the time-sequence of nine standardized residuals from an individual pig is typically much less than 1, suggesting that τ^2 is small relative to σ^2, say $\tau^2 \approx 1$, and therefore $\sigma^2 \approx 5$. These crude calculations imply the following working variance matrix,

$$W^{-1} = \begin{pmatrix} 6.4 & 5.8 & 6.2 & 6.6 & 7 & 7.4 & 7.8 & 8.2 & 8.6 \\ & 7.6 & 7.4 & 8.2 & 9.0 & 9.8 & 10.6 & 11.4 & 12.2 \\ & & 9.6 & 9.8 & 11.0 & 12.2 & 13.4 & 14.6 & 15.8 \\ & & & 12.4 & 13.0 & 14.6 & 16.2 & 17.8 & 19.4 \\ & & & & 16.0 & 17.0 & 19.0 & 21.0 & 23.0 \\ & & & & & 20.4 & 21.8 & 24.2 & 26.6 \\ & & & & & & 25.6 & 27.4 & 30.2 \\ & & & & & & & 31.6 & 33.8 \\ & & & & & & & & 38.4 \end{pmatrix}.$$

Using a block-diagonal weight matrix with non-zero blocks W in the weighted least-squares estimator (4.6.1) then gives estimates $\hat{\alpha} = 19.36$ and $\hat{\beta} = 6.21$.

The REML estimator (4.6.4), which in this simple example coincides with the sample variance matrix, is

$$\hat{V}_0 = \begin{pmatrix} 6.1 & 6.3 & 7.0 & 7.3 & 8.4 & 7.7 & 8.0 & 8.4 & 8.7 \\ & 7.8 & 9.0 & 9.5 & 11.1 & 10.4 & 10.8 & 10.8 & 11.7 \\ & & 12.6 & 12.7 & 14.9 & 14.3 & 14.9 & 15.7 & 17.3 \\ & & & 13.9 & 16.3 & 15.5 & 16.1 & 16.8 & 18.6 \\ & & & & 20.6 & 18.6 & 19.3 & 19.9 & 22.6 \\ & & & & & 19.8 & 21.3 & 22.4 & 25.1 \\ & & & & & & 24.7 & 25.9 & 28.9 \\ & & & & & & & 29.4 & 33.3 \\ & & & & & & & & 40.1 \end{pmatrix}.$$

Using a block-diagonal matrix with non-zero blocks $\hat{V}_0$ as the consistent estimate of V in (4.6.2), we obtain the variance matrix of $(\hat{\alpha}, \hat{\beta})$ as

$$\hat{R}_W = \begin{bmatrix} 0.1631 & -0.0049 \\ & 0.0085 \end{bmatrix}.$$

In particular, the respective standard errors of $\hat{\alpha}$ and $\hat{\beta}$ are 0.40 and 0.09.

In this example, the reasonably close agreement between W^{-1} and $\hat{V}_0$ suggests that the assumed form of the working variance matrix has successfully captured the essential structure of the true covariance. However, we emphasize that whilst this is desirable from the point of view of efficiency of estimation of β, it is not necessary for consistency of estimation.

Another implication of the close agreement between W^{-1} and $\hat{V}_0$ is that the estimated variance matrix of $(\hat{\alpha}, \hat{\beta})$ will be close to the estimate, $(X'WX)^{-1}$ that would have been obtained had we simply assumed the working variance matrix to be correct. This latter estimate is

$$\begin{bmatrix} 0.1151 & -0.0017 \\ & 0.0087 \end{bmatrix}.$$

However, we again emphasize that in general, $(X'WX)^{-1}$ is *not* a valid estimate of the variance matrix of the regression parameters.

The robust approach described in this section is extremely simple to implement. The REML estimates of the covariance structure are simple to compute provided that the experimental design allows the fitting of a saturated model for the mean response, and the remaining calculations involve only standard matrix manipulations. By design, consistent inferences for the mean response parameters follow from a correct specification of the mean structure, whatever the true covariance structure.

However, there are good reasons why we should nevertheless consider careful, explicit modelling of the covariance structure.

One argument, that of efficiency of estimation, has two distinct strands. Firstly, the theoretically optimal weighted least-squares estimate uses a weight matrix whose inverse is proportional to the true variance matrix, so it would seem reasonable to use the data to estimate this optimal weight matrix. Secondly, when there are n measurements per experimental unit, the robust approach uses $\frac{1}{2}n(n+1)$ parameters to describe the variance matrix, all of which must be estimated from the data. In contrast, the true covariance structure may involve many fewer parameters, which can themselves be estimated more accurately than the unconstrained variance matrix. Taken together, these arguments constitute a case for likelihood-based inference within an explicit parametric model for both the mean and covariance structure. However, as we have already argued, the resulting gains in efficiency are often modest, and may well be outweighed by the potential loss of consistency when the covariance structure is wrongly specified.

A more basic practical argument concerns the number, n, of measurements per experimental unit. When n is large, the objection to estimating $\frac{1}{2}n(n+1)$ parameters in the covariance structure gains force. In extreme cases, n can exceed the available replication.

A third argument concerns missing values. The robust approach uses the replication across experimental units to estimate the covariance structure non-parametrically, and this becomes problematical when there are many missing values, or when the times of measurement are not common to all the experimental units. In contrast, a parametric modelling approach can accommodate general patterns of missing values within a likelihood-based inferential framework. This does assume that the missing value mechanism is uninformative about the parameters of interest; the whole issue of *informative missing values* will be addressed in Chapter 13.

Finally, although robustly implemented OLS will usually give estimators which are reasonably efficient, we saw in the crossover example of Section 4.3 that this is not guaranteed. This argues in favour of using robust *weighted* least squares, in which the weighting matrix is chosen to reflect qualitatively reasonable assumptions about the covariance structure.

To summarize, the robust approach is usually satisfactory when the data consist of short, essentially complete, sequences of measurements observed at a common set of times on many experimental units, and care is taken in the choice of a working variance matrix. In other circumstances, it is worth considering a more careful parametric modelling. The next chapter takes up this theme.

5

Parametric models for covariance structure

5.1 Introduction

In this chapter, we continue with the general linear model (GLM) (4.2.1) for the data, but assume that the covariance structure of the sequence of measurements on each experimental unit is to be specified by the values of a few unknown parameters. Examples include the uniform correlation model (4.2.2) and the exponential correlation model (4.2.4), each of which uses two parameters to define the covariance structure.

As discussed in Section 4.6, a parametric modelling approach is particularly useful for data in which the measurements on different units are not made at a common set of times. For this reason, we use a slightly more general notation than in Chapter 4. Let $\boldsymbol{y}_i = (y_{i1}, \ldots, y_{in_i})$ be the vector of n_i measurements on the ith unit and $\boldsymbol{t}_i = (t_{i1}, \ldots, t_{in_i})$ the corresponding set of times at which these measurements are made. If there are m units altogether, write $\boldsymbol{y} = (\boldsymbol{y}_1, \ldots, \boldsymbol{y}_m)$, $\boldsymbol{t} = (\boldsymbol{t}_1, \ldots, \boldsymbol{t}_m)$ and $N = \sum_{i=1}^{m} n_i$.

We assume that the $\boldsymbol{y}_i$ are realizations of mutually independent Gaussian random vectors $\boldsymbol{Y}_i$, with

$$\boldsymbol{Y}_i \sim MVN\{X_i\boldsymbol{\beta}, V_i(\boldsymbol{t}_i, \boldsymbol{\alpha})\}. \tag{5.1.1}$$

In (5.1.1), X_i is an $n_i \times p$ matrix of explanatory variables. The unknown parameters are $\boldsymbol{\beta}$ of dimension p, and $\boldsymbol{\alpha}$ of dimension q. Note that the mean and covariance structures are parametrized separately. Also, when convenient we shall write the model for the entire set of data $\boldsymbol{y}$ as

$$\boldsymbol{Y} \sim MVN\{X\boldsymbol{\beta}, V(\boldsymbol{t}, \boldsymbol{\alpha})\}. \tag{5.1.2}$$

In (5.1.2), the $N \times p$ matrix X is obtained by stacking the unit-specific matrices X_i, and the $N \times N$ matrix $V(\cdot)$ is block-diagonal, with non-zero blocks $V_i(\cdot)$.

Our notation emphasizes that the natural setting for most longitudinal data is in continuous time. Because of this, we shall derive specific models by assuming that the sequences, Y_{ij}, $j = 1, \ldots, n_i$, are sampled from independent copies of an underlying continuous-time stochastic process, $\{Y(t),\ t \in R\}$. Thus, $Y_{ij} = Y_i(t_{ij}),\ j = 1, \ldots, n_i;\ i = 1, \ldots, m$. In the next section, we give examples of models which fall within the general framework of (5.1.1), and show how different kinds of stationary and non-stationary behaviour arise naturally. In later sections, we develop methods for fitting the models to data and describe several applications.

The principal tools which we shall use to describe the properties of each model for the stochastic process $\{Y(t)\}$ are the covariance function and its close relation, the variogram. Recall from Section 3.4 that the *variogram* of a stochastic process $\{Y(t)\}$ is the function

$$\gamma(u) = \tfrac{1}{2}\mathrm{E}\left[\{Y(t) - Y(t-u)\}^2\right], \quad u \geq 0.$$

For a *stationary process* $Y(t)$, if $\rho(u)$ denotes the correlation between $Y(t)$ and $Y(t-u)$, and $\sigma^2 = \mathrm{Var}\{Y(t)\}$, then

$$\gamma(u) = \sigma^2\{1 - \rho(u)\}.$$

5.2 Models

In order to develop a useful set of models we need to understand, at least qualitatively, what are the likely sources of random variation in longitudinal data. In the earlier chapters, we have shown several examples of the kinds of random variation which occur in practice. Our experience with these and many other sets of data leads us to the view that we would wish to be able to include in our models at least three qualitatively different sources of random variation.

1. **Random effects**: When units are sampled at random from a population, various aspects of their behaviour may show stochastic variation between units. Perhaps the simplest example of this is when the general level of the response profile varies between units, that is, some units are intrinsically high responders, others low responders. For example, this was very evident in the data of Example 1.3 concerning the growth of Sitka spruce trees.
2. **Serial correlation**: At least part of any unit's observed measurement profile may be a response to time-varying stochastic processes operating within that unit. For example, in the data of Example 1.4 concerning the protein content of milk samples, the measured sequences of protein contents must, to some extent, reflect the biochemical processes operating within each cow. This type of stochastic variation results in a correlation between pairs of measurements on the same unit which depends on the time separation between the pair of measurements. Typically, the correlation becomes weaker as the time separation increases.

3. **Measurement error**: Especially when the individual measurements involve some kind of sampling *within* units, the measurement process may itself add a component of variation to the data. The data on protein content of milk samples again illustrate the point. Here, two samples taken simultaneously from a cow would have different measured protein contents, because the measurement process involves an assay technique which itself introduces a component of random variation.

There are many different ways in which these qualitative features could be incorporated into specific models. The following additive formulation is tractable and, in our experience, useful.

First, we make explicit the separation between mean and covariance structures by writing (5.1.2) as

$$\boldsymbol{Y} = X\boldsymbol{\beta} + \boldsymbol{\epsilon}. \tag{5.2.1}$$

It follows that

$$\boldsymbol{\epsilon} \sim MVN\{0, V(\boldsymbol{t}, \boldsymbol{\alpha})\}. \tag{5.2.2}$$

Now, using ϵ_{ij} to denote the element of $\boldsymbol{\epsilon}$ which corresponds to the jth measurement on the ith unit, we assume an additive decomposition of ϵ_{ij} into random effects, serially correlated variation and measurement error. This can be expressed formally as

$$\epsilon_{ij} = \boldsymbol{d}'_{ij}\boldsymbol{U}_i + W_i(t_{ij}) + Z_{ij}. \tag{5.2.3}$$

In this decomposition, the Z_{ij} are a set of N mutually independent Gaussian random variables, each with mean zero and variance τ^2. The $\boldsymbol{U}_i$ are a set of m mutually independent r-element Gaussian random vectors, each with mean vector zero and covariance matrix G, say. The $\boldsymbol{d}_{ij}$ are r-element vectors of explanatory variables attached to individual measurements. The $W_i(t_{ij})$ are sampled from m independent copies of a stationary Gaussian process with mean zero, variance σ^2 and correlation function $\rho(u)$. Note that the $\boldsymbol{U}_i$, the $\{W_i(t_{ij})\}$ and the Z_{ij} correspond to random effects, serial correlation and measurement error, respectively.

In applications, the assumed additive structure may be more reasonable after a transformation of the data. For example, a logarithmic transformation would convert an underlying multiplicative structure to an additive one.

To say anything more useful about (5.2.3) we need some more notation. Write $\boldsymbol{\epsilon}_i = (\epsilon_{i1}, \ldots, \epsilon_{in_i})$ for the vector of random variables, ϵ_{ij}, associated with the ith unit. Let D_i be the $n_i \times r$ matrix with jth row $\boldsymbol{d}_{ij}$. Let H_i be the $n_i \times n_i$ matrix with (j,k)th element $h_{ijk} = \rho(\,|\,t_{ij} - t_{ik}\,|\,)$, that is, h_{ijk} is the correlation between $W_i(t_{ij})$ and $W_i(t_{ik})$. Finally, let I_i be the

$n_i \times n_i$ identity matrix. Then, the covariance matrix of $\boldsymbol{\epsilon}_i$ is

$$\text{Var}(\boldsymbol{\epsilon}_i) = D_i G D_i' + \sigma^2 H_i + \tau^2 I_i. \tag{5.2.4}$$

In the rest of this section, we look at particular examples of (5.2.4). Because all of our models have the property that measurements from different units are independent, we drop the subscript i, and write (5.2.4) as

$$\text{Var}(\boldsymbol{\epsilon}) = DGD' + \sigma^2 H + \tau^2 I. \tag{5.2.5}$$

In (5.2.5), $\boldsymbol{\epsilon} = (\epsilon_1, \ldots, \epsilon_n)$ denotes a generic sequence of n measurements from one unit. In what follows, we write $\boldsymbol{t} = (t_1, \ldots, t_n)$ for the corresponding set of times at which the measurements are made.

5.2.1 *Pure serial correlation*

For our first example we assume that neither random effects nor measurement errors are present, so that (5.2.3) reduces to

$$\epsilon_j = W(t_j),$$

and (5.2.5) correspondingly simplifies to

$$\text{Var}(\boldsymbol{\epsilon}) = \sigma^2 H.$$

Now, σ^2 is the variance of each ϵ_j, and the correlations amongst the ϵ_j are determined by the autocorrelation function $\rho(u)$. Specifically,

$$\text{Cov}(\epsilon_j, \epsilon_k) = \sigma^2 \rho(\,|\,t_j - t_k\,|\,).$$

The corresponding variogram is

$$\gamma(u) = \sigma^2\{1 - \rho(u)\}. \tag{5.2.6}$$

Thus, $\gamma(0) = 0$ and $\gamma(u) \to \sigma^2$ as $u \to \infty$. Typically, $\gamma(u)$ is an increasing function of u because the correlation, $\rho(u)$, decreases with increasing time-separation, u.

A popular choice for $\rho(u)$ is the exponential correlation model,

$$\rho(u) = \exp(-\phi u), \tag{5.2.7}$$

for some value of $\phi > 0$. Figure 5.1 shows the variogram (5.2.6) of this model for $\sigma^2 = 1$ and $\phi = 0.1, 0.25,$ and 1.0, together with a simulation of a sequence of $n = 25$ measurements at times $t_j = 1, 2, \ldots, 25$. As ϕ increases, the strength of the autocorrelation decreases; in the three examples shown, the autocorrelation between successive measurements is approximately 0.905, 0.779, and 0.368, respectively. The corresponding variograms and

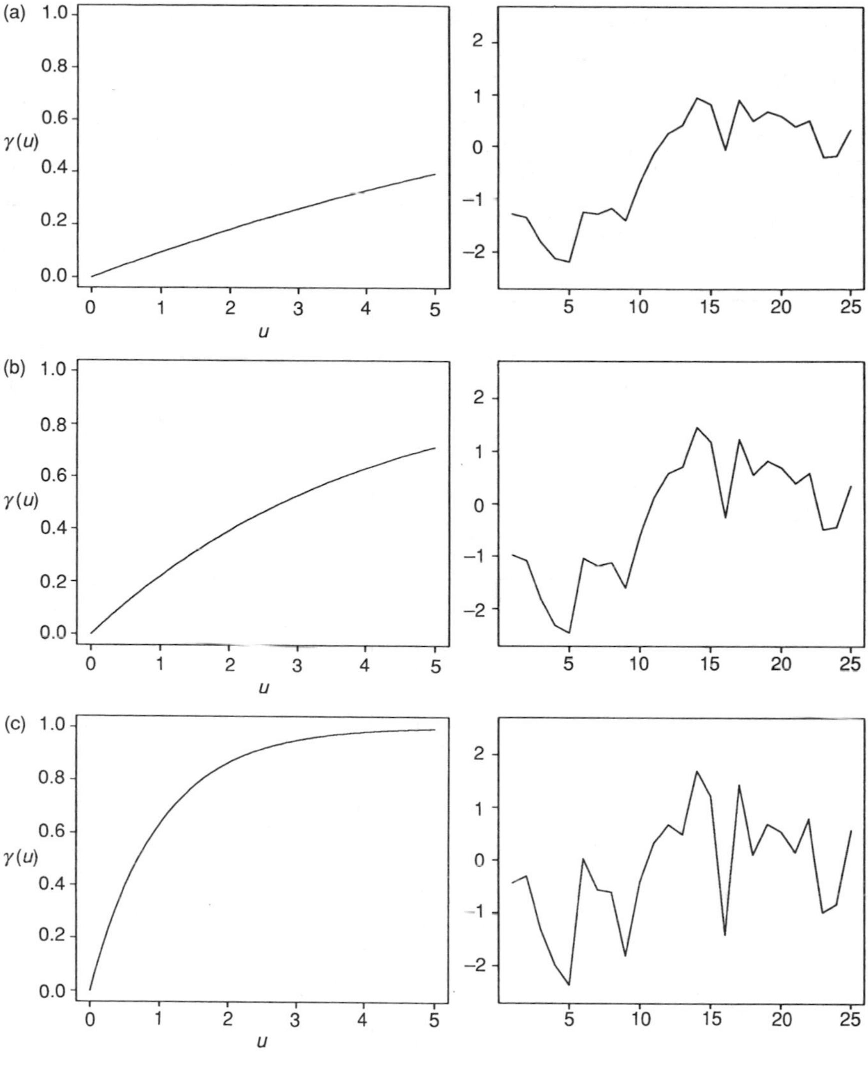

Fig. 5.1. Variograms (left-hand panels) and simulated realizations (right-hand panels) for the exponential correlation model: (a) $\phi = 0.1$; (b) $\phi = 0.25$; (c) $\phi = 1.0$.

simulated realizations reflect this; as ϕ increases, the variograms approach their asymptote more quickly and the simulated realizations appear less smooth.

In many applications the empirical variogram differs from the exponential correlation model by showing an initially slow increase as u increases from zero, then a sharp rise and finally a slower increase again as it approaches its asymptote. A model which captures this behaviour is the so-called Gaussian correlation function,

$$\rho(u) = \exp(-\phi u^2), \tag{5.2.8}$$

for some $\phi > 0$. Figure 5.2 shows the variogram and a simulated realization for $\sigma^2 = 1$ and each of $\phi = 0.1, 0.25$, and 1.0, with times of observation $t_j = 1, 2, \ldots, 25$, as in Fig. 5.1.

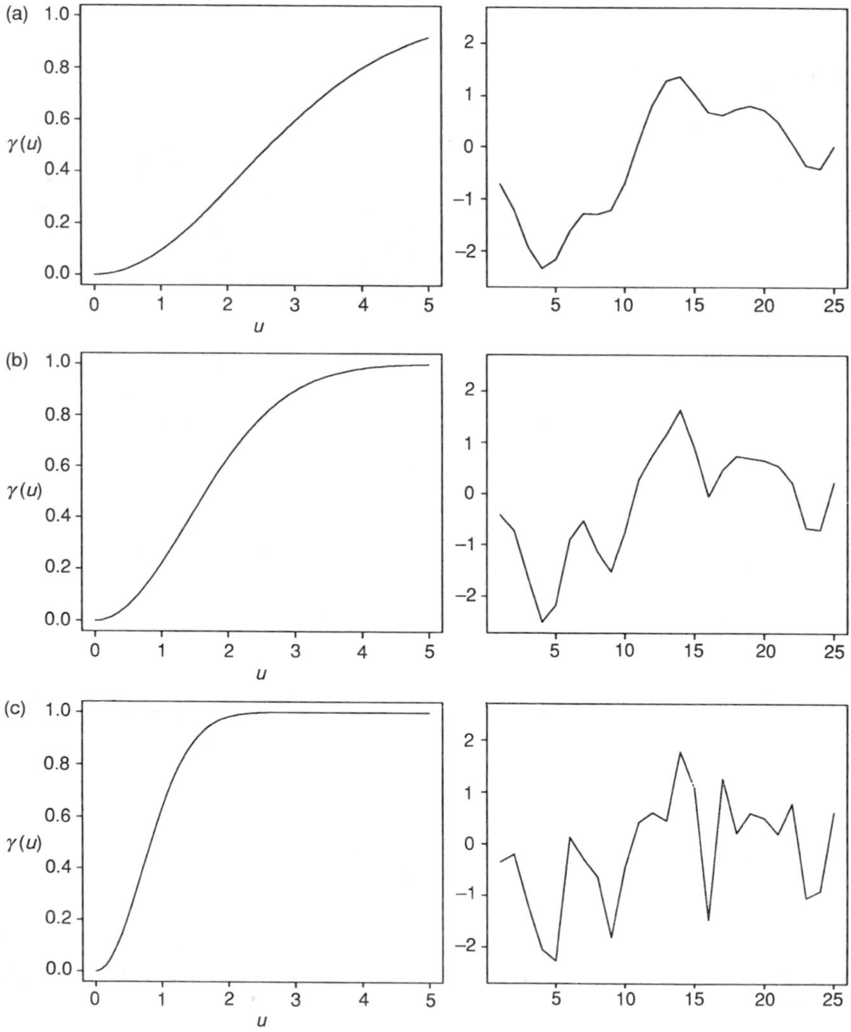

Fig. 5.2. Variograms (left-hand panels) and simulated realizations (right-hand panels) for the Gaussian correlation model: (a) $\phi = 0.1$; (b) $\phi = 0.25$; (c) $\phi = 1.0$.

A panel-by-panel comparison between Figs 5.1 and 5.2 is interesting. For both models the parameter ϕ has a qualitatively similar effect: as ϕ increases the variogram rises more sharply and the simulated realizations are less smooth. Also, for each value of ϕ, the correlation between successive unit-spaced measurements is the same for the two models. When $\phi = 1.0$ the correlations at larger time-separations decay rapidly to zero and the corresponding simulations of the two models are almost identical (the same underlying random number stream is used for all the simulations). For smaller values of ϕ the simulated realization of the Gaussian model has a smoother appearance than its exponential counterpart.

The most important qualitative difference between the Gaussian and exponential correlation functions is their behaviour near $u = 0$. Note that the domain of the correlation function is extended to all real u by the requirement that $\rho(-u) = \rho(u)$. Then, the exponential model (5.2.7) is continuous but not differentiable at $u = 0$, whereas the Gaussian model (5.2.8) is infinitely differentiable. The same remarks apply to the variogram, which is given by $\gamma(u) = \sigma^2\{1 - \rho(u)\}$. If we now recall the definition of the variogram as $\gamma(u) = \frac{1}{2}\mathrm{E}[\{\epsilon(t) - \epsilon(t-u)\}^2]$, we see why these considerations of mathematical smoothness in the correlation functions translate to physical smoothness in the simulated realizations. In particular, if we consider a Gaussian model with correlation parameter ϕ_1, and an exponential model with correlation parameter ϕ_2, then whatever the values of ϕ_1 and ϕ_2, there is some positive value, u_0 say, such that for time-separations less than u_0, the mean squared difference between $R(t)$ and $R(t-u_0)$ is smaller for the Gaussian than for the exponential. In other words, on a sufficiently small time-scale the Gaussian model will appear to be smoother than the exponential.

Another way to build pure serial correlation models is to assume an explicit dependence of the current ϵ_j on a limited number of its predecessors, $\epsilon_{j-1}, \ldots, \epsilon_1$. This approach has a long history in time series analysis, going back at least to Yule (1927). For longitudinal data, the approach was proposed by Kenward (1987), who adopted Gabriel's (1962) terminology of *ante-dependence of order p* to describe a model in which the conditional distribution of ϵ_j given its predecessors $\epsilon_{j-1}, \ldots, \epsilon_1$ depends only on $\epsilon_{j-1}, \ldots, \epsilon_{j-p}$. A sequence of random variables ϵ_j with this property is more usually called a pth *order Markov model*, after the Russian mathematician who first studied stochastic processes of this kind. Ante-dependence modelling therefore has close links with the study of Markov processes (Cox and Miller, 1965), and with recent developments in the graphical modelling of multivariate data (Whittaker, 1990).

The simplest example of an ante-dependence model for a zero-mean sequence is the *first-order autoregressive process*. In this model, the ϵ_j can be generated from the relationship

$$\epsilon_j = \alpha\epsilon_{j-1} + Z_j, \tag{5.2.9}$$

where the Z_j are a sequence of mutually independent $N(0, \sigma^2)$ random variables, and the process is initiated by $\epsilon_0 \sim N\{0, \sigma^2/(1-\alpha^2)\}$. An equivalent formulation, with the same initial conditions, specifies the conditional distribution of ϵ_j given ϵ_{j-1} as

$$\epsilon_j \,|\, \epsilon_{j-1} \sim N(\alpha\epsilon_{j-1}, \sigma^2).$$

Care needs to be taken in defining the analogous ante-dependence models for the time-sequences of responses, Y_j. To take a very simple illustration, suppose that we wish to incorporate a linear relationship between the response, Y, and an explanatory variable, x, with serially correlated random variation about the mean response. One possibility is to assume that

$$Y_j = \beta_1 x_j + \epsilon_j,$$

where the ϵ_js follow the first-order autoregressive process defined by (5.2.9), with parameters α_1 and σ_1^2. Another is to assume that the conditional distribution of Y_j given Y_{j-1} is

$$Y_j \,|\, Y_{j-1} \sim N(\beta_2 x_j + \alpha_2 Y_{j-1}, \sigma_2^2).$$

Both are valid models, but they are not equivalent and cannot be made so by any choices for the two sets of parameter values. The conditional version of the first model is obtained by writing

$$Y_j - \beta x_j = \alpha(Y_{j-1} - \beta x_{j-1}) + Z_j,$$

and re-arranging to give

$$Y_j|Y_{j-1} \sim N(\beta x_j - \alpha x_{j-1} + \alpha Y_{j-1}, \sigma^2).$$

We take up this point again in Chapter 7.

One very convenient feature of ante-dependence models is that the joint probability density function of $\boldsymbol{\epsilon}$ follows easily from the specified form of the conditional distributions. Let $f_c(\epsilon_j \,|\, \epsilon_{j-1}, \ldots, \epsilon_{j-p}; \boldsymbol{\alpha})$ be the conditional probability density function of ϵ_j given $\epsilon_{j-k}, k = 1, \ldots, p$, and $f_0(\epsilon_1, \ldots, \epsilon_p; \boldsymbol{\alpha})$ the implied joint probability density function of $(\epsilon_1, \ldots, \epsilon_p)$. Then the joint probability density function of $\boldsymbol{\epsilon}$ is

$$f(\epsilon_1, \ldots, \epsilon_n; \boldsymbol{\alpha}) = f_0(\epsilon_1, \ldots, \epsilon_p; \boldsymbol{\alpha}) \prod_{j=p+1}^{n} f_c(\epsilon_j \,|\, \epsilon_{j-1}, \ldots, \epsilon_{j-p}; \boldsymbol{\alpha}).$$

Typically, $f_c(\cdot)$ is specified explicitly, from which it may or may not be easy to deduce $f_0(\cdot)$. However, if p is small and n large, there is usually only a small loss of information in conditioning on $\epsilon_1, \ldots, \epsilon_p$, in which case the contribution to the overall likelihood function is simply the product of the $n - p$ conditional densities, $f_c(\cdot)$. This makes estimation of $\boldsymbol{\alpha}$ very straightforward. For example, if $f_c(\cdot)$ is specified as a Gaussian probability density function with mean depending linearly on the conditioning variables, so that the conditional distribution of ϵ_j, given $\epsilon_{j-k}, k = 1, \ldots, p$, is $N\left(\sum_{k=1}^{p} \alpha_k \epsilon_{j-k}, \alpha_0^2\right)$ then the conditional maximum likelihood estimates of the α_k are obtained simply by ordinary least-squares (OLS) regression, treating the observed values of $\epsilon_{j-1}, \ldots, \epsilon_{j-p}$ as a set of p explanatory variables attached to the response, ϵ_j.

Ante-dependence models are appealing for equally spaced data, less so for unequally spaced data. For example, it would be hard to give a natural interpretation to the α_k parameters in the above model if the measurements were not equally spaced in time. Similarly, ante-dependence models do not cope easily with data for which the times of measurement are not common to all units.

One exception to the above remark is the exponential correlation model, which can also be interpreted as an ante-dependence model of order 1. Specifically, if $\boldsymbol{\epsilon} = (\epsilon_1, \ldots, \epsilon_n)$ has a multivariate Gaussian distribution with covariance structure

$$\text{Cov}(\epsilon_j, \epsilon_k) = \sigma^2 \exp(-\phi \mid t_j - t_k \mid),$$

then the conditional distribution of ϵ_j given all its predecessors depends only on the value of ϵ_{j-1}. Furthermore

$$\epsilon_j \mid \epsilon_{j-1} \sim N\left(\alpha_j \epsilon_{j-1}, \sigma^2(1 - \alpha_j^2)\right), \quad j = 2, \ldots, n,$$

where

$$\alpha_j = \exp\left(-\phi \mid t_j - t_{j-1} \mid\right),$$

and

$$\epsilon_1 \sim N(0, \sigma^2).$$

As a final comment on ante-dependence models, we note that their Markovian structure is not preserved if we superimpose measurement error or random effects. For example, if a sequence Y_t is Markov but we observe the sequence $Y_t^* = Y_t + Z_t$, where Z_t is a sequence of mutually independent measurement errors, then Y_t^* is not Markov.

5.2.2 *Serial correlation plus measurement error*

These are models for which there are no random effects in (5.2.3), so that $Y_j = W(t_j) + Z_j$, and (5.2.5) reduces to

$$\text{Var}(\boldsymbol{\epsilon}) = \sigma^2 H + \tau^2 I.$$

Now, the variance of each ϵ_j is $\sigma^2 + \tau^2$, and if the elements of H are specified by a correlation function $\rho(u)$, so that $h_{ij} = \rho(\mid t_i - t_j \mid)$, then the

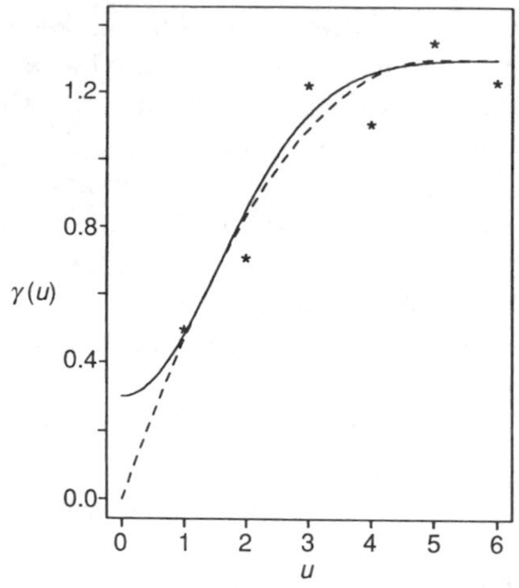

Fig. 5.3. A sample variogram and two different fitted models. $\star$: sample variogram; ——: fitted model with a non-zero intercept; – – –: fitted model with a zero intercept.

variogram becomes

$$\gamma(u) = \tau^2 + \sigma^2\{1 - \rho(u)\}. \tag{5.2.10}$$

A characteristic property of models with measurement error is that $\gamma(u)$ does not tend to zero as u tends to zero. If the data include duplicate measurements at the same time, we can estimate $\gamma(0) = \tau^2$ directly as one-half the average squared difference between such duplicates. Otherwise, estimation of τ^2 involves explicit or implicit extrapolation based on an assumed parametric model, and the estimate $\gamma(0)$ may be strongly model-dependent. Figure 5.3 illustrates this point. It shows an empirical variogram calculated from measurements at unit time-spacing, and two theoretical variograms which fit the data equally well but show very different extrapolations to $u = 0$.

5.2.3 *Random intercept plus serial correlation plus measurement error*

The simplest example of our general model (5.2.3) in which all three components of variation are present takes U to be a univariate, zero-mean Gaussian random variable with variance ν^2, and $d_j = 1$. Then, the realized value of U represents a random intercept, that is, an amount by which *all* measurements on the unit in question are raised or lowered relative to the population average. The variance matrix (5.2.5) becomes

$$\text{Var}(\boldsymbol{\epsilon}) = \nu^2 J + \sigma^2 H + \tau^2 I,$$

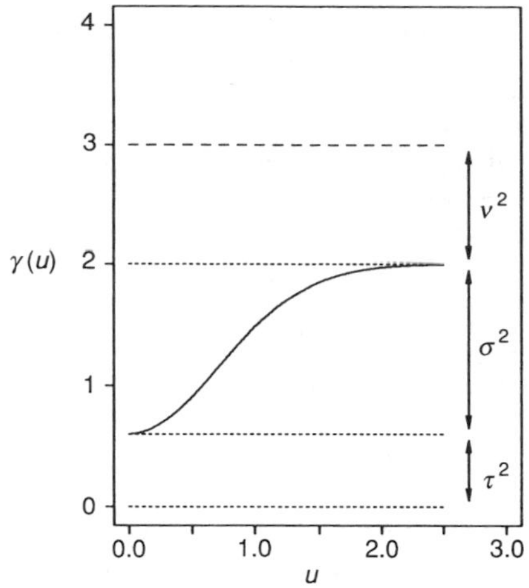

Fig. 5.4. The variogram for a model with a random intercept, serial correlation, and measurement error.

where J is an $n \times n$ matrix with all of its elements equal to 1. The variogram has the same form (5.2.10) as for the serial correlation plus measurement error model,

$$\gamma(u) = \tau^2 + \sigma^2\{1 - \rho(u)\},$$

except that now the variance of each ϵ_j is $\text{Var}(\epsilon_j) = \nu^2 + \sigma^2 + \tau^2$ and the limit of $\gamma(u)$ as $u \to \infty$ is *less* than $\text{Var}(\epsilon_j)$. Figure 5.4 shows this behaviour, using $\rho(u) = \exp(-u^2)$ as the correlation function of the serially correlated component.

The first explicit formulation of this model, with all three components of variation in a continuous-time setting, appears to be in Diggle (1988). Note that in fitting the model to data, the information on ν^2 derives from the replication of units within treatment groups.

5.2.4 *Random effects plus measurement error*

It is interesting to speculate on reasons for the relatively late infiltration of time series models into longitudinal data-analysis. Perhaps the explanation is the following. Whilst serial correlation would appear to be a natural feature of any longitudinal data model, in specific applications its effects may be dominated by the combination of random effects and measurement error. In terms of Fig. 5.4, if σ^2 is much smaller than either τ^2 or ν^2, the increasing curve of the variogram is squeezed between the two horizontal dotted lines, and becomes an unnecessary refinement of the model.

If we eliminate the serially correlated component altogether, (5.2.3) reduces to

$$\epsilon_j = \boldsymbol{d}_j'\boldsymbol{U} + Z_j.$$

The simplest model of this kind incorporates a scalar random intercept, U, with $d_j = 1$ for all j, to give

$$\mathrm{Var}(\boldsymbol{\epsilon}) = \nu^2 J + \tau^2 I.$$

The variance of each ϵ_j is $\nu^2 + \tau^2$, and the correlation between any two measurements on the same unit is

$$\rho = \nu^2/(\nu^2 + \tau^2).$$

As noted earlier, this uniform correlation structure is sometimes called a 'split-plot model' because of its formal equivalence with the correlation structure induced by the randomization for a classical split-plot experiment. However, the randomization argument gives no justification for its use with longitudinal data.

More general specifications of the random effect component lead to models with non-stationary structure. For example, if $\boldsymbol{U}$ is a pair of independent Gaussian random variables with variances ν_1^2 and ν_2^2, and $\boldsymbol{d}_j = (1, t_j)$, specifying a model with a linear time-trend for each unit but random intercept and slope between units, then $\mathrm{Var}(\epsilon_j) = \nu_1^2 + t_j^2\nu_2^2 + \tau^2$, and for $j \neq k$,

$$\mathrm{Cov}(\epsilon_j, \epsilon_k) = \nu_1^2 + t_j t_k \nu_2^2.$$

Figure 5.5 shows a simulated realization of this model with $\tau^2 = 0.25, \nu_1^2 = 0.5$, and $\nu_2^2 = 0.01$. The fanning out of the collection of response profiles over time is a common characteristic of growth data, for which non-stationary random effects models of this kind are often appropriate. Indeed, this kind of random effects model is often referred to as *the* growth curve model, following its systematic development in a seminal paper by Rao (1965) and many subsequent papers including Fearn (1977), Laird and Ware (1982), Verbyla (1986) and Verbyla and Venables (1988).

Sandland and McGilchrist (1979) advocate a different kind of non-stationary model for growth data. If $S(t)$ denotes the 'size' of an animal or plant at time t, measured on a logarithmic scale, then the relative growth rate (RGR) is defined to be the first derivative of $S(t)$. Sandland and McGilchrist argue that the RGR is often well modelled by a stationary random process. For models of this kind, the variance of $S(t)$ increases linearly over time, in contrast to the quadratic increase of the random slope and intercept model. Also, the source of the increasing variability is within, rather than between, units. In practice, quite long sequences of measurements may be needed to distinguish these two kinds of behaviour. Cullis and

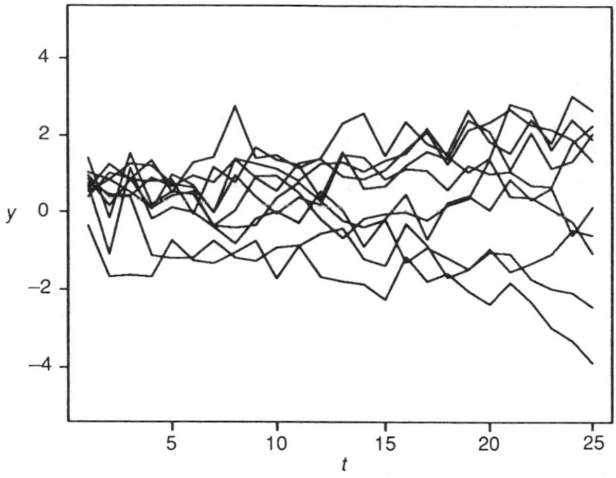

Fig. 5.5. A simulated realization of a model with random intercepts and random slopes.

McGilchrist (1990) advocate using the Sandland and McGilchrist model routinely in the longitudinal data setting. Note that for equally spaced data the model can be implemented by analysing successive differences, $R_t = S(t) - S(t-1)$, using a stationary model for the sequence $\{R_t\}$.

Random effects plus measurement error models as here defined can be thought of as incorporating *two* distinct *levels of variation* – between and within subjects – and might also be called *two-level models* of random variation. In some areas of application, the subjects may also be grouped in some way, and we may want to add a third level of random variation to describe the variability between groups. For example, in the context of animal experiments we might consider random variation between litters, between animals within litters, and between times within animals. Studies with more than two levels of variation, in this sense, are also common in social surveys. For example, in educational research we may wish to investigate variation between education authorities, between schools within authorities, between classes within schools, and between children within classes, with random sampling at every level of this hierarchy. Motivated by problems of this kind, Goldstein (1986) proposed a class of multi-level random effects models, which has since been further developed by Goldstein and co-workers into a systematic methodology with an associated software package, MLn.

5.3 Model-fitting

In fitting a model to a set of data, our objective is typically to answer questions about the process which generated the data. Note that 'model' and 'process' are not synonymous. We expect only that the former will be a useful approximation to the latter in the sense that it will contain a small number of parameters whose values can be interpreted as answers to the scientific questions posed by the data. Typically, the model will contain further parameters which are not of interest in themselves, but whose values affect the inferences which we make about the parameters of direct interest.

In many applications, inference about the model parameters is an end in itself. In others, we may wish to use the fitted model for prediction of the underlying continuous-time response profile associated with an individual unit. We take up this issue in Section 5.6. Here, we consider only the model-fitting process, which we divide into four stages:

(1) *formulation* – choosing the general form of the model;
(2) *estimation* – attaching numerical values to parameters;
(3) *inference* – calculating confidence intervals or testing hypotheses about parameters of direct interest;
(4) *diagnostics* – checking that the model fits the data.

5.3.1 *Formulation*

Formulation of a model is essentially a continuation of the exploratory data analysis considered in Chapter 3, but directed towards the specific aspects of the data which our model aims to describe. In particular, we assume here that any essentially model-independent issues such as the identification and treatment of outliers have already been resolved. The focus of attention is then the mean and covariance structure of the data.

With regard to the mean, time-plots of observed averages within treatment groups are simple and effective aids to model formulation for well-replicated data. When there are few measurements at any one time, non-parametric smoothing of the data is helpful.

For the covariance structure, we use residuals obtained by subtracting from each measurement the OLS estimate of the corresponding mean response, based on the most elaborate model we are prepared to contemplate for the mean response. As discussed in Section 4.4, for data from designed experiments in which the only relevant explanatory variables are the treatment labels we can use a saturated model, fitting a separate mean response for each combination of treatment and time. For data in which the times of measurement are not common to all units, or when there are continuously varying covariates which may affect the mean response non-linearly, the choice of a 'most elaborate model' is less obvious.

Time-plots, scatterplot matrices and empirical variogram plots of these residuals can then be used to give an idea of the underlying structure. Non-stationary variation in the time-plots of the residuals suggests the need for a transformation or an inherently non-stationary model such as a random effects model. When the pattern of variation appears to be stationary, the empirical variogram can be used to estimate the underlying covariance structure. In particular, if all units are observed at a common set of times the empirical variogram of the residuals is essentially unbiased for the underlying theoretical variogram (Diggle, 1990, Chapter 5). Diggle and Verbyla (1998) describe a version of the empirical variogram which can be used when the pattern of variation is non-stationary.

Note that if an incorrect parametric model is used to define the residuals, the empirical variogram will be biased to an unknown extent.

5.3.2 *Estimation*

Our objective in this second stage is to attach numerical values to the parameters in the model, whose general form is

$$\boldsymbol{Y} \sim MVN\{X\boldsymbol{\beta}, \sigma^2 V(\boldsymbol{\alpha})\}. \tag{5.3.1}$$

We write $\hat{\boldsymbol{\beta}}$, $\hat{\sigma}^2$, and $\hat{\boldsymbol{\alpha}}$ for the estimates of the model parameters, $\boldsymbol{\beta}$, σ^2, and $\boldsymbol{\alpha}$.

Particular methods of estimation have been derived for special cases of (5.3.1). However, it is straightforward to derive a general likelihood method. The resulting algorithm is computationally feasible provided that the sequences of measurements on individual units are not too long. If computing efficiency is paramount, more efficient algorithms can be derived to exploit the properties of special covariance structures. For example, estimation in ante-dependence models can exploit their Markovian structure.

The general method follows the same lines as the development in Section (4.4), but making use of the parametric structure of the variance matrix, $V(\boldsymbol{\alpha})$. Also as in Section 4.5 we favour restricted maximum likelihood (REML) estimates over classical maximum likelihood estimates to reduce the bias in the estimation of $\boldsymbol{\alpha}$, although this is less important if the dimensionality of $\boldsymbol{\beta}$ is small.

For given $\boldsymbol{\alpha}$, equation (4.5.5) holds in a modified form as

$$\hat{\boldsymbol{\beta}}(\boldsymbol{\alpha}) = \left(X'V(\boldsymbol{\alpha})^{-1}X\right)^{-1} X'V(\boldsymbol{\alpha})^{-1}\boldsymbol{y}, \tag{5.3.2}$$

and (4.5.6) likewise holds in the form

$$\hat{\sigma}^2(\boldsymbol{\alpha}) = \mathrm{RSS}(\boldsymbol{\alpha})/(N-p), \tag{5.3.3}$$

where

$$\mathrm{RSS}(\boldsymbol{\alpha}) = \{\boldsymbol{y} - X\hat{\boldsymbol{\beta}}(\boldsymbol{\alpha})\}'V(\boldsymbol{\alpha})^{-1}\{\boldsymbol{y} - X\hat{\boldsymbol{\beta}}(\boldsymbol{\alpha})\}, \tag{5.3.4}$$

and $N = \sum_{i=1}^m n_i$ is the total number of measurements on all m units. Finally, the REML estimate of $\boldsymbol{\alpha}$ maximizes

$$L^*(\boldsymbol{\alpha}) = -\tfrac{1}{2}\left[N \log\{\mathrm{RSS}(\boldsymbol{\alpha})\} + \log|\,V(\boldsymbol{\alpha})\,| \right. \\ \left. + \log|\,X'V(\boldsymbol{\alpha})^{-1}X\,|\right], \tag{5.3.5}$$

and the resulting REML estimate of $\boldsymbol{\beta}$ is $\hat{\boldsymbol{\beta}} = \hat{\boldsymbol{\beta}}(\hat{\boldsymbol{\alpha}})$.

The nature of the computations involved in maximizing $L^*(\boldsymbol{\alpha})$ becomes clear if we recognize explicitly the block-diagonal structure of $V(\boldsymbol{\alpha})$. Write $\boldsymbol{y}_i$ for the vector of n_i measurements on the ith unit and $\boldsymbol{t}_i$ for the corresponding vector of times at which these measurements are taken. Write $V_i(\boldsymbol{t_i};\boldsymbol{\alpha})$ for the non-zero $n_i \times n_i$ block of $V(\boldsymbol{\alpha})$ corresponding to the covariance matrix of $\boldsymbol{Y}_i$. The notation emphasizes that the source of the differences amongst the variance matrices of the different units is variation in the corresponding times of measurements. Finally, write X_i for the $n_i \times p$ matrix consisting of those rows of X which correspond to the explanatory variables measured on the ith unit. Then (5.3.4) and (5.3.5) can be written as

$$\mathrm{RSS}(\boldsymbol{\alpha}) = \sum_{i=1}^m \{\boldsymbol{y}_i - X_i\hat{\boldsymbol{\beta}}(\boldsymbol{\alpha})\}' V_i(\boldsymbol{t}_i;\boldsymbol{\alpha})^{-1}\{\boldsymbol{y}_i - X_i\hat{\boldsymbol{\beta}}(\boldsymbol{\alpha})\}, \tag{5.3.6}$$

and

$$L^*(\boldsymbol{\alpha}) = -\frac{1}{2}\left[N\log\{\mathrm{RSS}(\boldsymbol{\alpha})\} + \sum_{i=1}^m \log|\,V_i(\boldsymbol{t}_i;\boldsymbol{\alpha})\,| \right. \\ \left. + \sum_{i=1}^m \log|\,X_i'V_i(\boldsymbol{t}_i;\boldsymbol{\alpha})^{-1}X_i\,|\right]. \tag{5.3.7}$$

Each evaluation of $L^*(\boldsymbol{\alpha})$ therefore involves m determinants of order $p \times p$ for the second term in (5.3.7), and at most m determinants and inverses of the $V_i(\boldsymbol{t}_i;\,\boldsymbol{\alpha})$. In most applications, the number of distinct $V_i(\boldsymbol{t}_i;\boldsymbol{\alpha})$ is much fewer than m. Furthermore, the dimensionality of $\boldsymbol{\alpha}$ is typically very small, say three or four at most, and in our experience it is seldom necessary to use sophisticated optimization algorithms. Either the simplex algorithm of Nelder and Mead (1965) or a quasi-Newton algorithm, neither of which requires the user to provide information on the derivatives of $L^*(\boldsymbol{\alpha})$, usually works well. The only exceptions in our experience have been when an over-elaborate model is fitted to sparse data and the covariance parameters, $\boldsymbol{\alpha}$, are poorly determined. Finally in this subsection, note that whilst the REML estimates maximize $L^*(\boldsymbol{\alpha})$ given by (5.3.7), maximum likelihood estimates maximize

$$L(\boldsymbol{\alpha}) = -\frac{1}{2}\left[N\log\{\text{RSS}(\alpha)\} + \sum_{i=1}^{m}\log|V_i(\boldsymbol{t}_i;\boldsymbol{\alpha})|\right]. \tag{5.3.8}$$

5.3.3 *Inference*

Inference about $\boldsymbol{\beta}$ can be based on the result (5.3.2) which, in conjunction with (5.3.1), implies that

$$\hat{\boldsymbol{\beta}}(\boldsymbol{\alpha}) \sim MVN\{\boldsymbol{\beta}, \sigma^2(X'V(\boldsymbol{\alpha})^{-1}X)^{-1}\}. \tag{5.3.9}$$

We assume that (5.3.9) continues to hold, to a good approximation, if we substitute the REML estimates $\hat{\sigma}^2$ and $\hat{\boldsymbol{\alpha}}$ for the unknown values of σ^2 and $\boldsymbol{\alpha}$ in (5.3.9). This gives

$$\hat{\boldsymbol{\beta}} \sim MVN(\boldsymbol{\beta}, \hat{V}), \tag{5.3.10}$$

where

$$\hat{V} = \hat{\sigma}^2(X'V(\hat{\boldsymbol{\alpha}})^{-1}X)^{-1}.$$

The immediate application of (5.3.10) is to set standard errors on individual elements of $\boldsymbol{\beta}$. Almost as immediate is the calculation of confidence regions for general linear transformations of the form

$$\boldsymbol{\psi} = D\boldsymbol{\beta}, \tag{5.3.11}$$

where D is a full-rank, $r \times p$ matrix with $r \leq p$. Confidence regions for $\boldsymbol{\psi}$ follow from the result that if $\boldsymbol{\psi} = D\hat{\boldsymbol{\beta}}$, then

$$\hat{\boldsymbol{\psi}} \sim MVN(\boldsymbol{\psi}, D\hat{V}D'),$$

from which it follows in turn that

$$T(\boldsymbol{\psi}) = (\hat{\boldsymbol{\psi}} - \boldsymbol{\psi})'(D\hat{V}D')^{-1}(\hat{\boldsymbol{\psi}} - \boldsymbol{\psi}), \tag{5.3.12}$$

is distributed as χ^2_r. Let $c_r(q)$ denote the q-critical value of χ^2_r, so that $P\{\chi^2_r \geq c_r(q)\} = q$. Then, a $100(1-q)$ per cent confidence region for $\boldsymbol{\psi}$ is

$$\{\boldsymbol{\psi} : T(\boldsymbol{\psi}) \leq c_r(q)\}. \tag{5.3.13}$$

Using the well known duality between hypothesis tests and confidence regions, a test of a hypothesized value for $\boldsymbol{\psi}$, say H_0: $\boldsymbol{\psi} = \boldsymbol{\psi}_0$, consists of rejecting H_0 at the $100q$ per cent level if $T(\boldsymbol{\psi}_0) > c_r(q)$. Note in particular that a statistic to test H_0: $\boldsymbol{\psi} = \mathbf{0}$ is

$$T_0 = \hat{\boldsymbol{\psi}}'(D\hat{V}D')^{-1}\hat{\boldsymbol{\psi}}, \tag{5.3.14}$$

whose null sampling distribution is χ^2_r.

In implementing the above method of inference, the nuisance parameters, σ^2 and $\boldsymbol{\alpha}$, are estimated once only, from the maximal model for $\boldsymbol{\beta}$. The choice of the maximal model is sometimes difficult, especially when the times of measurement are highly variable between units or when there are continuously varying covariates. An alternative, 'step-up' approach may then be useful, beginning with a very simple model for $\boldsymbol{\beta}$ and considering the maximized log-likelihoods from a sequence of progressively more elaborate models. At each stage, the maximized log-likelihood is $L(\hat{\boldsymbol{\alpha}})$, where $L(\boldsymbol{\alpha})$ is defined by (5.3.8) with the current design matrix X, and $\hat{\boldsymbol{\alpha}}$ maximizes $L(\boldsymbol{\alpha})$. Let L_k be the maximized log-likelihood associated with the kth model in this nested sequence, and p_k the number of columns in the corresponding design matrix. The log-likelihood ratio statistic to test the adequacy of the kth model within the $(k+1)$st is

$$W_k = 2(L_{k+1} - L_k). \tag{5.3.15}$$

If the kth model is correct, W_k is distributed as chi-squared on $p_{k+1} - p_k$ degrees of freedom.

This likelihood ratio testing approach to inference is convenient when the data are unbalanced and there is no obvious maximal model. However, the earlier approach based on the multivariate Gaussian distribution for $\hat{\boldsymbol{\beta}}$ is in our view preferable when it is feasible because it more clearly separates the inferences about $\boldsymbol{\beta}$ and $\boldsymbol{\alpha}$.

5.3.4 *Diagnostics*

Diagnostic checking of the model against the data completes the model-fitting process. The aim of diagnostic checking is to compare the data with the fitted model in such a way as to highlight any systematic discrepancies. Since our models are essentially models for the mean and covariance structure of the data, simple and highly effective checks are to superimpose the fitted mean response profiles on a time-plot of the average observed response within each combination of treatment and time, and to superimpose the fitted variogram on a plot of the empirical variogram.

Simple plots of this kind can be very effective in revealing inconsistencies between data and model which were missed at earlier stages. If so, these can be incorporated into a revised model, and the fitting process repeated.

More formal diagnostic criteria for regression models are discussed by Cook and Weisberg (1982) and Atkinson (1985) in the context of linear models for cross-sectional data and, in a non-parametric setting, by Hastie and Tibshirani (1990).

5.4 Examples

In this section we give three applications of the model-based approach. These involve:

(1) the data set of Example 1.4 on the protein content of milk samples from cows on each of three different diets;

(2) a set of data on the body-weights of cows in a 2 by 2 factorial experiment;

(3) the data set of Example 1.1 on CD4+ cell numbers.

Example 5.1. Protein contents of milk samples

These data were shown in Fig. 1.4. They consist of measurements of protein content in up to 19 weekly samples taken from each of 79 cows allocated to one of three different diets: 25 cows received a barley diet, 27 cows a mixed diet of barley and lupins, and 27 cows a diet of lupins only. The initial inspection of the data reported in Chapter 1 suggested that the mean response profiles are approximately parallel, showing an initial sharp drop associated with a settling-in period, followed by an approximately constant mean response over most of the experimental period and a possible gentle rise towards the end. The empirical variogram, shown in Fig. 3.16, exhibits a smooth rise with increasing lag, levelling out within the range spanned by the data. Both the mean and covariance structure therefore seem amenable to parametric modelling.

Our provisional model for the mean response profiles takes the form

$$\mu_g(t) = \begin{cases} \beta_{0g} + \beta_1 t, & t \leq 3, \\ \beta_{0g} + 3\beta_1 + \beta_2(t-3) + \beta_3(t-3)^2, & t > 3, \end{cases} \qquad (5.4.1)$$

where $g = 1, 2, 3$ denotes treatment group, and time, t, is measured in weeks. Our provisional model for the covariance structure takes the form of (5.2.10) with an exponential correlation function. For the model-fitting, it is convenient to extract σ^2 as a scale parameter and reparametrize to $\alpha_1 = \tau^2/\sigma^2$ and $\alpha_2 = \nu^2/\sigma^2$. With this parametrization the theoretical variance of each measurement is $\sigma^2(1 + \alpha_1 + \alpha_2)$ and the theoretical variogram is

$$\gamma(u) = \sigma^2\{\alpha_1 + 1 - \exp(-\alpha_3 u)\}.$$

The REML estimates of the model parameters, with estimated standard errors and correlation matrix of the mean parameters, are given in Table 5.1. This information can now be used to make inferences about the mean response profiles as discussed in Section 5.3.3. We give two examples.

Because our primary interest is in whether the diets affect the mean response profiles, we first test the hypothesis that $\beta_{01} = \beta_{02} = \beta_{03}$. To do

Table 5.1. REML estimates for the model fitted to data on protein content of milk samples: (a) Mean response; (b) Covariance structure.

(a)

$$\mu_i(t) = \begin{cases} \beta_{0g} + \beta_1 t, & t \le 3, \\ \beta_{0g} + 3\beta_1 + \beta_2(t-3) + \beta_3(t-3)^2, & t > 3. \end{cases}$$

Parameter	Estimate	SE	Correlation matrix				
β_{01}	4.15	0.054	1.00				
β_{02}	4.05	0.053	0.52	1.00			
β_{03}	3.94	0.053	0.52	0.53	1.00		
β_1	−0.229	0.016	−0.61	−0.62	−0.62	1.00	
β_2	0.0078	0.0079	−0.60	−0.06	−0.06	−0.33	1.00
β_3	−0.00056	0.00050	0.01	0.01	0.02	0.24	−0.93

(b)

$$\gamma(u) = \sigma^2\{\alpha_1 + 1 - \exp(-\alpha_3 u)\},$$
$$\mathrm{Var}(Y) = \sigma^2(1 + \alpha_1 + \alpha_2).$$

Parameter	Estimate
σ^2	0.0635
α_1	0.3901
α_2	0.1007
α_3	0.1674

this, we need only consider the REML estimates and variance submatrix of $\boldsymbol{\beta}_0 = (\beta_{01}, \beta_{02}, \beta_{03})$. This submatrix is

$$\hat{V}_1 = \begin{bmatrix} 0.0029 & 0.0015 & 0.0015 \\ 0.0015 & 0.0028 & 0.0014 \\ 0.0015 & 0.0014 & 0.0028 \end{bmatrix}.$$

Now, using (5.3.11) and (5.3.12) on this three-parameter system, we proceed as follows. The hypothesis of interest is $\boldsymbol{\psi} = D\boldsymbol{\beta}_0 = \mathbf{0}$, where

$$D = \begin{bmatrix} 1 & -1 & 0 \\ 0 & 1 & -1 \end{bmatrix}.$$

The REML estimate of $\boldsymbol{\psi}$ is

$$\hat{\boldsymbol{\psi}} = D\hat{\boldsymbol{\beta}}_0 = (0.10, 0.11).$$

From (5.3.12), the test statistic is

$$T_0 = \hat{\boldsymbol{\psi}}'(D\hat{V}_1 D')^{-1}\boldsymbol{\psi} = 15.98,$$

which we refer to critical values of χ_2^2. Since $P\{\chi_2^2 > 15.98\} = 0.0003$, we clearly reject $\boldsymbol{\psi} = \mathbf{0}$ and conclude that diet affects the mean response profile. Furthermore, the ordering of the three estimates, $\hat{\beta}_{og}$, is sensible, with the parameter estimate for the mixed diet lying between those for the two pure diets.

A question of secondary interest is whether there is a rise in the mean response towards the end of the experiment. The hypothesis to test this is $\beta_2 = \beta_3 = 0$. The variance submatrix of $\hat{\boldsymbol{\beta}} = (\hat{\beta}_2, \hat{\beta}_3)$ is $\hat{V}_2$, where

$$10^6 \hat{V}_2 = \begin{bmatrix} 62.094 & -3.631 \\ -3.631 & 0.246 \end{bmatrix}.$$

The test statistic is

$$T_0 = \hat{\boldsymbol{\beta}}\hat{V}_2^{-1}\hat{\boldsymbol{\beta}} = 1.29,$$

which we again refer to critical values of χ_2^2. Since $P\{\chi_2^2 > 1.29\} = 0.525$, we do not reject the null hypothesis in favour of a late rise in the mean response. Refitting the simpler model with $\beta_2 = \beta_3 = 0$ leaves the other parameter estimates essentially unchanged, and does not alter the conclusions about the treatment effects. Results for the model with $\beta_2 = \beta_3 = 0$, but using maximum likelihood estimation, are given in Diggle (1990, Section 5.6).

Verbyla and Cullis (1990) suggest that the mean response curves in the three treatment groups may not be parallel, and fit a model in which the difference, $\mu_1(t) - \mu_3(t)$, is linear in t. A model which allows the difference in mean response between any two treatments to be linear in t replaces β_{02} and β_{03} in (5.4.1) by $\beta_{021} + \beta_{022}t$ and $\beta_{031} + \beta_{032}t$, respectively. Using this eight-parameter specification of the mean response profiles as our working model, a hypothesis of possible interest in that $\beta_{022} = \beta_{032} = 0$, that is that (5.4.1) gives an adequate description of the data. Fitting this enlarged model, we obtain

$$(\hat{\beta}_{022}, \hat{\beta}_{032}) = (-0.0042, -0.0095),$$

with estimated variance matrix, $\hat{V}_3$, where

$$10^6 \hat{V}_3 = \begin{bmatrix} 33.41 & 18.92 \\ 18.92 & 41.22 \end{bmatrix}.$$

The statistic to test $\beta_{022} = \beta_{032} = 0$ is $T_0 = 2.210$, which is to be compared with critical values of χ_2^2. Since $P\{\chi_2^2 > 2.210\} = 0.33$, there is no real evidence against $\beta_{022} = \beta_{032} = 0$. Even if we consider $\hat{\beta}_{032}$ alone, the statistic to test $\beta_{032} = 0$ is $T_0 = 2.208$, on one degree of freedom, which is still not significant. This analysis is not directly comparable with the one reported in Verbyla and Cullis (1990), as they consider only the last 16 time-points and use a non-parametric description of the mean response profile, $\mu_1(t)$, for cows on the barley diet.

Our provisional model for the data is summarized by the parameter estimates in Table 5.1 but with the simplification that $\beta_2 = \beta_3 = 0$. Figure 5.6 compares the empirical and fitted mean response profiles and

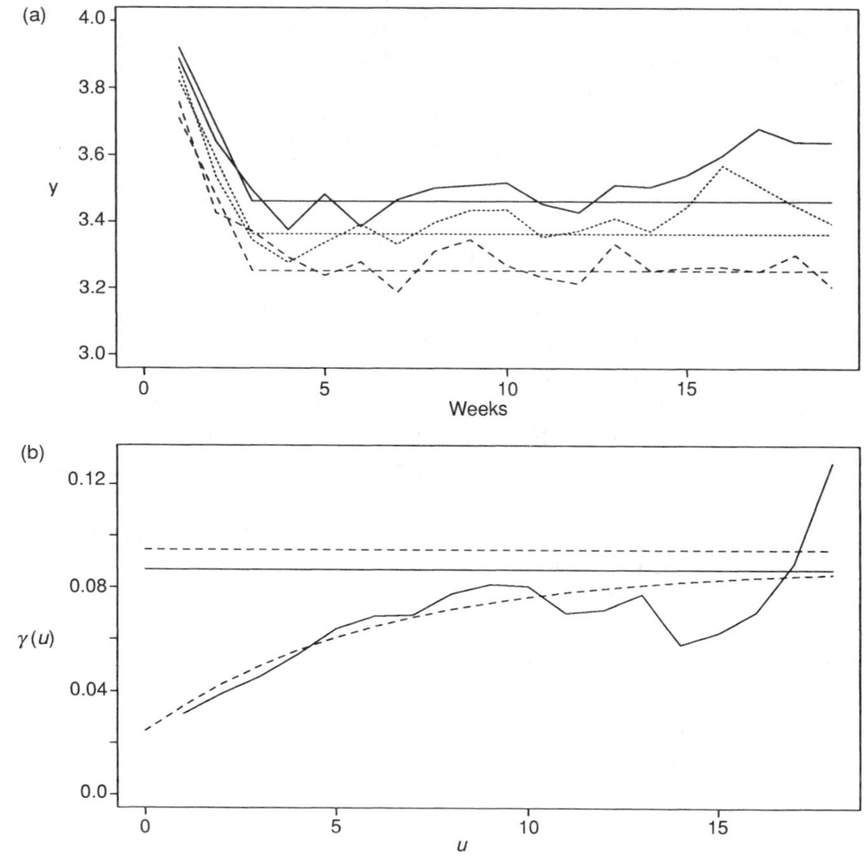

Fig. 5.6. Milk protein data: comparison between observed and fitted mean response profiles and variograms: (a) mean response profiles ——: barley diet; ....: mixed diet; – – –: lupins diet; (b) variograms ——: sample variogram; – – –: fitted variogram.

variograms. The fit to the variogram appears to be satisfactory. The rise in the empirical variogram at $u = 18$ can be discounted as it is based on only 41 observed pairwise differences. Since these pairwise differences derive from 41 different animals and are therefore approximately independent, elementary calculations give a 95% per cent confidence interval for the mean of $\hat{\gamma}(18)$ as 0.127 ± 0.052, which includes the fitted value, $\gamma(18) = 0.085$.

At first sight, the fit to the mean response profiles appears less satisfactory. However, the apparent lack of fit is towards the end of the experiment, by which time the responses from almost half of the animals are missing. Clearly, this increases the variability in the observed mean responses. Also the strong positive correlations between successive measurements mean that a succession of positive residuals is less significant than it would be for uncorrelated data. Finally, and most interestingly, we might question whether calving date is independent of the measurement process. If later-calving cows are also more likely to produce milk with a lower protein content, we would expect the observed mean responses to rise towards the end of the study. The implications for the interpretation of the fitted model are subtle, and will be pursued in Chapter 13.

Example 5.2. Body-weights of cows

These data, provided by Dr Andrew Lepper (CSIRO Division of Animal Health, Melbourne) consist of body-weights of 27 cows, measured at 23 unequally spaced times over a period of about 22 months. They are listed in Table 5.2. For the analysis, we use a time-scale which runs from 0 to 66, each unit representing 10 days. One animal showed an abnormally low weight-gain throughout the experiment and we have

Table 5.2. Data on log-bodyweights of cows. The original experiment was a 2 by 2 factorial with 27 animals allocated to experimental groups as follows: first 4 animals – control; next 4 – iron dosing; next 9 – infection with *M. paratuberculosis*; next 10 – iron dosing and infection. Data below are from the first two groups only.

Time in days											
122	150	166	179	219	247	276	296	324	354	380	445
4.7	4.905	5.011	5.075	5.136	5.165	5.298	5.323	5.416	5.438	5.541	5.652
4.868	5.075	5.193	5.22	5.298	5.416	5.481	5.521	5.617	5.635	5.687	5.768
4.868	5.011	5.136	5.193	5.273	5.323	5.416	5.46	5.521	5.58	5.617	5.687
4.828	5.011	5.136	5.193	5.273	5.347	5.438	5.561	5.541	5.598	5.67	5.521
4.787	4.977	5.043	5.136	5.106	5.298	5.298	5.371	5.438	5.501	5.561	5.652
4.605	4.828	4.942	5.011	5.106	5.165	5.22	5.298	5.273	5.298	5.371	5.394
4.745	4.868	5.043	5.106	5.22	5.298	5.347	5.347	5.416	5.501	5.561	5.58
4.745	4.905	5.011	5.106	5.165	5.273	5.371	5.416	5.416	5.521	5.541	5.635

removed it from the model-fitting analysis. The remaining 26 animals were allocated amongst treatments in a 2 by 2 factorial design. The two factors were presence/absence of iron dosing and of infection by the organism *M. paratuberculosis*. The replications in the four groups were: $4\times$ control, $3\times$ iron only, $9\times$ infection only, $10\times$ iron and infection. For further details of the biological background to these data, see Lepper *et al.* (1989).

We use a log-transformation of the bodyweights as the response variable, to stabilize the variance over time. The resulting data are shown in Fig. 5.7. The empirical variogram of OLS residuals from a saturated model for the mean response, that is, fitting a separate parameter for each combination of time and treatment, is shown in Fig. 5.8. As in the previous

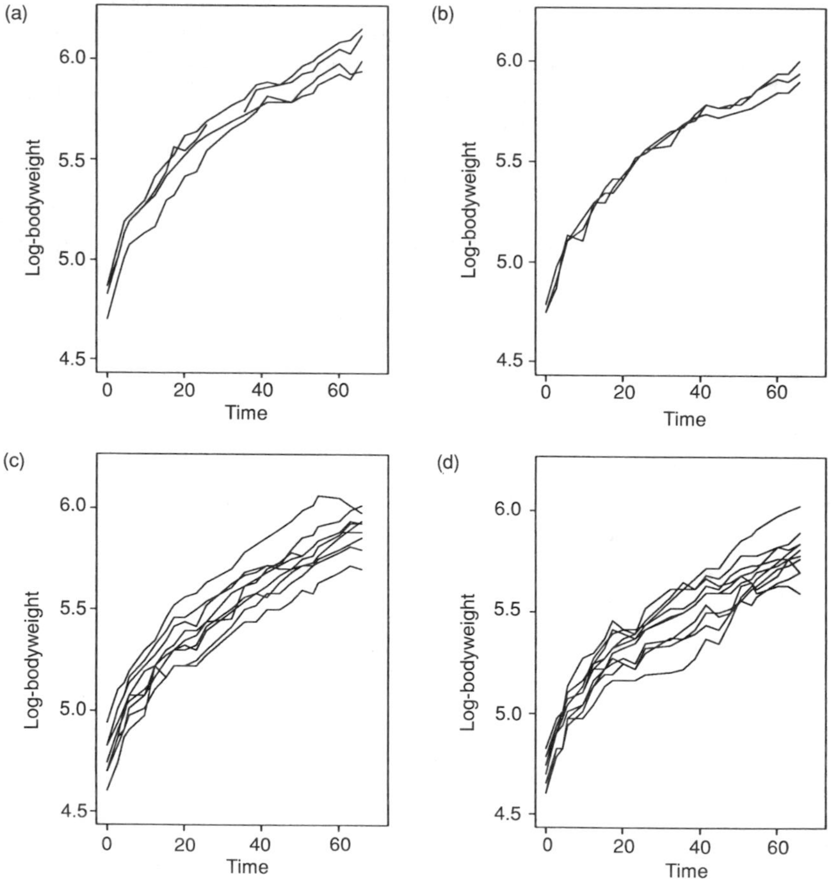

Fig. 5.7. Log-bodyweights of cows in a 2 by 2 factorial experiment: (a) control; (b) iron dosing; (c) infection; (d) iron dosing and infection.

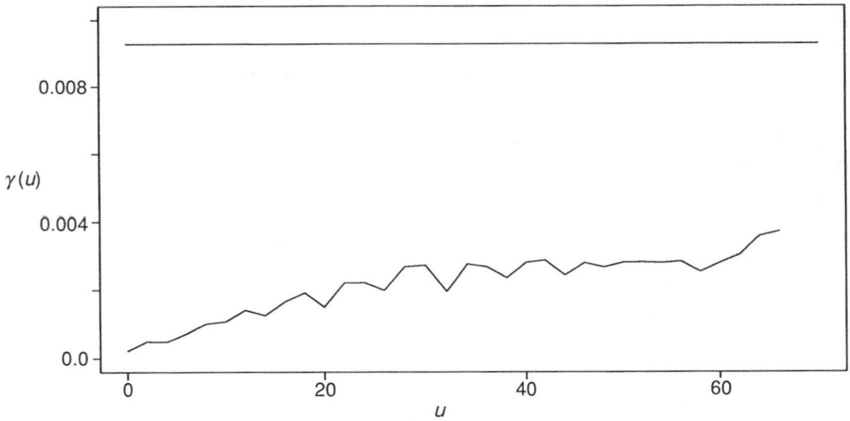

Fig. 5.8. Log-bodyweights of cows: sample variogram of residuals.

section, the model described in Section 5.2.3 seems reasonable, although the detailed behaviour is rather different than that of the milk protein data. For these data, the measurement error variance, τ^2, seems to be relatively small, as we would expect, whereas the between-animal variance, ν^2, is very large. Also, the behaviour of the empirical variogram near the origin suggests that a Gaussian correlation function might be more appropriate than an exponential. With a reparametrization to $\alpha_1 = \tau^2/\sigma^2$ and $\alpha_2 = \nu^2/\sigma^2$, this suggests a model in which the theoretical variance of log-weight is $\sigma^2(1 + \alpha_1 + \alpha_2)$ and the theoretical variogram takes the form

$$\gamma(u) = \sigma^2\{\alpha_1 + 1 - \exp(-\alpha_3 u^2)\}.$$

Fitting the mean response profiles into the framework of the general linear model, $\boldsymbol{\mu} = X\boldsymbol{\beta}$, proves to be difficult. This is not untypical of growth studies, in which the mean response shows an initially sharp increase before gradually levelling off as it approaches an asymptote. Low-degree polynomials provide poor approximations to this behaviour. A way forward is to use 23 parameters to describe the control mean response at each of the 23 time-points, and to model the factorial effects, or differences between groups, parametrically. This would not be sensible if the mean response profile were of intrinsic interest, but this is not so here. Interest focuses on the factorial effects. This situation is not uncommon, and the approach of modelling only contrasts between treatments, rather than treatment means themselves, has been advocated by a number of authors including Evans and Roberts (1979), Cullis and McGilchrist (1990) and Verbyla and Cullis (1990).

Figure 5.9 shows the observed mean response in the control group, and the differences in mean response for the other three groups relative to the

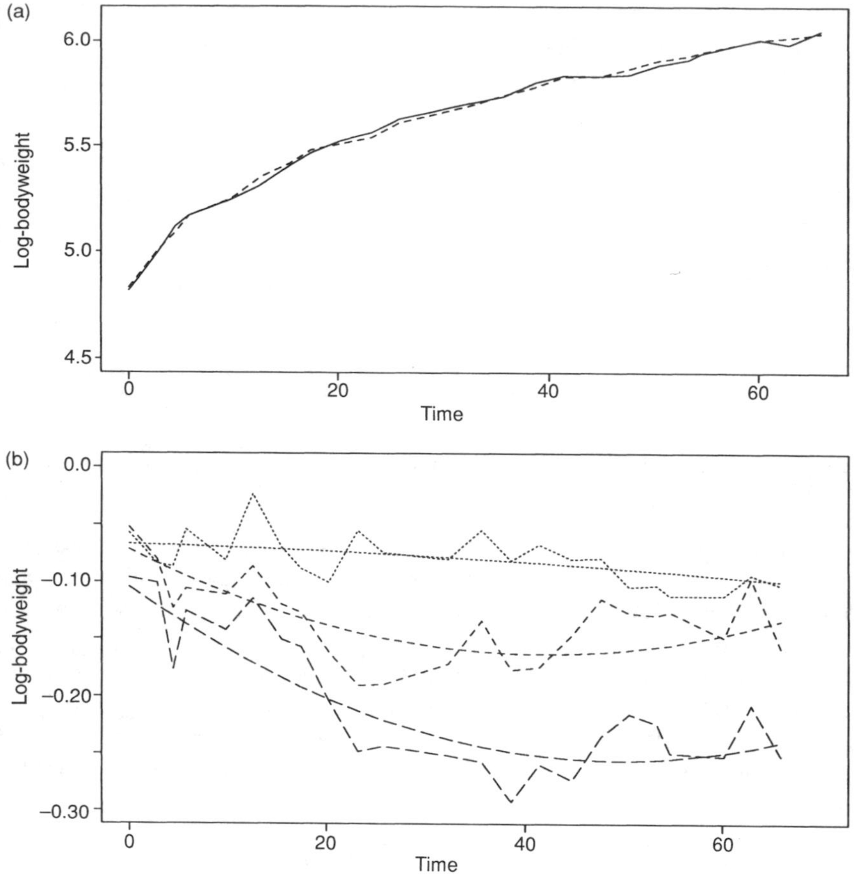

Fig. 5.9. Log-bodyweights of cows: observed and fitted mean response profiles: (a) control ——: observed; – – –: fitted; (b) difference between control and treated, with fitted contrasts shown as smooth curves ....: iron; – – –: infection; — —: both.

control. These differences do seem amenable to a linear modelling approach. The fitted curves are based on a model in which each treatment contrast is a quadratic function of time, whereas the control mean is described by a separate parameter at each of the 23 time-points. Note that the fit to the observed control mean is nevertheless not exact because it includes indirect information from the other three treatment groups, as a consequence of our using a parametric model for the treatment contrasts. The standard errors of the fitted control means range from 0.044 to 0.046. Figure 5.10 shows the fit to the empirical variogram. This seems to be satisfactory, and confirms that the dominant component of variation is between animals;

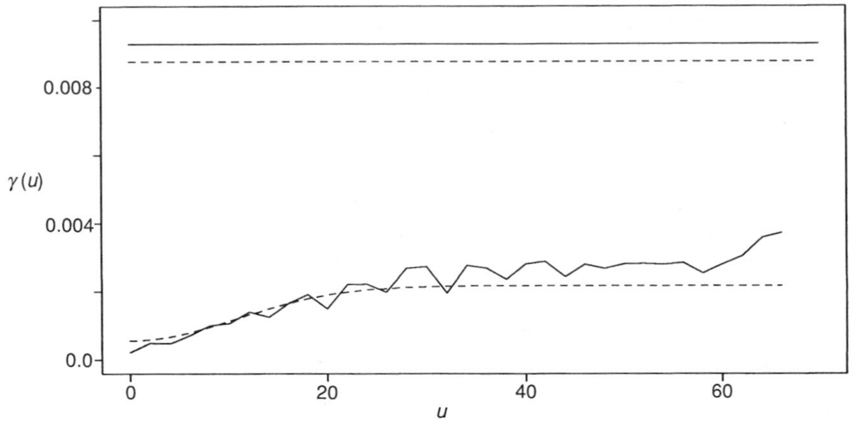

Fig. 5.10. Log-bodyweights of cows: observed and fitted variograms. ——: sample variogram; – – –: fitted model.

the estimated parameters in the covariance structure are $\hat{\sigma}^2 = 0.0016$, $\hat{\alpha}_1 = 0.353, \hat{\alpha}_2 = 4.099$, and $\hat{\alpha}_3 = 0.0045$.

Table 5.3 gives the parameter estimates of direct interest, with their estimated standard errors. For these data, the principal objective is to describe the main effects of the two factors and the interaction between them. Note that in our provisional model for the data, each factorial effect is a quadratic function of time, representing the difference in mean log-bodyweight between animals treated at the higher and lower levels of the effect in question.

One question is whether we could simplify the description by using linear rather than quadratic effects. Using the notation of Table 5.3, this amounts to a test of the hypothesis that $\beta_{21} = \beta_{22} = \beta_{23} = 0$. The chi-squared test statistic to test this hypothesis is $T_0 = 10.785$ on three degrees of freedom, corresponding to a p-value of 0.020; we therefore retain the quadratic description of the factorial effects. Attention now focuses on the significance of the two main effects and of the interaction between them. Again using the notation of Table 5.2, the hypothesis of no main effect for iron is $\beta_{01} = \beta_{11} = \beta_{21} = 0$, that of no main effect for infection is $\beta_{02} = \beta_{12} = \beta_{22} = 0$, and that of no interaction is $\beta_{03} = \beta_{01}+\beta_{02}$; $\beta_{13} = \beta_{11}+\beta_{12}$; $\beta_{23} = \beta_{21}+\beta_{22}$. The chi-squared statistics, T_0, each on three degrees of freedom, and their associated p-values, are as follows: Iron $- T_0 = 1.936$, $p = 0.586$; Infection $- T_0 = 14.32$, $p = 0.003$; Interaction $- T_0 = 0.521$, $p = 0.914$.

The conclusion is that there is a highly significant main effect of infection, whereas the main effect of iron and, not surprisingly, the interaction effect are not significant, that is iron dosing has failed to alleviate the

Table 5.3. Estimates of parameters defining the treatment contrasts between the model fitted to data on log-bodyweights of cows. The contrast between the mean response in treatment group g and the control group is $\mu_g(t) = \beta_{0g} + \beta_{1g}(t-33) + \beta_{2g}(t-33)^2$.

Treatment	Parameter	Estimates	SE
Iron	β_{01}	−0.079	0.067
	β_{11}	−0.00050	0.00071
	β_{21}	−0.0000040	0.000033
Infection	β_{02}	−0.159	0.053
	β_{12}	−0.00098	0.00056
	β_{22}	0.0000516	0.00026
Both	β_{03}	−0.239	0.052
	β_{13}	−0.0020	0.00055
	β_{23}	0.000062	0.000025

adverse effect of infection. Refitting a reduced model with only an infection effect, we obtain the following estimate for the contrast between the mean response with and without infection:

$$\hat{\mu}(t) = -0.167 - 0.00134(t-33) + 0.0000566(t-33)^2.$$

This equation and the associated standard errors of the three parameters provide a compact summary of the conclusions about treatment effects. The estimated standard errors for the intercept, linear, and quadratic coefficients are 0.042, 0.00044, and 0.00002, respectively.

Example 5.3. Estimation of the population mean CD4+ curve

For the CD4+ data of Example 1.1 there are $N = 2376$ observations of CD4+ cell numbers on $m = 369$ men infected with the HIV virus. Time is measured in years with the origin at the date of seroconversion, which is known approximately for each individual. In this example, our primary interest is in the progression of mean CD4+ count as a function of time since seroconversion, although in Section 5.5 we will also consider these data from the point of view of predicting the CD4+ trajectories of individual subjects. Our parametric model uses square-root-transformed CD4+ count as the response variable and specifies the mean time-trend, $\mu(t)$, as constant prior to seroconversion and quadratic in time thereafter. In the linear model for the mean response, we also include as explanatory variables: smoking (packs per day); recreational drug use (yes/no); numbers of sexual partners; and depressive symptoms as measured by the CESD scale.

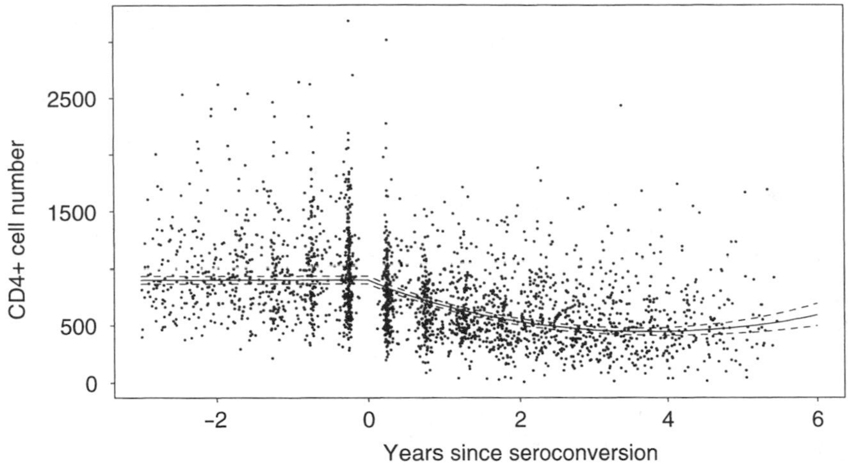

Fig. 5.11. CD4+ cell counts with parametric estimate and pointwise confidence limits (plus and minus two standard errors) for the mean time-trend.

Figure 5.11 shows the data with the estimated mean time-trend and pointwise confidence limits calculated as plus and minus two standard errors, re-expressed on the original scale. The standard errors were calculated from a parametric model for the covariance structure of the kind introduced in Section 5.2.3. Specifically, we assume that the variance of each measurement is $\tau^2 + \sigma^2 + \nu^2$ and that the variogram within each unit is $\gamma(u) = \tau^2 + \sigma^2\{1 - \exp(-\alpha u)\}$. Figure 5.12 shows the empirical variogram, using a grouping interval of 0.25 years, and a parametric fit obtained by maximum likelihood, which gave estimates $\hat{\tau}^2 = 10.7$, $\hat{\sigma}^2 = 25.0$, $\hat{\nu}^2 = 2.3$, and $\hat{\alpha} = 0.23$.

Figure 5.11 suggests that the mean number of CD4+ cells is approximately constant at close to 1000 cells prior to seroconversion. Within the first six months after seroconversion, the mean drops to around 700. Subsequently, the rate of loss is much slower. For example, it takes nearly three years before the mean number reaches 500, the level at which, when these data were collected, it was recommended that prophylactic AZT therapy should begin (Volberding *et al.*, 1990). As with Example 5.1 on the protein contents of milk samples, the interpretation of the fitted mean response is complicated by the possibility that subjects who become very ill may drop out of the study, and these subjects may also have unusually low CD4+ counts. In Chapter 13 we shall discuss ways of handling potentially informative dropout in longitudinal studies.

The upturn in the estimated mean time-trend from approximately four years after seroconversion is, of course, an artificial by-product of the assumption that the time-trend is quadratic. As in our earlier discussions

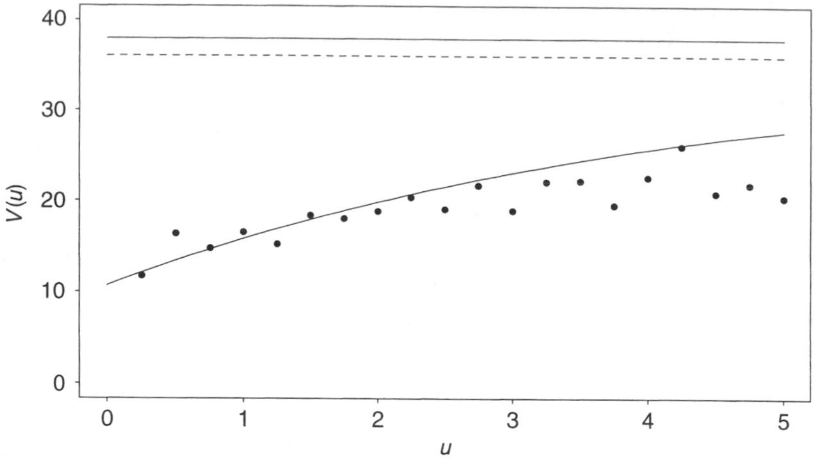

Fig. 5.12. CD4+ cell counts: observed and fitted variograms •: empirical variogram – – –: empirical variance ——: fitted model.

of these data a non-parametric, or at least non-linear, treatment of $\mu(t)$ would be preferable, and we shall take this up in Chapter 14.

5.5 Estimation of individual trajectories

The CD4+ data provide an example in which the mean response is of interest, but not of sole interest. For counselling individual patients, it is that individual's history of CD4+ levels which is relevant. However, because observed CD4+ levels are highly variable over time, in part because of a substantial component of variation due to measurement error, the individual's observed trajectory is not reliable. This problem could arise in either a non-parametric or a parametric setting. Because our motivation is the CD4+ data, we will use the same modelling framework as in the previous section.

The data again consist of measurements, y_{ij}, $j = 1, \ldots, n_i$; $i = 1, \ldots, m$, and associated times, t_{ij}. The model for the data is that

$$Y_{ij} = \mu(t_{ij}) + U_i + W_i(t_{ij}) + Z_{ij},$$

where the U_i are mutually independent $N(0, \nu^2)$, the Z_{ij} are mutually independent $N(0, \tau^2)$ and the $\{W_i(t)\}$ are mutually independent, zero-mean stationary Gaussian processes with covariance function $\sigma^2\rho(u)$. Our objective is to construct a predictor for the CD4+ number of an individual, i, at time t. Because the Z_{ij} represent measurement error, they make no direct contribution to the predictor, $\hat{Y}(t)$, although, as we shall see, they do affect the prediction variance of $\hat{Y}(t)$. Our predictor therefore takes the form

$$\begin{aligned}\hat{Y}_i(t) &= \hat{\mu}(t) + \hat{U} + \hat{W}_i(t) \\ &= \hat{\mu}(t) + \hat{R}_i(t),\end{aligned}$$

say.

For the time being, we shall assume that $\mu(t)$ is specified by a general linear model, and can therefore be estimated using the methods described in Section 5.3. To construct $\hat{R}_i(t)$ we proceed as follows. For an arbitrary set of times, $\boldsymbol{u} = (u_1, \ldots, u_p)$, let $\boldsymbol{R}_i$ be the p-element random vector with rth element $R_i(u_r)$. Let $\boldsymbol{Y}_i$ be the n_i-element vector with jth element $Y_{ij} = \mu(t) + R_i(t_{ij}) + Z_{ij}$, and write $\boldsymbol{t}_i = (t_{i1}, \ldots, t_{in_i})$. Then, as our predictor for $\boldsymbol{R}_i$ we use the conditional expectation

$$\hat{\boldsymbol{R}}_i = \mathrm{E}(\boldsymbol{R}_i \,|\, \boldsymbol{Y}_i).$$

Under our assumed model, $\boldsymbol{R}_i$ and $\boldsymbol{Y}_i$ have a joint multivariate Gaussian distribution. Furthermore, for any two vectors, $\boldsymbol{u}$ and $\boldsymbol{t}$ say, we can define a matrix, $G(\boldsymbol{u}, \boldsymbol{t})$, whose (r, j)th element is the covariance between $R_i(u_r)$ and $R_i(t_j)$, namely $\nu^2 + \sigma^2\rho(\,|\,u_r - t_j\,|\,)$. Then, the covariance matrix of $\boldsymbol{Y}_i$ is $\tau^2 I + G(\boldsymbol{t}_i, \boldsymbol{t}_i)$ and the complete specification of the joint distribution of $\boldsymbol{R}_i$ and $\boldsymbol{Y}_i$ is

$$\begin{bmatrix}\boldsymbol{R}_i \\ \boldsymbol{Y}_i\end{bmatrix} \sim MVN\left\{\begin{bmatrix}0 \\ \boldsymbol{\mu}_i\end{bmatrix}\begin{bmatrix}G(\boldsymbol{u}, \boldsymbol{u}) & G(\boldsymbol{u}, \boldsymbol{t}_i) \\ G(\boldsymbol{t}_i, \boldsymbol{u}) & \tau^2 I + G(\boldsymbol{t}_i, \boldsymbol{t}_i)\end{bmatrix}\right\},$$

where $\boldsymbol{\mu}_i$ has jth element $\mu(t_{ij})$.

Using standard properties of the multivariate Gaussian distribution it now follows that

$$\hat{\boldsymbol{R}}_i = G(\boldsymbol{u}, \boldsymbol{t}_i)\{\tau^2 I + G(\boldsymbol{t}_i, \boldsymbol{t}_i)\}^{-1}(\boldsymbol{Y}_i - \boldsymbol{\mu}_i), \tag{5.5.1}$$

with variance matrix $\mathrm{Var}(\hat{\boldsymbol{R}}_i)$ defined as

$$\mathrm{Var}(\boldsymbol{R}_i \,|\, \boldsymbol{Y}_i) = G(\boldsymbol{u}, \boldsymbol{u}) - G(\boldsymbol{u}, \boldsymbol{t}_i)\{\tau^2 I + G(\boldsymbol{t}_i, \boldsymbol{t}_i)\}^{-1} G(\boldsymbol{t}_i, \boldsymbol{u}). \tag{5.5.2}$$

Note that when $\tau^2 = 0$ and $\boldsymbol{u} = \boldsymbol{t}_i$, the predictor, $\hat{\boldsymbol{R}}_i$, reduces to $\boldsymbol{Y}_i - \boldsymbol{\mu}_i$ with zero variance, as it should – when there is no measurement error the data are a perfect prediction of the true CD4+ numbers at the observation times. More interestingly, when $\tau^2 > 0$, $\hat{\boldsymbol{R}}_i$ reflects a compromise between $\boldsymbol{Y}_i - \boldsymbol{\mu}_i$ and zero, tending towards the latter as τ^2 increases. Again, this makes intuitive sense – if measurement error variance is large, an individual's observed CD4+ counts are unreliable and the prediction for that individual should be moved away from the individual's data and towards the population mean trajectory.

In practice, formulae (5.5.1) and (5.5.2) would be evaluated replacing $\boldsymbol{\mu}$ by the fitted linear model with $\hat{\boldsymbol{\mu}} = X\hat{\boldsymbol{\beta}}$. They therefore assume that $\mu(t), \boldsymbol{\beta}$ and the covariance matrix, V, are known exactly. They should hold approximately in large samples when $\mu(t), \boldsymbol{\beta}$, and V are estimated. It is possible to adjust the prediction standard errors to reflect the uncertainty in $\hat{\boldsymbol{\beta}}$ but the corresponding adjustment for the uncertainty in the estimated covariance structure is analytically intractable.

Example 5.4. Prediction of individual CD4+ trajectories

We now apply these ideas to the CD4+ data using the same estimates of $\mu(t)$ and V as in Example 5.3. Figure 5.13 shows the estimated mean time-trend as a thick solid curve together with the data for two men and their predicted trajectories. The predictions were calculated from (5.5.1) in conjunction with the estimated population mean trajectory $\hat{\mu}(t)$ and covariance matrix $\hat{V}$. These predicted curves are referred to as *empirical Bayes estimates.* Note that the predicted trajectories smooth out the big fluctuations in observed CD4+ numbers, reflecting the substantial measurement error variance, τ^2. In particular, for individual A the predicted trajectory stays above the 500 threshold for AZT therapy throughout, whereas the observed CD4+ count dipped below this threshold during the fourth year post-seroconversion. For individual B, the fluctuations in observed CD4+ numbers are much smaller and the prediction tracks the data closely. Note that in both cases the general level of the observed data is preserved in the predicted trajectories. This reflects the effect of the component of variance, ν^2, between individuals; the model recognizes that some men are

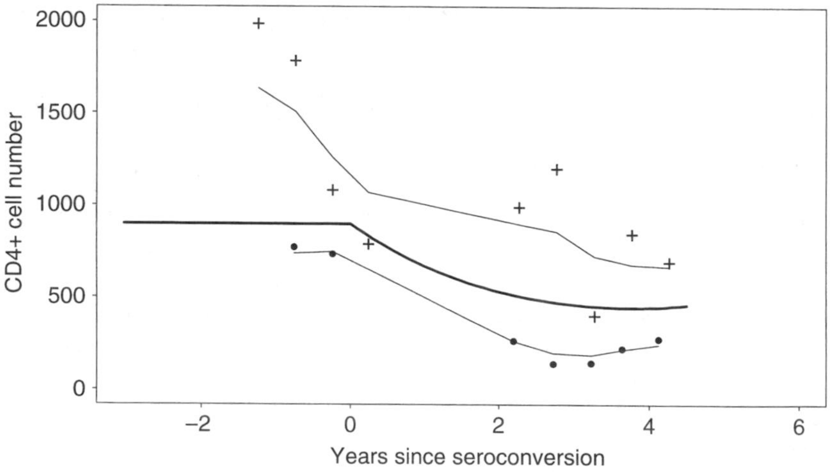

Fig. 5.13. CD4+ cell counts and empirical Bayes predictions for two subjects, with parametric estimate of population mean response profile.

intrinsically high responders and some low responders, and does not force the predictions towards the population mean level.

5.6 Further reading

The subject of parametric modelling for longitudinal data continues to generate an extensive literature. Within the scope of the linear model with correlated errors, most of the ideas are now well established, and the specific models proposed by different authors often amount to sensible variations on a familiar theme. Contributions not cited earlier include Pantula and Pollock (1985), Ware (1985), Jones and Ackerson (1990), Munoz *et al.* (1992) and Pourahmadi (1999). Jones (1993) describes a state–space approach to linear modelling of longitudinal data with serial correlation, drawing on the ideas of Kalman filtering (Kalman, 1960). Goldstein (1995) reviews the multi-level modelling approach. A comprehensive discussion of the linear mixed model can be found in Verbeke and Molenberghs (2000). Non-linear regression models with correlated error structure are considered in Chapter 14.

6

Analysis of variance methods

6.1 Preliminaries

In this chapter we describe how simple methods for the analysis of data from designed experiments, in particular the analysis of variance (ANOVA) can be adapted to longitudinal studies. ANOVA has limitations which prevent its recommendation as a general approach for longitudinal data. The first is that it fails to exploit the potential gains in efficiency from modelling the covariance among repeated observations. A second is that, to a greater or lesser extent, ANOVA is a simple method only with a complete, balanced array of data. This second limitation has been substantially diminished by the development of general methodolodgy for incomplete data problems (Little and Rubin, 1987), but the first is fundamental. Whether it is crucial in practice depends on the details of the particular application, for example the size and shape of the data array. As noted in Section 4.1, modelling the covariance structure is most valuable for data consisting of a small number of long sequences of measurements.

Throughout this chapter, we denote the data by a triply subscripted array,

$$y_{hij}, \quad h = 1, \ldots, g; \; i = 1, \ldots, m_h; \; j = 1 \ldots, n, \tag{6.1.1}$$

in which each y_{hij} denotes the jth observation from the ith unit within the hth treatment group. Furthermore, we assume a common set of times of observation, $t_j, j = 1, \ldots, n$, for all of the $m = \sum_{h=1}^{g} m_h$ sequences of observations. An emphasis on designed experiments is implicit in this choice of notation, although in principle we could augment the data-array by covariate vectors, $\boldsymbol{x}_{hij}$, attached to each y_{hij}, and so embrace many observational studies.

We write $\mu_{hj} = \mathrm{E}(Y_{hij})$ for the mean response at time t_j in treatment group h, and define the *mean response profile* in group h to be the vector $\boldsymbol{\mu}_h = (\mu_{h1}, \ldots, \mu_{hn})$. The primary objective of the analysis is to make inferences about the μ_{hj} with particular reference to differences amongst the g mean response profiles, $\boldsymbol{\mu}_h$.

6.2 Time-by-time ANOVA

A time-by-time ANOVA consists of n separate analyses, one for each subset of data corresponding to each time of observation, t_j. Each analysis is a conventional ANOVA, based on the appropriate underlying experimental design and incorporating relevant covariate information. Details can be found in any standard text, for example Snedecor and Cochran (1989), Winer (1977), and Mead and Curnow (1983).

The simplest illustration is the case of a one-way ANOVA for a completely randomized design. For the ANOVA table, we use the dot notation to indicate averaging over the relevant subscripts, so that

$$y_{h \cdot j} = m_h^{-1} \sum_{i=1}^{m_h} y_{hij}$$

and

$$\begin{aligned} y_{\cdot \cdot j} &= m^{-1} \sum_{h=1}^{g} \sum_{i=1}^{m_h} y_{hij} \\ &= m^{-1} \sum_{h=1}^{g} m_h y_{h \cdot j}. \end{aligned}$$

Then, the ANOVA table for the jth time-point is

Source of variation	Sum of squares	df
Between treatments	$\text{BTSS} = \sum_{h=1}^{g} m_h (y_{h \cdot j} - y_{\cdot \cdot j})^2$	$g - 1$
Residual	$\text{RSS} = \text{TSS} - \text{BTSS}$	$m - g$
Total	$\text{TSS} = \sum_{h=1}^{g} \sum_{i=1}^{m_h} (y_{hij} - y_{\cdot \cdot j})^2$	$m - 1$

The F-statistic to test the hypothesis of no treatment effects is $F = \{\text{BTSS}/(g-1)\}/\{\text{RSS}/(m-g)\}$. Note that j is fixed throughout the analysis and should *not* be treated as a second indexing variable in a two-way ANOVA.

Whilst a time-by-time ANOVA has the virtue of simplicity, it suffers from two major weaknesses. Firstly, it cannot address questions concerning treatment effects which relate to the longitudinal development of the mean response profiles; for example, growth rates between successive t_j. This can be overcome in part by using observations, y_{hik}, at earlier times as covariates for the response y_{hij}. Kenward's (1987) ante-dependence models, which we discussed in Section 5.2.1, are a logical development of this idea.

Secondly, the inferences made within each of the n separate analyses are not independent, nor is it clear how they should be combined. For example, a succession of marginally significant group-mean differences may be collectively compelling with weakly correlated data, but much less so if there are strong correlations between successive observations on each unit.

Example 6.1. Weights of calves in a trial on intestinal parasites

Kenward (1987) describes an experiment to compare two different treatments, A and B say, for controlling intestinal parasites of calves. The data consist of the weights of 60 calves, 30 in each group, at each of 11 times of measurement, as listed in Table 6.1.

Figure 6.1 shows the two observed mean response profiles. The observed mean response for treatment B is initially below that for treatment A, but the order is reversed between the seventh and eighth measurement times.

A time-by-time analysis of these data consists of a two-sample t-test at each of the 11 times of measurement. Table 6.2 summarizes the results of these t-tests. None of the 11 tests attains conventional levels of significance and the analysis would appear to suggest that the two mean response profiles are identical. An alternative analysis is a time-by-time analysis of successive weight-gains, $d_{hij} = y_{hij} - y_{hij-1}$. The results of this second analysis are also given in Table 6.2. The striking features of the second analysis are the highly significant negative difference between the mean responses on treatments A and B at time eight, and the positive difference at time 11. This simple analysis leads to essentially the same conclusions as the more sophisticated ante-dependence analysis reported in Kenward (1987).

The overall message of Example 6.1 is that a simple analysis of longitudinal data can be highly effective *if* it focuses on exactly the right feature of the data, which in this case was the weight-gain between successive two-week periods rather than the weight itself. This leads us to a discussion of *derived variables* for longitudinal data analysis.

6.3 Derived variables

Given a vector of observations, $\boldsymbol{y}_{hi} = (y_{hi1}, \dots, y_{hin})$, on a particular unit, a *derived variable* is a scalar-valued function, $u_{hi} = u(\boldsymbol{y}_{hi})$. The motivation for analysing a derived variable is two-fold. From a pragmatic point of view it reduces a multivariate problem to a univariate one; in particular applications, a single derived variable may convey the essence of the substantive issues raised by the data. For example, in growth studies the detailed growth process for each unit may be complex, yet for some purposes the interest may focus on something as simple as the average growth rate during the course of the experiment. By reducing each $\boldsymbol{y}_{hi}$ to a scalar quantity, u_{hi}, we avoid the issue of correlation within each sequence, and can again use standard ANOVA or regression methods for the data analysis. When there are two or more derived variables of interest, the problem of combined inference which we encountered with the time-by-time ANOVA

Table 6.1. Weights (kg) of calves in a trial on the control of intestinal parasites. The original experiment involved 60 calves, 30 in each of two groups. Data below are for the first group only.

Time in weeks										
0	2	4	6	8	10	12	14	16	18	19
233	224	245	258	271	287	287	287	290	293	297
231	238	260	273	290	300	311	313	317	321	326
232	237	245	265	285	298	304	319	317	334	329
239	246	268	288	308	309	327	324	327	336	341
215	216	239	264	282	299	307	321	328	332	337
236	226	242	255	263	277	290	299	300	308	310
219	229	246	265	279	292	299	299	298	300	290
231	245	270	292	302	321	322	334	323	337	337
230	228	243	255	272	276	277	289	289	300	303
232	240	247	263	275	286	294	302	308	319	326
234	237	259	289	311	324	342	347	355	368	368
237	235	258	263	282	304	318	327	336	349	353
229	234	254	276	294	315	323	341	346	352	357
220	227	248	273	290	308	322	326	330	342	343
232	241	255	276	293	309	310	330	326	329	330
210	225	242	260	272	277	273	295	292	305	306
229	241	252	265	274	285	303	308	315	328	328
204	198	217	233	251	258	272	283	279	295	298
220	221	236	260	274	295	300	301	310	318	316
233	234	250	268	280	298	308	319	318	336	333
234	234	254	274	294	306	318	334	343	349	350
200	207	217	238	252	267	284	282	282	284	288
220	213	229	252	254	273	293	289	294	292	298
225	239	254	269	289	308	313	324	327	347	344
236	245	257	271	294	307	317	327	328	328	325
231	231	237	261	274	285	291	301	307	315	320
208	211	238	254	267	287	306	312	320	337	338
232	248	261	285	292	307	312	323	318	328	329
233	241	252	273	301	316	332	336	339	348	345
221	219	231	251	270	272	287	294	292	292	299

again needs to be addressed. However, it is arguable that the practical importance of the combined inference question is reduced if the separate derived variables address substantially different questions and each one has a natural interpretation in its own right.

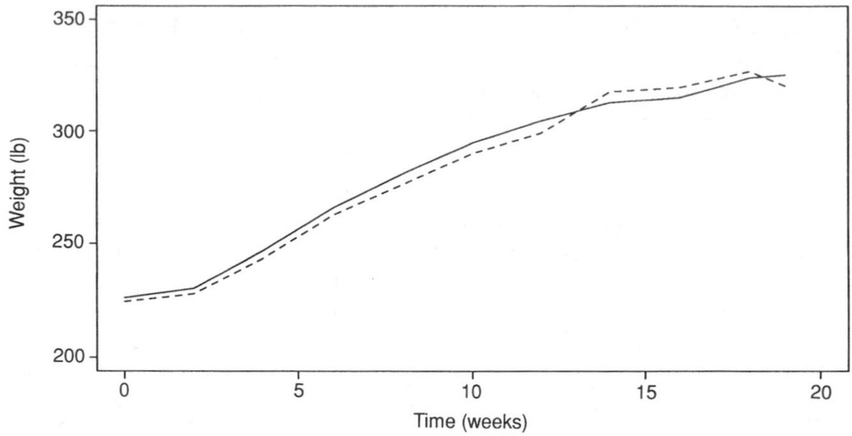

Fig. 6.1. Observed mean response profiles for data on weights of calves. ——: treatment A; – – –: treatment B.

Table 6.2. Time-by-time analysis of weights of calves. The analysis at each time is a two-sample t-test, using either the weights, y_{hij}, or the weight-gains, d_{hij}, as the response. The 5%, 1%, and 0.1% critical values of t_{58} are 2.00, 2.16 and 3.47.

	Test statistic at time										
	1	2	3	4	5	6	7	8	9	10	11
y	0.60	0.82	1.03	0.88	1.21	1.12	1.28	−1.10	−0.95	−0.53	0.85
d		0.51	0.72	−0.15	1.21	0.80	0.55	−6.85	0.21	0.72	4.13

The derived variable approach goes back at least to Wishart (1938), and was systematized by Rowell and Walters (1976). Rowell and Walters set out the details of an analysis for data recorded at equally spaced time-points, t_j, in which the n-dimensional response, $\boldsymbol{y}_{hi}$, is transformed to a set of orthogonal polynomial coefficients of degree, $0, 1, \ldots, n-1$. The first two of these are immediately interpretable in terms of average response and average rate of change, respectively, during the course of the experiment. It is less clear what tangible interpretation can be placed on higher degree coefficients. Also, from an inferential point of view, it is important to recognize that the 'orthogonal' sums of squares associated with the polynomial decomposition are *not* orthogonal in the statistical sense, that is, *not* independent, because the observations within $\boldsymbol{y}_{hi}$ are in general correlated.

A more imaginative use of derived variables is to fit scientifically interpretable *non-linear* models to each time-sequence, $\boldsymbol{y}_{hi}$, and to use the parameter estimates from these fits as a natural set of derived variables. For example, we might decide that the individual time-sequences can be well described by a logistic growth model of the form

$$\mu_{hi}(t) = \alpha_{hi}[1 + \exp\{-\beta_{hi}(t - \delta_{hi})\}]^{-1},$$

in which case estimates of the asymptotes α_{hi}, slope parameters β_{hi} and points of inflection δ_{hi} form a natural set of derived variables. Note that non-linear least squares could be used to estimate the α_{hi}, β_{hi}, and δ_{hi}, and that no assumptions about the correlation structure are needed to validate the subsequent derived variable analysis. However, whilst validity is one thing, efficiency is quite another. The small-sample behaviour of ordinary least squares (OLS) estimation in non-linear regression modelling is often poor, and this can only be exacerbated by correlations amongst the y_{hij}. Furthermore, the natural parametrization from a scientific point of view may not correspond to a good parametrization from a statistical point of view. In the simpler context of uncorrelated data, these issues are addressed in Bates and Watts (1988) and in Ratkowsky (1983).

Strictly, the derived variable approach breaks down when the array, y_{hij}, is incomplete because of missing values, or when the m times of observation are not common to all units. This is because the derived variable no longer satisfies the standard ANOVA assumption of a common variance for all observations. Also, we cannot simply weight the values of the derived variables according to the numbers of observations contained in the corresponding vectors, $\boldsymbol{y}_{hi}$, because of the unknown effects of the correlation structure in the original data. In practice, derived variables appear to be used somewhat optimistically with moderately incomplete data. The consequences of this are unclear, although the randomization justification for the ANOVA is available if we are prepared to assume that the mechanisms leading to the incompleteness of the data are independent of both the experimental treatments applied and the measurement process itself. As we shall see in Chapter 11, this is often not so.

Example 6.2. Growth of Sitka spruce with and without ozone

To illustrate the use of derived variables we consider the 1989 growth data on Sitka spruce. Recall that these consist of 79 trees grown in four controlled environment chambers in which the first two chambers are treated with introduced ozone at 70 ppb. The respective numbers of trees in the four chambers are 27, 27, 12 and 13. The objective of the experiment was to investigate the effect of ozone on tree growth, and the response from each tree was a sequence of eight measurements of $y = \log(d^2h)$ on days 103, 130, 162, 190, 213, 247, 273, and 308 where day one is first January 1989, and d and h refer to stem diameter and height, respectively.

In Section 4.6 we saw that the dominant source of variation in these data was a random shift in the response profile for each tree. This suggests that the observed mean response would be a suitable derived variable. The appropriate analysis is then a one-way ANOVA estimating a separate mean response parameter, μ_h, in each of the four chambers, followed by estimation of the treatment versus control contrast,

$$c = (\mu_1 + \mu_2) - (\mu_3 + \mu_4).$$

The ANOVA table is as follows:

Source of variation	Sum of squares	df	Mean square
Between chambers	2.2448	3	0.7483
Residual	31.0320	75	0.4136
Total	33.2768	78	0.4266

Note that the F-statistic to test for chamber effects is not significant ($F_{3,75} = 1.81$, p-value $\simeq 0.15$). However, the estimate of the treatment versus control contrast is

$$\hat{c} = (5.89 + 5.87) - (6.17 + 6.29) = -0.70,$$

with estimated standard error

$$\mathrm{se}(\hat{c}) = \left\{\sqrt{0.4136}\left(\frac{1}{27} + \frac{1}{27} + \frac{1}{12} + \frac{1}{13}\right)\right\} = 0.31,$$

corresponding to a t-statistic of 2.26 on 75 df, which is significant (p-value $\simeq$ 0.03). The conclusion from this analysis is that introduced ozone suppresses growth of Sitka spruce, although the evidence is not overwhelming.

Example 6.3. Effect of pH on drying rate of holly leaves

This example concerns an experiment to investigate the effect of different pH treatments on the drying rate of holly leaves. The treatment was administered by intermittent spraying during the plant's life. Ten plants were allocated to each of four pH levels, 2.5, 3.5, 4.5, and 5.6, the last being a control. Leaves from the plant were then allowed to dry, and were weighed at each of 13 times, irregularly spaced over a three-day period. The recorded variable was the ratio of current to initial fresh weight. Thus, if $w(t)$ denotes the weight at time t, the recorded sequence of values from each plant is

$$x_j = w(t_j)/w(0), \quad j = 1, \ldots, 13.$$

Note that $t_1 = 0$, and $x_1 = 1$ for every plant.

A plausible model for the drying process is one of exponential decay towards a lower bound which represents the dry weight of the plant material. If this lower bound is a small fraction of the initial weight, a convenient approximation is to assume exponential decay towards zero. This gives $w(t) = w(0)\exp(-\beta t)$ or, dividing by $w(0), x_j = \exp(-\beta t_j)$. Taking $y_j = \log(x_j)$, this in turn gives a linear regression through the origin,

$$y_j = -\beta t_j + \epsilon_j.$$

Figure 6.2 shows the 40 sequences of measurements, y_j, plotted against t_j. The linear model gives a good approximation, but with substantial variation in the slope, $-\beta$, for the different plants. This suggests using a least-squares estimate of β from each of the 40 plants as a derived variable. Note that β has a direct interpretation as a *drying rate*. Table 6.3 shows the resulting values, $b_{hi}, h = 1, \ldots, 4; i = 1, \ldots, 10$, the subscripts h and i referring to pH level and replicate within pH level, respectively.

To analyse this derived variable, we would assume that the b_{hi} are realizations of Gaussian random variables, with constant variance and means dependent on pH level. However, the pattern of the standard errors in Table 6.3 casts doubt on the constant variance assumption. For this reason, we transform the b_{hi} to $z_{hi} = \log(b_{hi})$ and assume that $z_{hi} \sim N(\mu_h, \sigma^2)$, where μ_h denotes the mean value of the derived variable within pH

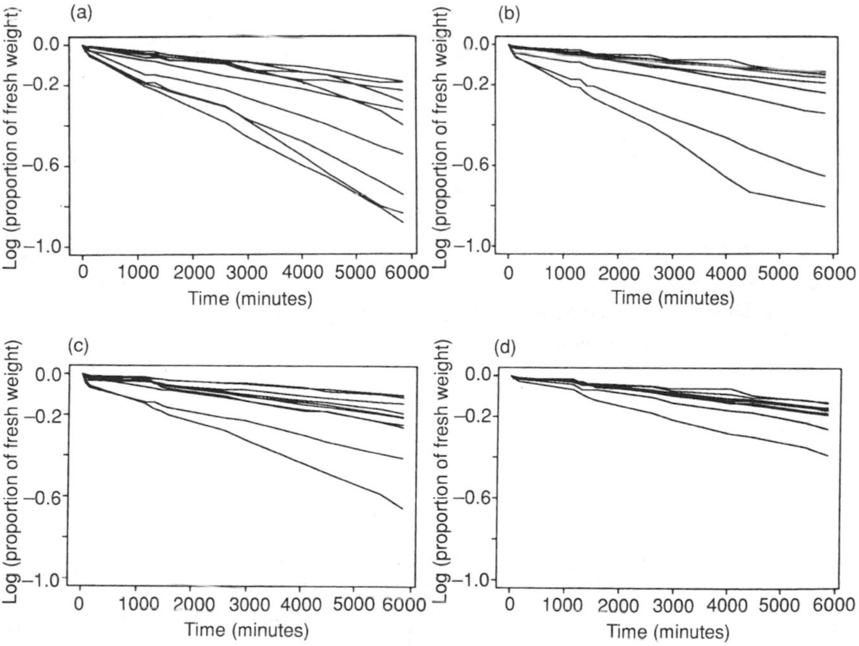

Fig. 6.2. Data on drying rates of holly leaves: (a) pH = 2.5; (b) pH = 3.5; (c) pH = 4.5; (d) pH = 5.6 (control).

Table 6.3. Derived data (b_{hi}) for analysis of the drying rates of holly leaves.

	pH			
Replication	2.5	3.5	4.5	5.6
1	0.33	0.27	0.76	0.23
2	0.30	0.35	0.43	0.68
3	0.91	0.26	0.18	0.28
4	1.41	0.10	0.21	0.32
5	0.41	0.24	0.17	0.21
6	0.41	1.51	0.32	0.43
7	1.26	1.17	0.35	0.31
8	0.57	0.26	0.43	0.26
9	1.51	0.29	1.11	0.28
10	0.55	0.41	0.36	0.28
Mean	0.77	0.54	0.44	0.33
SE	(0.15)	(0.14)	(0.09)	(0.04)

level h. The means and standard errors of the log-transformed drying rate, corresponding to the last two rows of Table 6.3, are

Mean	−0.44	−1.03	−1.01	−1.17
SE	0.19	0.25	0.19	0.11

In contrast to the direct relationship observed in Table 6.3 between mean and variance for the estimated drying rates, b_{hi}, a constant variance model does seem reasonable for the log-transformed rates, z_{hi}.

We now consider three possible models for μ_h, the mean log-drying-rate within pH level, h. These are

(1) $\mu_h = \mu$ (no pH effect);

(2) μ_h arbitrary;

(3) $\mu_h = \theta_0 + \theta_1 u_h$ where u_h denotes pH level in treatment group h.

A comparison between models one and two involves a one-way ANOVA of the data in Table 6.3. The F-statistic is 3.14 on three and 35 degrees of freedom, corresponding to a p-value of 0.037 which is indicative of differences in mean response between pH levels. Model three is motivated by the observation that the log-transformed rates of drying seem to depend on pH in a roughly linear fashion. The F-statistic to test the hypothesis

$\theta_1 = 0$ within model three, using the residual mean square from the saturated model two, is 9.41 on 1 and 36 degrees of freedom. This corresponds to a p-value of 0.004, representing strong evidence against $\theta_1 = 0$. The F-statistic to test lack of fit of model three within model two is 0.31 on two and 36 degrees of freedom, which is clearly not significant (p-value $=$ 0.732).

The conclusion from this analysis is that log-drying-rate decreases, approximately linearly, with increasing pH.

6.4 Repeated measures

A *repeated measures* ANOVA can be regarded as a first attempt to provide a single analysis of a complete longitudinal data set. The rationale for the analysis is to regard time as a factor on n levels in a hierarchial design with units as sub-plots. In agricultural research, this type of experiment is usually called a *split-plot* experiment. However, the usual randomization justification for the split-plot analysis is not available because there is no sense in which the allocation of times to the n observations within each unit can be randomized. We therefore have to assume an underlying model for the data, namely,

$$y_{hij} = \beta_h + \gamma_{hj} + U_{hi} + Z_{hij}, \quad j = 1, \ldots, n; \; i = 1, \ldots, m_h; \; h = 1, \ldots, g \tag{6.4.1}$$

in which the β_h represent main effects for treatments and the γ_{hj} interactions between treatments and times with the constraint that $\sum_{j=1}^{n} \gamma_{hj} = 0$, for all h. Also, the U_{hi} are mutually independent random effects for units and the Z_{hij} mutually independent random measurement errors.

In the model (6.4.1), $\mathrm{E}(Y_{hij}) = \beta_h + \gamma_{hj}$. If we assume that $U_{hi} \sim N(0, \nu^2)$ and $Z_{hij} \sim N(0, \sigma^2)$, then the resulting distribution of $\boldsymbol{Y}_{hi} = (Y_{hi1}, \ldots, Y_{hin})$ is multivariate Gaussian with covariance matrix

$$\boldsymbol{V} = \sigma^2 I + \nu^2 J,$$

where I is the identity matrix and J a matrix all of whose elements are 1. This implies a constant correlation, $\rho = \nu^2/(\nu^2 + \sigma^2)$, between any two observations on the same unit.

The split-plot ANOVA for the model (6.4.1) is given by the following table: In this ANOVA table, we again use the dot notation for averaging, so that $y_{hi\cdot} = n^{-1} \sum_{j=1}^{n} y_{hij}$, $y_{h\cdot\cdot} = (m_h n)^{-1} \sum_{i=1}^{m_h} \sum_{j=1}^{n} y_{hij}$, and so on. Also, $m = \sum_{h=1}^{g} m_h$ denotes the total number of units. The first F-statistic associated with the table is

$$F_1 = \{\mathrm{BTSS}_1/(g-1)\}/\{\mathrm{RSS}_1/(m-g)\},$$

Source of variation	Sum of squares	df
Between treatments	$\text{BTSS}_1 = m\sum_{h=1}^{g} m_h(y_{h\cdot\cdot} - y_{\cdots})^2$	$g-1$
Whole plot residual	$\text{RSS}_1 = \text{TSS}_1 - \text{BTSS}_1$	$m-g$
Whole plot total	$\text{TSS}_1 = m\sum_{h=1}^{g}\sum_{i=1}^{m_h}(y_{hi\cdot} - y_{\cdots})^2$	
Between times	$\text{BTSS}_2 = n\sum_{j=1}^{n}(y_{\cdot\cdot j} - y_{\cdots})^2$	$n-1$
Treatment by time interaction	$\text{ISS}_2 = \sum_{j=1}^{n}\sum_{h=1}^{g} n_h(y_{h\cdot j} - y_{\cdot\cdot})^2 - \text{BTSS}_1 - \text{BTSS}_2$	$(g-1)\times(n-1)$
Split-plot residual	$\text{RSS}_2 = \text{TSS}_2 - \text{ISS}_2 - \text{BTSS}_2 - \text{TSS}_1$	$(m-g)\times(n-1)$
Split-plot total	$\text{TSS}_2 = \sum_{h=1}^{g}\sum_{i=1}^{m_h}\sum_{j=1}^{n}(y_{hij} - y_{\cdots})^2$	$nm-1$

which tests the hypothesis that $\beta_h = \beta, h = 1, \ldots, g$. The second is

$$F_2 = \{\text{ISS}_2/[(g-1)(n-1)]\}/\{\text{RSS}_2/[(m-g)(n-1)]\},$$

which tests the hypothesis that $\gamma_{hj} = \gamma_j$, $h = 1, \ldots, g$ for each of $j = 1, \ldots, n$, that is, that all g group mean response profiles are parallel.

The split-plot ANOVA strictly requires a complete data array. As noted in Section 6.1, recent developments in methodology for incomplete data relax this requirement. Alternatively, and in our view preferably, we can analyse incomplete data under the split-plot *model* (6.4.1) by the general likelihood-based approach given in Chapters four and five with the assumption of a constant correlation between any two measurements on the same unit and, incidentally, a general linear model for the mean response profiles.

Example 6.4. Growth of Sitka spruce with and without ozone (continued) The following table presents a split-plot ANOVA for the 1989 sitka spruce data. We ignore possible chamber effects to ease comparison with the results from the robust analysis given in Section 4.6.

Source of variation	Sum of squares	df	Mean square
Between treatments	17.106	1	17.106
Whole plot residuals	249.108	77	3.235
Whole plot total	266.214	78	3.413
Between times	41.521	7	5.932
Treatment by time interaction	0.045	7	0.0064
Split-plot residual	5.091	539	0.0094
Split-plot total	312.871	631	

The F-statistic for differences between control and treated mean response is $F_1 = 5.29$ on one and 77 degrees of freedom, corresponding to a p-value of approximately 0.02. The F-statistic for departure from parallelism is $F_2 = 0.68$ on seven and 539 degrees of freedom, corresponding to a p-value of approximately 0.69. The analysis therefore gives moderate evidence of a difference in mean response between control and treated trees, and no evidence of departure from parallelism.

6.5 Conclusions

The principal virtue of the ANOVA approach to longitudinal data analysis is its technical simplicity. The computational operations involved are elementary and there is an apparently reassuring familiarity in the solution of a complex class of problems by standard methods. However, we believe that this virtue is outweighed by the inherent limitations of the approach as noted in Section 6.1.

Provided that the data are complete, the method of derived variables can give a simple and easily interpretable analysis with a strong focus on particular aspects of the mean response profiles. Furthermore, it provides a feasible method of analysing inherently non-linear models for the mean response profiles, notwithstanding the statistical difficulties which arise with non-linear least-squares estimation in small samples. The method runs into trouble if the data are seriously incomplete, or if no single derived variable can address the relevant scientific questions. In the former case, the inference is strictly invalidated whilst in the latter there are difficulties in making a correct combined inference for the complete analysis. The method is not applicable if a key subject-specific covariate varies over time.

Time-by-time ANOVA can be viewed as a special case of a derived variable analysis in which the problem of combined inference is seen in an acute form. Additionally, the implicitly cross-sectional view of the data fails to address the question of evolution over time which is usually of fundamental importance in longitudinal studies.

The split-plot ANOVA embodies strong assumptions about the covariance structure of the data. If these are reasonable, a model-based analysis under the assumed uniform correlation structure achieves the same ends, while coping naturally with missing values and allowing a structured linear model for the mean response profiles.

In summary, whilst ANOVA methods are undoubtedly useful in particular circumstances, they do not constitute a generally viable approach to longitudinal data analysis.

7

Generalized linear models for longitudinal data

This chapter surveys approaches to the analysis of discrete and continuous longitudinal data using extensions of generalized linear models (GLMs). We have shown in Chapter 4 how regression inferences using *linear* models can be made robust to assumptions about the correlation, especially when the number of observations per person, n_i, is small relative to the number of individuals, m. With linear models, although the *estimation* of the regression parameters must take into account the correlations in the data, their *interpretation* is essentially independent of the correlation structure. With non-linear models for discrete data, such as logistic regression, different assumptions about the source of correlation can lead to regression coefficients with distinct interpretations. The data-analyst must therefore think even more carefully about the objectives of the analysis and the source of correlation in choosing an approach.

In this chapter we discuss three extensions of GLMs for longitudinal data: *marginal*, *random effects*, and *transition* models. The objective is to present the ideas underlying each model as well as their domains of application. We focus on the interpretation of regression coefficients. Chapters 8–10 present details about each method and examples of their use.

7.1 Marginal models

In a marginal model, the regression of the response on explanatory variables is modelled separately from within-person (within-unit) correlation. In the regression, we model the marginal expectation, $\mathrm{E}(Y_{ij})$, as a function of explanatory variables. By marginal expectation, we mean the average response over the sub-population that shares a common value of x. The marginal expectation is what we model in a cross-sectional study. Specifically, a marginal model has the following assumptions:

(1) the marginal expectation of the response, $\mathrm{E}(Y_{ij}) = \mu_{ij}$, depends on explanatory variables, $\boldsymbol{x_{ij}}$, by $h(\mu_{ij}) = \boldsymbol{x_{ij}}'\beta$ where h is a known *link* function such as the logit for binary responses or log for counts;

(2) the marginal variance depends on the marginal mean according to $\text{Var}(Y_{ij}) = v(\mu_{ij})\phi$ where v is a known variance function and ϕ is a scale parameter which may need to be estimated;

(3) the correlation between Y_{ij} and Y_{ik} is a function of the marginal means and perhaps of additional parameters $\boldsymbol{\alpha}$, that is $\text{Corr}(Y_{ij}, Y_{ik}) = \rho(\mu_{ij}, \mu_{ik}; \boldsymbol{\alpha})$ where $\rho(\cdot)$ is a known function.

Marginal regression coefficients, $\boldsymbol{\beta}$, have the same interpretation as coefficients from a cross-sectional analysis. Marginal models are natural analogues for correlated data of GLMs for independent data.

Nearly all of the linear models introduced in Chapters 4–6 can be formulated as marginal models since they have as part of their specification an equation of the form $\text{E}(Y_{ij}) = \boldsymbol{x}'_{ij}\boldsymbol{\beta}$ for some set of explanatory variables, $\boldsymbol{x}_{ij}$. For example, consider a linear regression whose errors follow the exponential correlation model introduced in Section 4.2.2. Responses, Y_{ij}, are taken at integer times, $t_j = 1, 2, \ldots, n$, on each of m subjects. The mean responses are $\text{E}(Y_{ij}) = \boldsymbol{x}'_{ij}\boldsymbol{\beta}$. The covariance structure is given by $\text{Cov}(Y_{ij}, Y_{ik}) = \sigma^2 \exp(-\phi \mid t_j - t_k \mid)$ and the variance is assumed to be independent of the mean.

To illustrate a logistic marginal model, consider the problem of assessing the dependence of respiratory infection on vitamin A status in the Indonesian Children's Health Study (ICHS). Let x_{ij} indicate whether or not child i is vitamin A deficient (1 yes; 0-no) at visit j. Let Y_{ij} denote whether the child has respiratory infection (1-yes; 0-no) and let $\mu_{ij} = \text{E}(Y_{ij})$. One marginal model is given by the following assumptions:

- $\text{logit}(\mu_{ij}) = \log \dfrac{\mu_{ij}}{1 - \mu_{ij}} = \log \dfrac{\Pr(Y_{ij} = 1)}{\Pr(Y_{ij} = 0)} = \beta_0 + \beta_1 x_{ij}$,
- $\text{Var}(Y_{ij}) = \mu_{ij}(1 - \mu_{ij})$,
- $\text{Corr}(Y_{ij}, Y_{ik}) = \alpha$.

Here, the transformed regression coefficient $\exp(\beta_0)$ is the ratio of the frequency of infected to uninfected children among the sub-population that is not vitamin A deficient. The parameter $\exp(\beta_1)$ is the odds of infection among vitamin A deficient children divided by the odds among children replete with vitamin A. When the prevalence of the response is low as in the Indonesian example, the odds ratio is approximately the ratio of frequencies of infection among the vitamin A deficient and replete sub-groups. Note that $\exp(\beta_1)$ is a ratio of population frequencies so we refer to it as a *population-averaged* parameter. If all individuals with the same x have the same probability of disease, the population frequency is the same as the individual's probability. However, when there is heterogeneity in the risk of disease among subjects with a common x, the population frequency is the average of the individual risks.

The variance of a binary response is a known function of its mean as given in the second assumption above. The correlation between two observations for a child is assumed to be α regardless of the times or expectations of the observations. For continuous data, this form of correlation derives from a random intercept in the linear model. It can only be a first order approximation for binary outcomes. To see why, note that the correlation between two binary responses, Y_1 and Y_2 with means μ_1 and μ_2, is given by

$$\mathrm{Corr}(Y_1, Y_2) = \frac{\Pr(Y_1 = 1, Y_2 = 1) - \mu_1\mu_2}{\{\mu_1(1-\mu_1)\mu_2(1-\mu_2)\}^{1/2}}. \tag{7.1.1}$$

The joint probability, $\Pr(Y_1 = 1, Y_2 = 1)$, is constrained to satisfy

$$\max(0,\ \mu_1 + \mu_2 - 1) < \Pr(Y_1 = 1, Y_2 = 1) < \min(\mu_1, \mu_2), \tag{7.1.2}$$

so that the correlation must satisfy a constraint which depends in a complicated way on the means μ_1 and μ_2 (Prentice, 1988). For this reason many authors, including Lipsitz (1989), Lipsitz *et al.* (1991) and Liang *et al.* (1992) have modelled the association among binary data using the odds ratio

$$\mathrm{OR}(Y_1, Y_2) = \frac{\Pr(Y_1 = 1, Y_2 = 1)\Pr(Y_1 = 0, Y_2 = 0)}{\Pr(Y_1 = 1, Y_2 = 0)\Pr(Y_1 = 0, Y_2 = 1)}, \tag{7.1.3}$$

which is not constrained by the means. For example, in the Indonesian study, we might assume that the odds ratios rather than correlations among all pairs of responses for a child are equal to an unknown constant, α. Specifying the means, variances and odds ratios fully determines the covariances among repeated outcomes for one child. Modelling odds ratios instead of correlations is further discussed in Chapter 8.

7.2 Random effects models

Section 5.2 introduced the linear random effects model where the response is assumed to be a linear function of explanatory variables with regression coefficients that vary from one individual to the next. This variability reflects natural heterogeneity due to unmeasured factors. An example is a simple linear regression for infant growth where the coefficients represent birth weight and growth rate. Children obviously are born at different weights and have different growth rates due to genetic and environmental factors which are difficult or impossible to quantify. A random effects model is a reasonable description if the set of coefficients from a population of children can be thought of as a sample from a distribution. Given the actual coefficients for a child, the linear random effects model further assumes that repeated observations for that person are independent. The correlation among repeated observations arises because we cannot observe the underlying growth curve, that is, the true regression coefficients, but have only imperfect measurements of weight on each infant.

This idea extends naturally to regression models for discrete and non-Gaussian continuous responses. It is assumed that the data for a subject are independent observations following a GLM, but that the regression coefficients can vary from person to person according to a distribution, F. To illustrate, once again consider a logistic model for the probability of respiratory infection in the ICHS. We might assume that the propensity for respiratory infection varies across children, reflecting their different genetic predispositions and unmeasured influences of environmental factors. The simplest model would assume that every child has its own propensity for respiratory disease but that the effect of vitamin A deficiency on this probability is the same for every child. This model takes the form

$$\text{logit}\,\Pr(Y_i = 1 \mid U_i) = (\beta_0^* + U_i) + \beta_1^* x_{ij}, \tag{7.2.1}$$

where x_{ij} is 1 if child i is vitamin A deficient at visit j, and 0 otherwise. Given U_i, we further assume that the repeated observations for the ith child are independent of one another. Finally, the model requires an assumption about the distribution of the U_i across children in the population. Typically, a parametric model such as the Gaussian with mean zero and unknown variance, ν^2, is used.

In this example β_0^* is the log odds of respiratory infection for a typical child with random effect $U_i = 0$. The parameter β_1^* is the log-odds ratio for respiratory infection when a child is deficient relative to when that same child is not. The variance ν^2 represents the degree of heterogeneity across children in the propensity for disease, not attributable to x.

The general specification of the random effects GLM is as follows:

1. Given $\boldsymbol{U_i}$, the responses $Y_{i1}, \ldots, Y_{in_i}$ are mutually independent and follow a GLM with density $f(y_{ij} \mid \boldsymbol{U_i}) = \exp[\{(y_{ij}\theta_{ij} - \psi(\theta_{ij}))\}/\phi + c(y_{ij}, \phi)]$. The conditional moments, $\mu_{ij} = \mathrm{E}(Y_{ij} \mid \boldsymbol{U_i}) = \psi'(\theta_{ij})$ and $v_{ij} = \mathrm{Var}(Y_{ij} \mid \boldsymbol{U_i}) = \psi''(\theta_{ij})\phi$, satisfy $h(\mu_{ij}) = \boldsymbol{x_{ij}}'\boldsymbol{\beta}^* + \boldsymbol{d_{ij}}'\boldsymbol{U_i}$ and $v_{ij} = v(\mu_{ij})\phi$ where h and v are known link and variance functions, respectively, and $\boldsymbol{d}_{ij}$ is a subset of $\boldsymbol{x}_{ij}$.
2. The random effects, $\boldsymbol{U_i}$, $i = 1, \ldots, m$, are mutually independent with a common underlying multivariate distribution, F.

To summarize, the basic idea underlying a random effects model is that there is natural heterogeneity across individuals in their regression coefficients and that this heterogeneity can be represented by a probability distribution. Correlation among observations for one person arises from their sharing unobservable variables, $\boldsymbol{U_i}$. A model of this type is sometimes referred to as a *latent variable* model (Bartholomew, 1987).

The random effects model is most useful when the objective is to make inference about individuals rather than the population average. In the MACS example, a random effects approach will allow us to estimate the CD4+ status of an individual man. In the ICHS, the random effects model would permit inference about the propensity for a particular child to have respiratory infection. The regression coefficients, $\boldsymbol{\beta}^*$, represent the effects of the explanatory variables on an individual child's chance of infection. This is in contrast to the marginal model coefficients which describe the effect of explanatory variables on the population average.

7.3 Transition (Markov) models

Under a transition model, correlation among $Y_{i1}, \ldots, Y_{in_i}$ exists because the past values, $Y_{i1}, \ldots, Y_{ij-1}$, explicitly influence the present observation, Y_{ij}. The past outcomes are treated as additional predictor variables.

The *marginal* model with an exponential autocorrelation function considered in Section 7.1 can be re-interpreted as a *transition* model by writing it as

$$Y_{ij} = \boldsymbol{x}'_{ij}\boldsymbol{\beta} + \epsilon_{ij},$$

where

$$\epsilon_{ij} = \alpha\epsilon_{ij-1} + Z_{ij},$$

$\alpha = \exp(-\phi)$, the Z_{ij} are mutually independent, $N(0, \tau^2)$ random variables and $\tau^2 = \sigma^2(1-\alpha^2)$. By substituting $\epsilon_{ij} = Y_{ij} - \boldsymbol{x}'_{ij}\boldsymbol{\beta}$ into the second of these equations and re-arranging, we obtain the conditional distribution of Y_{ij}, given the preceding response, Y_{ij-1}, as

$$Y_{ij} \mid Y_{ij-1} \sim N\{\boldsymbol{x}'_{ij}\boldsymbol{\beta} + \alpha(Y_{ij-1} - \boldsymbol{x}'_{ij-1}\boldsymbol{\beta}), \tau^2\}.$$

This form treats both the explanatory variables and the prior response as explicit predictors of the current outcome.

The generalized linear transition model can be easily specified. We model the conditional distribution of Y_{ij} given the past as an explicit function of the q preceding responses. For example, in the Indonesian study, we might assume that the probability of respiratory infection for child i at visit j has a direct dependence on whether or not the child had infection at visit $j-1$, as well as on explanatory variables, $\boldsymbol{x}_{ij}$. One explicit formulation is

$$\text{logit}\,\Pr(Y_{ij} = 1 \mid Y_{ij-1}, Y_{ij-2}, \ldots, Y_{i1}) = \boldsymbol{x}'_{ij}\boldsymbol{\beta}^{**} + \alpha Y_{ij-1}. \qquad (7.3.1)$$

Here, the chance of respiratory infection at time t_{ij} depends on explanatory variables but also on whether or not the child had infection three months earlier. The parameter $\exp(\alpha)$ is the ratio of the odds of infection among children who did and did not have infection at the prior visit. A coefficient in $\boldsymbol{\beta}^{**}$ can be interpreted as the change per unit change in x in the log odds of infection, among children who were free of infection at the previous visit.

This transition model for respiratory infection is a first order Markov chain (Feller, 1968, volume 1, p. 372). With a dichotomous response, Y_{ij}, observed at equally spaced intervals, the process is described by the 2×2 transition matrix whose elements are $\Pr(Y_{ij} = y_{ij} \mid Y_{ij-1} = y_{ij-1})$ where each of y_{ij-1} and y_{ij} may take values 0 or 1. The logistic regression equation above specifies the transition matrix as

$$
\begin{array}{ccc}
 & & y_{ij} \\
 & 0 & 1 \\
y_{ij-1} \quad 0 & \dfrac{1}{1+\exp(\boldsymbol{x}'_{ij}\boldsymbol{\beta}^{**})} & \dfrac{\exp(\boldsymbol{x}'_{ij}\boldsymbol{\beta}^{**})}{1+\exp(\boldsymbol{x}'_{ij}\boldsymbol{\beta}^{**})} \\
\quad\quad 1 & \dfrac{1}{1+\exp(\boldsymbol{x}'_{ij}\boldsymbol{\beta}^{**}+\alpha)} & \dfrac{\exp(\boldsymbol{x}'_{ij}\boldsymbol{\beta}^{**}+\alpha)}{1+\exp(\boldsymbol{x}'_{ij}\boldsymbol{\beta}^{**}+\alpha)}.
\end{array}
\quad (7.3.2)
$$

Note that because the transition probabilities depend on explanatory variables, the transition matrix can vary across individuals.

To specify the general transition model, let $\mathcal{H}_{ij} = \{y_{i1}, \ldots, y_{ij-1}\}$ represent the past responses for the ith subject. Also, let $\mu_{ij}^{\mathrm{C}} = \mathrm{E}(Y_{ij} \mid \mathcal{H}_{ij})$ and $v_{ij}^{\mathrm{C}} = \mathrm{Var}(Y_{ij} \mid H_{ij})$ be the conditional mean and variance of Y_{ij} given past responses and the explanatory variables. Analogous to the GLM for independent data, we assume:

- $h(\mu_{ij}^{\mathrm{C}}) = \boldsymbol{x}'_{ij}\boldsymbol{\beta}^{**} + \sum_{r=1}^{s} f_r(\mathcal{H}_{ij}; \boldsymbol{\alpha})$
- $v_{ij}^{\mathrm{C}} = v(\mu_{ij}^{\mathrm{C}})\phi$.

Here, we are modelling the transition from the prior state as represented by the functions f_r, to the present response. The past outcomes, after transformation by the known functions, f_r, are treated as additional explanatory variables. It may also be important to include interactions among prior responses when predicting the current value. If the model for the conditional mean is correctly specified, we can treat the repeated transitions for a person as independent events and use standard statistical methods. Korn and Whittemore (1979), Ware *et al.* (1988), Wong (1986), Zeger and Qaqish (1988), and Kaufmann (1987) discuss specific examples of transition models for binary and count data. Transition models are reviewed in more detail in Chapter 10.

7.4 Contrasting approaches

To contrast further the three modelling approaches, we consider the hypothetical linear model for infant growth and the logistic model for the respiratory disease data from the ICHS.

In the linear case, it is possible to formulate the three regression approaches to have coefficients with the same interpretation. That is, coefficients from random effects and transition linear models can have marginal interpretations as well. To illustrate, consider the simple linear regression model for infant growth

$$Y_{ij} = \beta_0 + \beta_1 t_{ij} + \epsilon_{ij},$$

where t_{ij} is the age, in months, of child i at visit j, Y_{ij} is the weight at age t_{ij} and ϵ_{ij} is a mean-zero deviation. Because children do not all grow at the same rate, the residuals, $\epsilon_{i1}, \ldots, \epsilon_{in_i}$, for child i will likely be correlated with one another. The marginal modelling approach is to assume

(1) $\mathrm{E}(Y_{ij}) = \beta_0 + \beta_1 t_{ij}$;

(2) $\mathrm{Corr}(\epsilon_{ij}, \epsilon_{ik}) = \rho(t_{ij}, t_{ik}; \boldsymbol{\alpha})$.

Assumption (1) is that the average weight for all infants in the population at any time t is $\beta_0+\beta_1 t$. The parameter β_1 is therefore the change per month in the population-average weight. Assumption (2) specifies the nature of the autocorrelation; a specific example might be that

$$\rho(t_{ij}, t_{ik}; \boldsymbol{\alpha}) = \begin{cases} \alpha_0, & |t_{ij} - t_{ik}| < 6 \text{ months}, \\ \alpha_1, & |t_{ij} - t_{ik}| \geq 6 \text{ months}. \end{cases}$$

That is, residuals within six months of each other have correlation α_0, while those further apart in time have correlation α_1. In the marginal approach, we separate the modelling of the regression and the correlation; either can be changed without necessarily changing the other.

A linear random effects model for infant growth can be written as

$$Y_{ij} = \beta_0^* + U_{i0} + (\beta_1^* + U_{i1})t_{ij} + Z_{ij}, \tag{7.4.1}$$

where Z_{ij}, $j = 1, \ldots, n_i$ are independent, mean-zero deviations with variance σ^2 and (U_{i0}, U_{i1}) are independent realizations from a mean-zero distribution with covariance matrix whose elements are $\mathrm{Var}(U_{i0}) = G_{11}$, $\mathrm{Var}(U_{i1}) = G_{22}$ and $\mathrm{Cov}(U_{i0}, U_{i1}) = G_{12}$. For mathematical convenience, we typically assume that all random variables follow Gaussian distributions. Figure 7.1(a) shows a sample of 10 linear growth curves whose intercepts and slopes are simulated from a bivariate Gaussian distribution with means $\beta_0^* = 8$ lbs, $\beta_1^* = 10$ lbs/year, variances $G_{11} = 2.0$ lbs^2, $G_{22} = 0.4$ (lbs/year)^2 and correlation $\rho = 0.2$. Of course, we do not observe these curves, but only imprecise values, y_{ij}. One realization of the data is shown in Fig. 7.1(b) where the residual standard deviation is $\sigma = 0.5$.

In the linear random effects model, the regression coefficients also have a marginal interpretation since $\mathrm{E}(Y_{ij}) = \beta_0^* + \beta_1^* t_{ij}$. This is because the

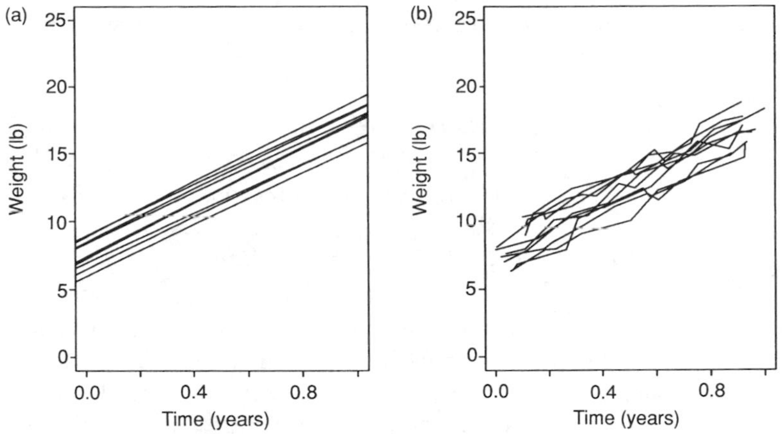

Fig. 7.1. Simulation of a random effects growth model: (a) underlying linear growth curves; (b) observed data.

average of the rates of growth for individuals is the same as the change in the population-average weight across time in a linear model.

The correlation for the linear growth model is given by

$$\operatorname{Corr}(Y_{ij}, Y_{ik}) = \frac{G_{11} + G_{22}t_{ij}t_{ik} + (t_{ij} + t_{ik})G_{12}}{\{(G_{11} + 2G_{12}t_{ij} + G_{22}t_{ij}^2 + \sigma^2)(G_{11} + 2G_{12}t_{ik} + G_{22}t_{ik}^2 + \sigma^2)\}^{1/2}}.$$

If there is no heterogeneity in the growth rates ($G_{22} = 0$), then $\operatorname{Corr}(Y_{ij}, Y_{ik}) = G_{11}/(G_{11}+\sigma^2)$. That is, the correlation is the same for any two observation times reflecting the fact that it derives from their sharing a common random intercept.

A transition model for infant growth might have the form

$$Y_{ij} = \beta_0^{**} + \beta_1^{**}t_{ij} + \epsilon_{ij}, \tag{7.4.2}$$

$$\epsilon_{ij} = \alpha\epsilon_{ij-1} + Z_{ij}, \tag{7.4.3}$$

where the Z_{ij} are independent mean-zero innovations with variance σ^2. This model can be re-expressed as

$$Y_{ij} = \beta_0^{**} + \beta_1^{**}t_{ij} + \alpha(Y_{ij-1} - \beta_0^{**} - \beta_1^{**}t_{ij-1}) + Z_{ij}. \tag{7.4.4}$$

Hence, $\mathrm{E}(Y_{ij} \mid y_{ij-1}, \ldots, y_{i1}) = \beta_0^{**} + \beta_1^{**}t_{ij} + \alpha(y_{ij-1} - \beta_0^{**} - \beta_1^{**}t_{ij-1})$. The expectation for the present response given the past depends explicitly on the previous observation. Note that (7.4.2) and (7.4.3) imply also that $\mathrm{E}(Y_{ij}) = \beta_0^{**} + \beta_1^{**}t_{ij}$ so that this form of a transition model has coefficients which also have a marginal interpretation.

Econometricians use autoregressive (transition) models for prediction. Some prefer the form

$$Y_{ij} = \boldsymbol{x}'_{ij}\boldsymbol{\beta}^{+} + \alpha Y_{ij-1} + Z_{ij}. \tag{7.4.5}$$

Here, the response is regressed on the covariates and on the previous outcome itself without adjusting for its expectation. The predictions from (7.4.4) and (7.4.5) are identical. However, the interpretation of $\boldsymbol{\beta}^{**}$ and $\boldsymbol{\beta}^{+}$ differ. Equation (7.4.5) implies that $\mathrm{E}(Y_{ij}) = \sum_{r=0}^{\infty} \alpha^r \boldsymbol{x}'_{ij-r}\boldsymbol{\beta}^{+}$ so that $\boldsymbol{\beta}^{+}$ does not have a marginal interpretation as the coefficient for $\boldsymbol{x}_{ij}$. The formula for the marginal mean will change as the model for the correlation changes, for example by adding additional lagged values of Y in the model. Hence, the interpretation of the regression coefficients $\boldsymbol{\beta}^{+}$ depends on the assumed form of the autocorrelation model. When the dependence of Y on x is the focus, we believe the formulation in (7.4.4) is preferable.

We have shown for the linear model that regression coefficients can have a marginal interpretation for each of the three approaches. With non-linear link functions, such as the logit, this is not the case. To expand on this point, we now consider the logistic regression model for the ICHS example of vitamin A and respiratory disease.

The random effects logistic model

$$\operatorname{logit} \Pr(Y_{ij} = 1 \mid U_i) = \beta_0^* + U_i + \beta_1^* x_{ij},$$

states that each child has its own baseline risk of infection, given by $\exp(\beta_0^* + U_i)/\{1 + \exp(\beta_0^* + U_i)\}$, and that a child's odds of infection are multiplied by $\exp(\beta_1^*)$ if they become vitamin A deficient. To illustrate this idea, Fig. 7.2 shows the risk of infection for 100 hypothetical children whose U_i's were chosen at random from a Gaussian distribution. Each child is represented by a vertical line connecting their risk with and without vitamin A deficiency plotted at the child's value for U_i. The Gaussian curve of the U_i is shown at the bottom. We used the parameter values $\beta_0 = -2.0$, $\beta_1 = 0.4$ and $\mathrm{Var}(U_i) = \nu^2 = 2.0$, so that a child with random effect $U_i = 0.0$ has a 17% chance of infection when deficient and a 12% chance when not. Since the random intercepts follow a Gaussian distribution, 95% of the children who are not deficient have risks in the range 0.8% to 68%. Note that the logistic model assumes that the odds ratio for vitamin A deficiency is the same for every child, equal to $\exp(0.4) = 1.5$. But the corresponding change in absolute risk differs depending on the baseline rate. Children with a lower propensity for infection ($U_i < 0$) at the left side of the figure have a smaller change in absolute risk than those with propensities near 0.5.

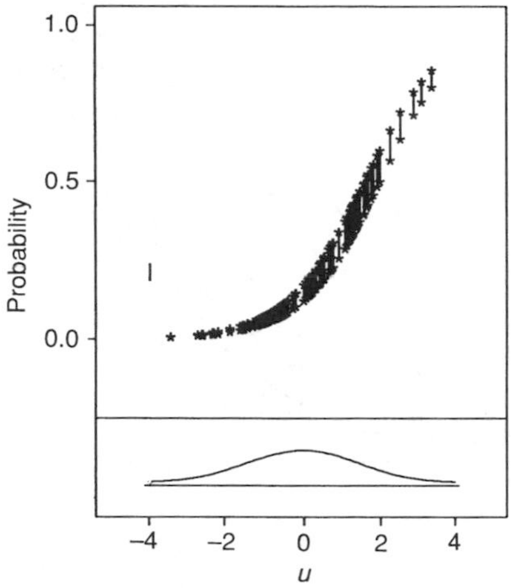

Fig. 7.2. Simulation of risk of infection with and without dichotomous risk factor, for 100 children in a logistic model with random intercept. Population-average risks with and without infection are indicated by the vertical line on the left. The Gaussian density for the random intercepts is shown.

The population rate of infection is the average risk, which is given by

$$\begin{aligned}\Pr(Y_{ij} = 1) &= \int \Pr(Y_{ij} = 1 \mid U_i) \mathrm{d}F(U_i) \\ &= \int \frac{\exp(\beta_0^* + U_i + \beta_1^* x_{ij})}{1 + \exp(\beta_0^* + U_i + \beta_1^* x_{ij})} f(U_i; \nu^2) \mathrm{d}U_i,\end{aligned}$$

where $f(\cdot)$ denotes the Gaussian density function with mean zero and variance ν^2. The marginal rates, $\Pr(Y_{ij} = 1)$, are 0.18 and 0.23 for the sub-groups that are vitamin A replete and deficient respectively under the parameter values above.

In the marginal model, we ignore the differences among children and model the population-average, $\Pr(Y_{ij} = 1)$, rather than $\Pr(Y_{ij} = 1 \mid U_i)$, by assuming that

$$\operatorname{logit} \Pr(Y_{ij} = 1) = \beta_0 + \beta_1 x_{ij}.$$

Here, the infection rate in the sub-group that has sufficient vitamin A is $\exp(\beta_0)/\{1 + \exp(\beta_0)\} = 0.18$ so that $\beta_0 = -1.23$. The odds ratio for vitamin A deficiency is $\exp(\beta_1) = \{0.23/(1.0-0.23)\}/\{0.18/(1.0-0.18)\} = 1.36$ so that $\beta_1 = 0.31$. We have now established an important point. The marginal and random effects model parameters differ in the logistic model. The former describes the ratio of population odds; the latter describes the ratio of an individual's odds. Note that the marginal parameter values are

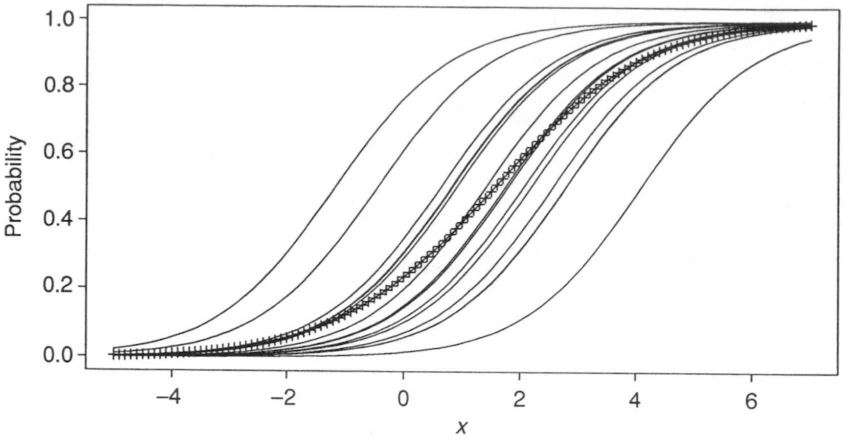

Fig. 7.3. Simulation of the probability of a positive response in a logistic model with random intercept and a continuous covariate. ——: sample curves; ++++++: average curve.

smaller in absolute value than their random effects analogues. The vertical line on the left side of Fig. 7.2 shows the change in the population rates with and without vitamin A for comparison with the person-specific rates which change size as a function of the random effect.

This attenuation of the parameter values in the marginal model also occurs if x is a continuous, rather than discrete, variable. Figure 7.3 displays $\Pr(Y_{ij} = 1 \mid U_i)$ as a function of x_{ij} in the simple model given by $\operatorname{logit} \Pr(Y_{ij} = 1 \mid U_i) = (\beta_0^* + U_i) + \beta_1^* x_{ij}$, for a number of randomly generated U_i from a mean-zero Gaussian distribution with $\nu^2 = 2.0$. Also shown is the average curve at each value of x. Notice how the steep rate of increase as a function of x in the individual curves is attenuated in the average curve. This phenomenon is well known in the related errors-in-variables regression problem; see for example Stefanski and Carroll (1985).

Neuhaus *et al.* (1991) show that if $\operatorname{Var}(U_i) > 0$, then the elements of the marginal ($\boldsymbol{\beta}$) and random effects ($\boldsymbol{\beta}^*$) regression vectors satisfy

(1) $|\beta_k| \leq |\beta_k^*|$, $k = 1, \ldots, p$;

(2) equality holds if and only if $\beta_k^* = 0$;

(3) the discrepancy between β_k and β_k^* increases with $\operatorname{Var}(U_i)$.

In particular, if U_i is assumed to follow a Gaussian distribution with mean zero and variance ν^2, Zeger *et al.* (1988) show that

$$\operatorname{logit} \mathrm{E}(Y_{ij}) \approx (c^2\nu^2 + 1)^{-1/2} x_{ij} \boldsymbol{\beta}^*, \tag{7.4.6}$$

where $c = 16\sqrt{3}/(15\pi)$ so that

$$\boldsymbol{\beta} \approx (c^2\nu^2 + 1)^{-1/2}\boldsymbol{\beta}^*, \tag{7.4.7}$$

where $c^2 \approx 0.346$. Note that (7.4.7) is consistent with the three properties listed above.

We have established the connection between random effects and marginal model parameters in logistic regression. The parameters in transition models such as (7.3.1) also differ from either the random effects or marginal parameters. The relationship between the marginal and transition parameters can be established, but only in limited cases. See Zeger and Liang (1992) for further discussion.

In log-linear models for counted data, random effects and marginal parameters can be equivalent in some important special cases. Consider the random effects model

$$\log \mathrm{E}(Y_{ij} \mid \boldsymbol{U}_i) = \boldsymbol{x}'_{ij}\boldsymbol{\beta}^* + \boldsymbol{d}'_{ij}\boldsymbol{U}_i, \tag{7.4.8}$$

where $\boldsymbol{d}_{ij}$ is a vector containing a subset of the variables in $\boldsymbol{x}_{ij}$. The marginal expectation has the form

$$\mathrm{E}(Y_{ij}) = \int \exp(\boldsymbol{x}'_{ij}\boldsymbol{\beta}^*)\exp(\boldsymbol{d}'_{ij}\boldsymbol{U}_i)f(\boldsymbol{U}_i)\mathrm{d}\boldsymbol{U}_i. \tag{7.4.9}$$

In the random intercept case with $d_{ij} = 1$, note that $\mathrm{E}(Y_{ij}) = \exp(\boldsymbol{x}'_{ij}\boldsymbol{\beta}^* + \nu^2/2)$, so that the marginal expectation has the same exponential form apart from an additive constant in the exponent. Hence, if we fit a marginal model which assumes that $\mathrm{E}(Y_{ij}) = \exp(\boldsymbol{x}'_{ij}\boldsymbol{\beta})$, all of the parameters except the intercept will have the same value and interpretation as in the random effects model.

7.5 Inferences

With random effects and transitional extensions of the GLM, it is possible to estimate unknown parameters using traditional maximum likelihood methods. Starting with random effects models, the likelihood of the data, expressed as a function of the unknown parameters, is given by

$$L(\boldsymbol{\beta}^*, \boldsymbol{\alpha}; \boldsymbol{y}) = \prod_{i=1}^{m} \int \prod_{j=1}^{n_i} f(y_{ij} \mid \boldsymbol{U}_i) f(\boldsymbol{U}_i; \boldsymbol{\alpha})\mathrm{d}\boldsymbol{U}_i, \tag{7.5.1}$$

where $\boldsymbol{\alpha}$ represents the parameters of the random effects distribution. The likelihood is the integral over the unobserved random effects of the joint distribution of the data and the random effects. With Gaussian data, the integral has a closed form and relatively simple methods exist for maximizing the likelihood or restricted likelihood, as discussed in

Chapter 5. With non-linear models, numerical integration techniques are often necessary to evaluate the likelihood. Techniques for finding maximum likelihood estimates are discussed further in Chapters 9 and 11.

Transition models can also be fitted using maximum likelihood. The joint distribution of the responses, $Y_{i1}, \ldots, Y_{in_i}$, can be written in the form

$$f(y_{i1}, \ldots, y_{in_i}) = f(y_{in_i} \mid y_{in_i-1}, \ldots, y_{i1}) f(y_{in_i-1} \mid y_{in_i-2}, \ldots, y_{i1}) \ldots$$
$$f(y_{i2} \mid y_{i1}) f(y_{i1}). \tag{7.5.2}$$

In a first-order Markov model,

$$f(y_{ij} \mid y_{ij-1}, \ldots, y_{i1}; \boldsymbol{\beta}^{**}, \boldsymbol{\alpha}) = f(y_{ij} \mid y_{ij-1}; \boldsymbol{\beta}^{**}, \boldsymbol{\alpha}),$$

so that the likelihood contribution from person i simplifies to

$$f(y_{i1}, \ldots, y_{in_i}; \boldsymbol{\beta}^{**}, \boldsymbol{\alpha}) = f(y_{i1}; \boldsymbol{\beta}^{**}, \boldsymbol{\alpha}) \prod_{j=2}^{n_i} f(y_{ij} \mid y_{ij-1}; \boldsymbol{\beta}^{**}, \boldsymbol{\alpha}). \tag{7.5.3}$$

Again, in the linear model this likelihood is easy to evaluate and maximize. For GLMs with non-linear link functions, one difficulty is that the marginal distribution of Y_{i1} often cannot be determined from the conditional distributions $f(y_{ij} \mid y_{ij-1})$ without additional assumptions. A simple alternative is to maximize the *conditional likelihood* of $Y_{i2}, \ldots, Y_{in_i}$ given Y_{i1}, which is obtained by omitting $f(y_{i1})$ from the equation above. Conditional maximum likelihood estimates can be found using standard GLM software, treating functions of the previous responses as explanatory variables. Inferences conditional on Y_{i1} are less efficient than maximum likelihoods, but are all that is available without additional assumptions about $f(Y_{i1})$. Inferences about transition models are discussed in more detail in Chapter 10.

In our marginal modelling approach, we specify only the first two moments of the responses for each person. With Gaussian data, the first two moments fully determine the likelihood, but this is not the case with other members of the GLM family. To specify the entire likelihood, additional assumptions about higher-order moments are also necessary. Examples for binary data are given by Prentice and Zhao (1991), Fitzmaurice *et al.* (1993) and Liang *et al.* (1992).

Even if additional assumptions are made, the likelihood is often intractable and involves many nuisance parameters in addition to $\boldsymbol{\alpha}$ and $\boldsymbol{\beta}$ that must be estimated. For this reason, a reasonable approach in many problems is to use *generalized estimating equations* or GEE, a multivariate analogue of quasi-likelihood which we now outline. The reader can find details in Liang and Zeger (1986), Zeger and Liang (1986) and Prentice (1988).

In the absence of a convenient likelihood function to work with, it is sensible to estimate $\boldsymbol{\beta}$ by solving a multivariate analogue of the quasi-score function (Wedderburn, 1974):

$$\boldsymbol{S}_{\boldsymbol{\beta}}(\boldsymbol{\beta},\boldsymbol{\alpha}) = \sum_{i=1}^{m} \left(\frac{\partial \boldsymbol{\mu_i}}{\partial \boldsymbol{\beta}}\right)' \mathrm{Var}(\boldsymbol{Y_i})^{-1}(\boldsymbol{Y_i} - \boldsymbol{\mu_i}) = \boldsymbol{0}. \tag{7.5.4}$$

In the multivariate case, there is the additional complication that $\boldsymbol{S}_{\boldsymbol{\beta}}$ depends on $\boldsymbol{\alpha}$ as well as on $\boldsymbol{\beta}$ since $\mathrm{Var}(\boldsymbol{Y_i}) = \mathrm{Var}(\boldsymbol{Y_i}; \boldsymbol{\beta}, \boldsymbol{\alpha})$. This can be overcome by replacing $\boldsymbol{\alpha}$ in the equation above by an $m^{1/2}$-consistent estimate, $\hat{\boldsymbol{\alpha}}(\hat{\boldsymbol{\beta}})$. Liang and Zeger (1986) and Gourieroux *et al.* (1984) show that the solution of the resulting equation is asymptotically as efficient as if $\boldsymbol{\alpha}$ were known.

The correlation parameters $\boldsymbol{\alpha}$ may be estimated by simultaneously solving $\boldsymbol{S}_{\boldsymbol{\beta}} = \boldsymbol{0}$ and

$$\boldsymbol{S}_{\boldsymbol{\alpha}}(\boldsymbol{\beta},\boldsymbol{\alpha}) = \sum_{i=1}^{m} \left(\frac{\partial \boldsymbol{\eta}_i}{\partial \boldsymbol{\alpha}}\right)' \boldsymbol{H}_i^{-1}(\boldsymbol{W}_i - \boldsymbol{\eta_i}) = \boldsymbol{0}, \tag{7.5.5}$$

where $\boldsymbol{W_i} = (R_{i1}R_{i2}, R_{i1}R_{i3}, \ldots, R_{in_i-1}R_{in_i}, R_{i1}^2, R_{i2}^2, \ldots, R_{in_i}^2)'$, the set of all products of pairs of residuals and squared residuals with $R_{ij} = \{Y_{ij} - \mu_{ij}\}/\{v(\mu_{ij})\}^{1/2}$, and $\boldsymbol{\eta_i} = \mathrm{E}(\boldsymbol{W_i}; \boldsymbol{\beta}, \boldsymbol{\alpha})$ (Prentice, 1988). The choice of the weight matrix, $\boldsymbol{H}_i$, depends on the type of responses. For binary response, the last n_i components of $\boldsymbol{W_i}$ can be ignored since the variance of a binary response is determined by its mean. In this case, we can use

$$\boldsymbol{H}_i = \begin{pmatrix} \mathrm{Var}(R_{i1}R_{i2}) & & & 0 \\ & \mathrm{Var}(R_{i1}R_{i3}) & & \\ & & \ddots & \\ 0 & & & \mathrm{Var}(R_{in_i-1}R_{in_i}) \end{pmatrix},$$

which ensures that $\boldsymbol{S}_{\boldsymbol{\alpha}}$ depends on $\boldsymbol{\beta}$ and $\boldsymbol{\alpha}$ only. For counted data, we suggest the use of the $n_i^* \times n_i^*$ identity matrix for $\boldsymbol{H}_i$ when solving $\boldsymbol{S}_{\boldsymbol{\alpha}} = \boldsymbol{0}$, where

$$n_i^* = \binom{n_i}{2} + n_i,$$

is the number of elements of $\boldsymbol{W_i}$.

The suggested $\boldsymbol{H}_i$ are not optimal (Godambe, 1960). However, our experience in applications has been that the choice of $\boldsymbol{H}_i$ has small impact on inference for $\boldsymbol{\beta}$ when m is large. See Hall and Severini (1998) for a comparative study of a diagonal $\boldsymbol{H}_i$ to alternative weight matrices. Furthermore, to use the most suitable weight, namely $\mathrm{Var}(\boldsymbol{W_i})$, we would need to make further assumptions about the third and the fourth joint moments of $\boldsymbol{Y_i}$. See Fitzmaurice and Laird (1993) and Liang *et al.* (1992) for details in the case of binary responses.

The solution, $(\hat{\boldsymbol{\beta}}, \hat{\boldsymbol{\alpha}})$, of $\boldsymbol{S_\beta} = \mathbf{0}$ and $\boldsymbol{S_\alpha} = \mathbf{0}$ is asymptotically Gaussian (Liang and Zeger, 1986), with variance consistently estimated by

$$\left(\sum_{i=1}^{m} C_i' B_i^{-1} D_i\right)^{-1} \left(\sum_{i=1}^{m} C_i' B_i^{-1} V_{0i} B_i^{-1} C_i\right) \left(\sum_{i=1}^{m} D_i' B_i^{-1} C_i\right)^{-1}, \quad (7.5.6)$$

evaluated at $(\hat{\boldsymbol{\beta}}, \hat{\boldsymbol{\alpha}})$, where

$$C_i = \begin{pmatrix} \frac{\partial \boldsymbol{\mu_i}}{\partial \boldsymbol{\beta}} & 0 \\ 0 & \frac{\partial \boldsymbol{\eta_i}}{\partial \boldsymbol{\alpha}} \end{pmatrix}, \quad B_i = \begin{pmatrix} \mathrm{Var}(\boldsymbol{Y_i}) & 0 \\ 0 & \boldsymbol{H}_i \end{pmatrix}, \quad D_i = \begin{pmatrix} \frac{\partial \boldsymbol{\mu_i}}{\partial \boldsymbol{\beta}} & \frac{\partial \boldsymbol{\mu_i}}{\partial \boldsymbol{\alpha}} \\ \frac{\partial \boldsymbol{\eta_i}}{\partial \boldsymbol{\beta}} & \frac{\partial \boldsymbol{\eta_i}}{\partial \boldsymbol{\alpha}} \end{pmatrix},$$

and

$$V_{0i} = \begin{pmatrix} \boldsymbol{y_i} - \boldsymbol{\mu_i} \\ \boldsymbol{w_i} - \boldsymbol{\eta_i} \end{pmatrix} \begin{pmatrix} \boldsymbol{y_i} - \boldsymbol{\mu_i} \\ \boldsymbol{w_i} - \boldsymbol{\eta_i} \end{pmatrix}'.$$

This variance estimate is consistent as the number of individuals contributing to each element of the matrix goes to infinity. For example, in an analysis of variance problem, the number of units in each treatment group must get large.

The proposed method of estimation enjoys two properties. First, $\hat{\boldsymbol{\beta}}$ is nearly efficient relative to the maximum likelihood estimates of $\boldsymbol{\beta}$ in many practical situations provided that $\mathrm{Var}(\boldsymbol{Y}_i)$ has been reasonably approximated (e.g. Liang and Zeger, 1986; Liang *et al.*, 1992). In fact, the GEE is the maximum likelihood score equation for multivariate Gaussian data and for binary data from a log-linear model when $\mathrm{Var}(\boldsymbol{Y}_i)$ is correctly specified (Fitzmaurice and Laird, 1993). Second, $\hat{\boldsymbol{\beta}}$ is consistent as $m \to \infty$, even if the covariance structure of $\boldsymbol{Y_i}$ is incorrectly specified. When regression coefficients are the scientific focus as in the examples here, one should invest the lion's share of time in modelling the mean structure, while using a reasonable approximation to the covariance. The robustness of the inferences about $\boldsymbol{\beta}$ can be checked by fitting a final model using different covariance assumptions and comparing the two sets of estimates and their robust standard errors. If they differ substantially, a more careful treatment of the covariance model may be necessary.

In this section, we have focused on inference for marginal models. Transition models can also be fitted using GEE. The reader is referred to Korn and Whittemore (1979), Ware *et al.* (1988), and references therein. Further discussion is provided in Chapter 10.

8
Marginal models

8.1 Introduction

This chapter describes regression methods that characterize the marginal expectation of a discrete or continuous response, Y, as a function of explanatory variables. The methods are designed to permit separate modelling of the regression of Y on $\boldsymbol{x}$, and the association among repeated observations of Y for each individual. Marginal models are appropriate when inferences about the population-average are the focus. For example, in a clinical trial the average difference between control and treatment is most important, not the difference for any one individual. Marginal models are also useful for epidemiological studies. For example, in the Indonesian Children's Health Study (ICHS), a marginal model can be used to address questions such as:

(1) what is the age-specific prevalence of respiratory infection in children?

(2) is the prevalence of respiratory infection greater in the sub-population of children with vitamin A deficiency?

(3) how does the association of vitamin A deficiency and respiratory infection change with age?

Note that the scientific objectives are to characterize and contrast populations of children.

In addition to modelling the effects of covariates on the marginal expectations, we must also specify a model for the association among observations from each subject. This is to be contrasted with random effects and transitional models where the covariate effects and within-subject association are modelled through a single equation. As discussed in Chapter seven, all three approaches lead to the same class of linear models for Gaussian data. But in the discrete data case, different (non-linear) models can lead to different interpretations for the regression coefficients. The choice of model should therefore depend on the scientific question being addressed.

This chapter discusses marginal models for categorical and count longitudinal data. Similar ideas apply to the analysis of skewed continuous

(Paik, 1992) and censored data which will not be covered here. Section 8.2 focuses on binary data contrasting traditional log-linear and marginal models. In Section 8.2.2, we compare three distinct parameterizations of the covariance among repeated binary observations, in terms of correlations, conditional odds ratios, and marginal odds ratios. Section 8.2.3 considers *generalized estimating equations* (GEE) for estimating regression and association parameters without specifying the entire likelihood. Examples of logistic models for binary longitudinal data are presented in Section 8.3. Discussion of ordered categorical and multinomial responses is delayed until Chapter 10. Section 8.4 treats models for count data.

8.2 Binary responses

8.2.1 *The log-linear model*

This section focuses on probability models for $\Pr(Y_{i1}, \ldots, Y_{in_i})$. To simplify the notation, we suppress for the moment the individual's subscript, i, as well as dependence on covariates, $\boldsymbol{x}_{ij}$.

The most widely used probability model for multivariate binary data is the log-linear model (Bishop *et al.*, 1975)

$$\begin{aligned}
&\Pr(\boldsymbol{Y} = \boldsymbol{y}) \\
&\quad = c(\boldsymbol{\theta}) \exp\left(\sum_{j=1}^{n} \theta_j^{(1)} y_j + \sum_{j_1 < j_2} \theta_{j_1 j_2}^{(2)} y_{j_1} y_{j_2} + \cdots + \theta_{1,\ldots,n}^{(n)} y_1 \cdots y_n \right),
\end{aligned}$$

where the $(2^n - 1)$-vector of canonical parameters is

$$\boldsymbol{\theta} = \left(\theta_1^{(1)}, \ldots, \theta_n^{(1)}, \theta_{12}^{(2)}, \ldots, \theta_{n-1n}^{(2)}, \ldots, \theta_{1,\ldots,n}^{(n)} \right).$$

The function $c(\boldsymbol{\theta})$ normalizes the probability distribution to sum to one. The equation above represents a saturated model in which the only constraint on the 2^n cell probabilities is that they add to one.

The canonical parameters facilitate calculation of cell probabilities but are less useful for describing $\Pr(\boldsymbol{Y} = \boldsymbol{y})$ as a function of the explanatory variables $\boldsymbol{x}$, because, for example, the parameter θ_{jk} describes the association between Y_j and Y_k *conditional* on all the other responses, $Y_l, l \neq j, k$. To establish this point, consider the quadratic exponential model (Zhao and Prentice, 1990; Gourieroux *et al.*, 1984), a log-linear model with third and higher-order terms equal to 0, so that

$$\Pr(\boldsymbol{Y} = \boldsymbol{y}) = c(\boldsymbol{\theta}) \exp\left(\sum_{j=1}^{n} \theta_j^{(1)} y_j + \sum_{j<k} \theta_{jk}^{(2)} y_j y_k \right).$$

For this model,

$$\log\left\{\frac{\Pr(Y_j=1 \mid Y_k=y_k, Y_l=0, l\neq j,k)}{\Pr(Y_j=0 \mid Y_k=y_k, Y_l=0, l\neq j,k)}\right\} = \theta_j^{(1)} + \theta_{jk}^{(2)} y_k.$$

Here, $\theta_j^{(1)}$ is the log-odds for $Y_j = 1$ given that the remaining responses $Y_l, l \neq j$ are all zero. Similarly, $\theta_{jk}^{(2)}$ is the log-odds ratio describing the association between Y_j and Y_k given that all the other responses are fixed, here set equal to zero. The log-linear canonical parameters, $\boldsymbol{\theta}$, may be undesirable if we now want to formulate a model in which they depend on explanatory variables by letting $\boldsymbol{\theta} = \boldsymbol{\theta}(\boldsymbol{x})$. Suppose that $Y_1, \ldots, Y_n$ indicate whether a child has respiratory infection each month and the key explanatory variable is an indicator of whether the child's mother smokes, $x = 1$ for smokers. If we now assume that the quadratic exponential model above has different parameter values for the smokers and non-smokers, we have a regression model. But the difference between $\theta_j^{(1)}(x=1)$ and $\theta_j^{(1)}(x=0)$ represents the effect of smoking on the conditional probability of respiratory infection at visit j given that there was no infection at any of the other visits. Since mother's smoking is likely to influence all visits, a part of the smoking effect will be conditioned away when we control for the other outcomes. A better formulation of the log-linear model is with parameters that describe the marginal probability $\Pr(Y_j = 1 \mid \boldsymbol{x})$ as a function of the smoking variable (Neuhaus and Jewell, 1990).

A second limitation of the canonical parameters is that their interpretation depends on the number of responses, n. Hence, if we add or delete an observation for an individual, the interpretation and value of the canonical parameters will change. In longitudinal studies, the number of observations commonly differs across subjects so that the applicability of models formulated in terms of $\boldsymbol{\theta}$ is limited.

8.2.2 *Log-linear models for marginal means*

We can still build a log-linear model by starting with the marginal parameters,

$$\mu_j = \Pr(Y_j = 1), \quad j = 1, \ldots, n. \tag{8.2.1}$$

The saturated log-linear model for an n-vector $\boldsymbol{Y}$ has $2^n - 1$ free parameters. If we start with the n μ_j's, we have $2^n - 1 - n$ parameters to be specified. This can be done in a number of useful ways; we briefly consider three of these.

The first is to use the μ_j's, plus the second- and higher-order canonical parameters, $\theta_{12}^{(2)}, \ldots, \theta_{n-1n}^{(2)}, \ldots, \theta_{12,\ldots,n}^{(n)}$, as proposed by Fitzmaurice and Laird (1993). If we let $\boldsymbol{w} = (y_1y_2, y_1y_3, \ldots, y_{n-1}y_n, y_1y_2y_3, \ldots, y_1y_2, \ldots, y_n)$,

$\boldsymbol{\theta}_1 = (\theta_1^{(1)}, \ldots, \theta_n^{(1)})$ and $\boldsymbol{\theta}_2 = (\theta_{12}^{(2)}, \theta_{13}^{(2)}, \ldots, \theta_{n-1n}^{(2)}, \ldots, \theta_{1,\ldots,n}^{(n)})$ then the log-linear model can be written as

$$\Pr(\boldsymbol{Y} = \boldsymbol{y}) = c(\boldsymbol{\theta_1}, \boldsymbol{\theta_2}) \exp(\boldsymbol{y}'\boldsymbol{\theta}_1 + \boldsymbol{w}'\boldsymbol{\theta_2}).$$

The parameters of interest are $\boldsymbol{\mu} = (\mu_1, \ldots, \mu_n) = \boldsymbol{\mu}(\boldsymbol{\theta_1}, \boldsymbol{\theta_2})$, so we can make a transformation from the canonical parameters, $(\boldsymbol{\theta_1}, \boldsymbol{\theta_2})$, to $(\boldsymbol{\mu}, \boldsymbol{\theta_2})$. In the regression context, we assume that the marginal means, μ_j, satisfy a model such as $\text{logit}\mu_j = \boldsymbol{x}_j'\boldsymbol{\beta}$. Interestingly, the score equation for $\boldsymbol{\beta}$ under this parameterization takes the GEE form

$$\left(\frac{\partial \boldsymbol{\mu}}{\partial \boldsymbol{\beta}}\right)' \text{Var}(\boldsymbol{Y})^{-1}(\boldsymbol{Y} - \boldsymbol{\mu}) = 0,$$

where the variance matrix of $\boldsymbol{Y}$ is determined by both $\boldsymbol{\beta}$ and $\boldsymbol{\theta_2}$. This demonstrates that the solution of the GEE is the maximum likelihood estimate under the log-linear model when the covariance assumption, $\text{Var}(\boldsymbol{Y}_i)$, is correct for all $i = 1, \ldots, m$.

The limitation of this parameterization is that the interpretation of $\boldsymbol{\theta_2}$ as a conditional odds ratio depends on the number of other responses in a cluster. Hence, this formulation is most useful when the number of observations per person is the same, at least by design, as for example is often the case in clinical trials. Also, the conditional odds ratios are not easily interpreted when the association among responses is itself a focus of the study.

The second parameterization of the log-linear model that uses marginal means was proposed by Bahadur (1961). Here, second-order moments are specified in terms of correlations. If we let $R_j = (Y_j - \mu_j)/\{\mu_j(1 - \mu_j)\}^{1/2}, \rho_{jk} = \text{Corr}(Y_j, Y_k) = \text{E}(R_j R_k), \rho_{jkl} = \text{E}(R_j R_k R_l)$ and so on, up to $\rho_{1,\ldots,n} = \text{E}(R_1, \ldots, R_n)$, then we can write the probability distribution $\Pr(\boldsymbol{Y} = \boldsymbol{y})$ as

$$\prod_{j=1}^{n} \mu_j^{y_j}(1 - \mu_j)^{(1-y_j)}$$

$$\times \left(1 + \sum_{j<k} \rho_{jk} r_j r_k + \sum_{j<k<l} \rho_{jkl} r_j r_k r_l + \cdots + \rho_{1,\ldots,n} r_1 r_2, \ldots, r_n\right).$$

Here, the joint distribution is expressed in terms of the marginal means, pairwise correlations, and higher moments of the standardized variables R_j.

The Bahadur representation is attractive because it uses marginal probabilities and correlations, which are familiar parameters from the analysis of continuous responses. The serious drawback, however, is that, unlike for Gaussian data, the correlations among binary responses are constrained in complicated ways by the marginal means. Hence, if we assume that the marginal means depend on covariates, $\boldsymbol{x}$, it may not be correct to assume that the correlations and higher-order moments are independent of $\boldsymbol{x}$, as would be convenient.

A compromise between conditional odds ratios which are unconstrained by the means but which have interpretations that depend on n, and correlations which are seriously constrained, is to parameterize the likelihood in terms of marginal odds ratios. These have weaker constraints and their interpretations are independent of n. The marginal odds ratio is defined as

$$\gamma_{jk} = \frac{\Pr(Y_j = 1, Y_k = 1)\Pr(Y_j = 0, Y_k = 0)}{\Pr(Y_j = 1, Y_k = 0)\Pr(Y_j = 0, Y_k = 1)}. \tag{8.2.2}$$

It takes values in $(0, \infty)$; a value greater than one indicates positive association. The odds ratio is a popular measure of association because it is unconstrained on the logarithmic scale and is in common use as the parameter in a logistic regression.

The full distribution of $\boldsymbol{Y}$ may be specified in terms of the means $\boldsymbol{\mu}$, the odds ratios $\boldsymbol{\gamma} = (\gamma_{12}, \ldots, \gamma_{n-1n})$ and contrasts of odds ratios, the first two given by

$$\begin{aligned}
\zeta_{j_1 j_2 j_3} &= \log \mathrm{OR}(y_{j_1}, y_{j_2} \mid y_{j_3} = 1) - \log \mathrm{OR}(y_{j_1}, y_{j_2} \mid y_{j_3} = 0), \\
\zeta_{j_1 j_2 j_3 j_4} &= \log \mathrm{OR}(y_{j_1}, y_{j_2} \mid y_{j_3} = 1, y_{j_4} = 1) \\
&\quad - \log \mathrm{OR}(y_{j_1}, y_{j_2} \mid y_{j_3} = 1, y_{j_4} = 0) \\
&\quad - \log \mathrm{OR}(y_{j_1}, y_{j_2} \mid y_{j_3} = 0, y_{j_4} = 1) \\
&\quad + \log \mathrm{OR}(y_{j_1}, y_{j_2} \mid y_{j_3} = 0, y_{j_4} = 0).
\end{aligned}$$

The general term has the somewhat complicated expression

$$\zeta_{j_1, \ldots, j_n} = \sum_{y_{j_3}, \ldots, y_{j_n} = 0,1} (-1)^{b(\boldsymbol{y})}, \log \mathrm{OR}(y_{j_1}, y_{j_2} \mid y_{j_3}, \ldots, y_{j_n}),$$

where $b(\boldsymbol{y}) = \sum_{\ell=3}^{n} y_{j_\ell} + n - 2$. Liang *et al.* (1992) discuss the evaluation of the likelihood function in terms of these odds ratios and their contrasts. This is not a simple matter except in cases with a small number of observations per person. For example, with two observations the joint distribution, $\Pr(Y_1 = y_1, Y_2 = y_2)$, can be written as

$$\mu_1^{y_1}(1 - \mu_1)^{1-y_1}\mu_2^{y_2}(1 - \mu_2)^{1-y_2} + (-1)^{(y_1 - y_2)}(\mu_{11} - \mu_1\mu_2),$$

where $\mu_{11} = \Pr(Y_1 = Y_2 = 1)$ is given in terms of μ_j and γ_{12} by

$$\mu_{11} = \begin{cases} \frac{1-(\mu_1+\mu_2)(1-\gamma_{12})-[\{1-(\mu_1+\mu_2)(1-\gamma_{12})\}^2-4(\gamma_{12}-1)\gamma_{12}\mu_1\mu_2]^{1/2}}{2(\gamma_{12}-1)}, & \gamma_{12} \neq 1, \\ \mu_1\mu_2, & \gamma_{12} = 1. \end{cases}$$

We note that there are $\binom{n_i}{2}$ pairs of odds ratios per subject, and this number becomes substantial when n_i increases. The problem of having a large number of nuisance parameters can be alleviated by using a regression model for the odds ratios as is done for the marginal expectations. The simplest model is $\gamma_{ijk} = \gamma$ for all i, j, k which says that the degree of association is the same for all pairs of observations from the same subject. Alternatively, we might assume that

$$\log \gamma_{ijk} = \alpha_0 + \alpha_1 \mid t_{ij} - t_{ik} \mid^{-1},$$

that is, the degree of association is inversely proportional to the time between observations. In general, we write

$$\gamma_{ijk} = \gamma(\boldsymbol{\alpha}), \tag{8.2.3}$$

where $\boldsymbol{\alpha}$ is a vector of q parameters to be estimated.

We often do not have sensible, simple models for third- and higher-order moments regardless of which formulation we adopt. Even when a probability model is fully specified, the likelihood can be complicated to evaluate except with small and constant n_i. For these reasons, we now apply the GEE approach discussed in Section 7.5 to logistic regression.

8.2.3 *Generalized estimating equations*

In the logistic regression model, we specify that the marginal expectations, $\mathrm{E}(Y_{ij}) = \mu_{ij}$, satisfy $\mathrm{logit}\mu_{ij} = \boldsymbol{x}'_{ij}\boldsymbol{\beta}$. We have seen that the GEE estimating function introduced in Section 7.5 is the score equation for $\boldsymbol{\beta}$ when the data follow a log-linear probability distribution and we correctly specify $\mathrm{Var}(\boldsymbol{Y}_i)$. Even when we must model the covariance, it seems sensible to estimate $\boldsymbol{\beta}$ by solving the GEE

$$S_{\boldsymbol{\beta}}(\boldsymbol{\beta}, \boldsymbol{\alpha}) = \sum_{i=1}^{m} \left(\frac{\partial \boldsymbol{\mu}_i}{\partial \boldsymbol{\beta}} \right)' \mathrm{Var}(\boldsymbol{Y_i})^{-1} (\boldsymbol{Y_i} - \boldsymbol{\mu}_i) = 0. \tag{8.2.4}$$

The quantity $S_{\boldsymbol{\beta}}(\boldsymbol{\beta}, \boldsymbol{\alpha})$ can be viewed as a multivariate version of the quasi-score function first proposed by Wedderburn (1974) with an additional complication that it depends not only on $\boldsymbol{\beta}$ but also on $\boldsymbol{\alpha}$, since $\mathrm{Var}(\boldsymbol{Y_i}) = \mathrm{Var}(\boldsymbol{Y_i}; \boldsymbol{\beta}, \boldsymbol{\alpha})$. The dependence on $\boldsymbol{\alpha}$ can be resolved by replacing $\boldsymbol{\alpha}$ in the GEE above with a $m^{1/2}$-consistent estimate, $\hat{\boldsymbol{\alpha}}(\hat{\boldsymbol{\beta}})$. Liang and Zeger (1986) and Gourieroux *et al.* (1984) have shown that the solution of the resulting equation is asymptotically as efficient as if $\boldsymbol{\alpha}$ were known.

With binary responses, the association parameters, $\boldsymbol{\alpha}$, may be formulated and estimated in a number of ways. Liang and Zeger (1986) parameterize $\mathrm{Var}(\boldsymbol{Y_i})$ in terms of correlations and use moment estimators for the unknown parameters. Fitzmaurice and Laird (1993) use conditional odds ratios for data sets with block designs and estimate the association parameters using maximum likelihood. Lipsitz *et al.* (1991), Liang *et al.* (1992) and Carey *et al.* (1993) formulate $\text{Var}(\boldsymbol{Y_i})$ in terms of marginal odds ratios.

Following Prentice (1988), we can estimate association parameters by adding a second set of estimating equations $S_{\boldsymbol{\alpha}}(\boldsymbol{\beta}, \boldsymbol{\alpha}) = 0$ and simultaneously solving the expanded equations for $\hat{\boldsymbol{\beta}}$ and $\hat{\boldsymbol{\alpha}}$. The $\boldsymbol{\alpha}$ equations take the form

$$S_{\boldsymbol{\alpha}}(\boldsymbol{\beta}, \boldsymbol{\alpha}) = \sum_{i=1}^{m} \left(\frac{\partial \boldsymbol{\eta}_i}{\partial \boldsymbol{\alpha}} \right)' \boldsymbol{H}_i^{-1}(\boldsymbol{W}_i - \boldsymbol{\eta}_i) = 0, \qquad (8.2.5)$$

where

$$\boldsymbol{W_i} = (R_{i1}R_{i2}, R_{i1}R_{i3}, \ldots, R_{in_i-1}R_{in_i}),$$

$H_i = \text{diag}\{\text{Var}(R_{i1}R_{i2}), \ldots, \text{Var}(R_{in_i-1}R_{in_i})\}$, $R_{ij} = \{Y_{ij} - \mu_{ij}\}/\{\mu_{ij}(1 - \mu_{ij})\}^{1/2}$ and $\boldsymbol{\eta}_i = \text{E}(\boldsymbol{W}_i)$. With binary responses, $\boldsymbol{\eta}_i$ and H_i are fully determined by the mean and correlation models without additional assumptions about higher-order moments. One simple example is if we assume that $\text{Corr}(Y_{ij}, Y_{ik}) = \alpha$ for all i and all $j \neq k$. Here, if we use the simpler identity weighting matrix in (8.2.5), we can estimate α by

$$\hat{\alpha} = (1/N^*) \sum_{i=1}^{m} \sum_{j<k} r_{ij} r_{ik},$$

where $N^* = \sum_i \binom{n_i}{2}$ and $r_{ij} = (y_{ij} - \hat{\mu}_{ij})/\{\hat{\mu}_{ij}(1 - \hat{\mu}_{ij})\}^{1/2}$.

When marginal odds ratios are used to model association, $\boldsymbol{\alpha}$ can be estimated by the approach introduced by Carey *et al.* (1993) and developed by Carey (1992). They estimate the odds ratios using an offset logistic regression. Let α_{ijk} be the log-odds ratio for responses Y_{ij} and Y_{ik} and let $\mu_{ijk} = \Pr(Y_{ij} = Y_{ik} = 1)$. Then, it can easily be shown that

$$\text{logit}\,\Pr(Y_{ij} = 1 \mid Y_{ik} = y_{ik}) = \alpha_{ijk} y_{ik} + \log \left(\frac{\mu_{ij} - \mu_{ijk}}{1 - \mu_{ij} - \mu_{ik} + \mu_{ijk}} \right).$$

Suppose that we now impose the model that all the odds ratios are the same, that is, $\alpha_{ijk} = \alpha$. Then α can be estimated by a logistic regression of y_{ij} on $y_{ik}, 1 \leq j < k \leq n_i, i = 1, \ldots, m$, using the second term on the right hand side of the equation above as an offset. Note that the offset depends on both $\boldsymbol{\beta}$ and $\boldsymbol{\alpha}$ so that iteration is required. More generally, we can assume a model $\alpha_{ijk} = \boldsymbol{d}'_{\boldsymbol{ijk}}\boldsymbol{\alpha}$, where $\boldsymbol{d_{ijk}}$ is a set of covariates that characterizes the log-odds ratio between observations j and k. We then estimate the vector $\boldsymbol{\alpha}$ by a logistic regression of y_{ij} on the product $\boldsymbol{d_{ijk}} y_{ik}$. Carey *et al.* (1993) give more details of this implementation of GEE, which they call 'alternating logistic regressions', or ALR.

8.3 Examples

In this section we demonstrate the use of marginal models for binary data from four biomedical studies. The first two examples are from clinical trials with crossover designs. Crossovers are commonly used in biomedical studies to compare treatments for chronic diseases such as asthma and hypertension. The third uses data from the schizophrenia trial described in Example 1.7. The fourth example is from the observational study of the association between vitamin A deficiency and respiratory infection in Indonesian children.

Example 8.1. A 2×2 crossover trial

The data shown in Table 8.1 are adapted from Jones and Kenward (1989, p. 90) who reported results from a crossover trial on cerebrovascular deficiency in which an active drug (A) and a placebo (B) were compared. Only data from centre two are used for illustration. Thirty-four patients received the active drug (A) followed by placebo (B); another 33 patients were treated in the reverse order. The response variable is defined to be 0 for an abnormal and 1 for a normal electrocardiogram reading. Table 8.1 shows, for example, that 22 patients in the AB group respond positively on both treatments, whereas four patients in the BA group respond negatively to the first treatment (B) but positively to the second treatment (A).

Also shown in Table 8.1 are the marginal distributions of responses at the two periods for both the AB and BA groups. Focusing on the data at period 1 for the moment, we observe that 82% (28/34) of patients receiving the active drug (A) were normal as opposed to 61% (20/33) of the patients receiving the placebo (B). This gives $(13 \times 28)/(20 \times 6) = 3.0$ as an estimate of the odds ratio comparing the chance of being normal for the active drug versus the placebo. The standard error for the estimated log-odds ratio, $\log 3.0 = 1.1$, is in turn estimated as $(28^{-1} + 6^{-1} + 20^{-1} + 13^{-1})^{1/2} = 0.57$.

Table 8.1. Data from a 2×2 crossover trial on cerebrovascular deficiency adapted from Jones and Kenward (1989, p. 90), where treatments A and B are active drug and placebo, respectively; the outcome indicates whether an electrocardiogram was judged abnormal (0) or normal (1).

	Responses					Period	
Group	(1, 1)	(0, 1)	(1, 0)	(0, 0)	Total	1	2
AB	22	0	6	6	34	28	22
BA	18	4	2	9	33	20	22

For an explanation of these calculations, see Appendix A, Example A.1. The estimate of the treatment effect, measured by the odds ratio, is greater than one, indicating that the active drug produces a higher proportion of normal readings. However, the treatment effect is not statistically significant at the 0.05 level due to the large standard error. It is therefore desirable to combine the odds ratio estimated from the first period with that from second period, $(22 \times 12)/(11 \times 22) = 1.1$, to reduce the sampling error. Two problems arise. First, this approach ignores the possible treatment-by-period interaction known as the *carry-over effect* whereby the effect of treatment in period 1 influences the response in the next period. Secondly, the two responses obtained from the same subject are likely to be dependent. In fact, both groups show strong degrees of within-subject dependence. The odds ratio defined in (8.2.2) to estimate within-subject association, is estimated to be $(22 \times 6)/(6 \times 0.5) = 44$ and $(18 \times 9)/(4 \times 2) = 20.3$ for groups AB and BA, respectively.

We now use the GEE method, together with a sensible choice of model, to make inferences about the treatment effect, combining the data from both periods. Conceptually, 2×2 crossover trials can be viewed as longitudinal studies with $n_i = n = 2$. In this example, $m = 67$. The two major covariates, treatment (x_1) and period (x_2), are both time-dependent, and are coded as

$$x_1 = \begin{cases} 1 & \text{active drug (A)}, \\ 0 & \text{placebo (B)}, \end{cases} \qquad x_2 = \begin{cases} 1 & \text{period 2}, \\ 0 & \text{period 1}. \end{cases}$$

We first fit a logistic regression model

$$\text{logit}\,\Pr(Y_{ij} = 1) = \beta_0 + \beta_1 x_{ij1} + \beta_2 x_{ij2} + \beta_3 x_{ij1} \cdot x_{ij2},$$

under the assumption of a constant odds ratio, γ, across subjects. Results from Table 8.2 show little support for a treatment-by-period interaction ($\hat{\beta}_3 = -1.02 \pm 0.98$) and a strong within-subject association ($\hat{\gamma} = \exp(3.54) = 34.5$). The association parameter indicates that subjects with normal responses at the first visit have odds of normal readings at the next visit that are almost 35 times higher than those whose first response was abnormal.

When dropping the interaction term from the model, we estimate a statistically significant treatment effect ($\hat{\beta}_1 = 0.57 \pm 0.23$). Thus, the overall odds of a normal electrocardiogram reading are estimated to be 77% higher ($0.77 = \exp(0.57) - 1$) when using the active drug as compared to the placebo. We note that if we incorrectly assume that there is no within-subject dependence, as was done in the last column of Table 8.2, the treatment effect is erroneously assessed to be statistically insignificant ($\hat{\beta}_1 = 0.56 \pm 0.38$). However, this potential pitfall can be avoided by

Table 8.2. Logistic regression coefficients (standard errors) from GEE for the 2×2 crossover trial on cerebrovascular deficiency. Models 1 and 2 are fitted using alternating logistic regressions (Carey *et al.*, 1993).

	Model		
Variable	1	2	3
Intercept	0.43	0.67	0.66
	(0.36)	(0.29)	(0.29)*
			[0.32]**
Treatment (x_1)	1.11	0.57	0.56
	(0.57)	(0.23)	(0.23)
			[0.38]
Period (x_2)	0.18	−0.30	−0.27
	(0.51)	(0.23)	(0.23)
			[0.38]
$x_1 \cdot x_2$	−1.02	—	—
	(0.98)	—	—
$\log \gamma$	3.54	3.56	—
	(0.82)	(0.81)	—

*robust SE.
**model-based SE.

using the robust standard error (0.23) instead of the model-based standard error (0.38).

Example 8.2. A three-treatment, three-period crossover trial

This example demonstrates how marginal models can be easily extended to more complicated designs. It also serves to contrast the results from using marginal and conditional parameters. Table 8.3, previously shown as Table 1.4, gives data from a crossover trial in which two treatments were compared with placebo for the relief of primary dysmenorrhoea (Jones and Kenward, 1987). The placebo is labelled treatment A, whilst treatments B and C are analgesic with low and high dose, respectively. The response variable, measured at the end of each period, is coded one for some relief and zero for no relief. Table 8.3 shows, for example, that among 15 patients randomized to the group receiving treatments A, B and C in order, 9 patients had the outcome (011) indicating no relief in period 1 followed by some relief for both the second and third periods.

Table 8.3. Data from a 3 × 3 crossover trial on primary dysmenorrhoea from Jones and Kenward (1987).

	Response								
Group	000	100	010	001	110	101	011	111	Total
ABC	0	0	2	2	1	0	9	1	15
ACB	2	1	0	0	0	0	9	4	16
BAC	0	1	1	1	0	8	3	1	15
BCA	0	1	1	1	8	0	0	1	12
CAB	3	0	0	0	1	7	2	1	14
CBA	1	5	0	0	4	3	1	0	14

Restricting attention to the data from the first period only, we notice that the fraction of patients with relief is considerably lower, 23 % = 7/31, in the placebo group than in the low, 74% = 20/27, or high, 75% = 21/28, analgesic groups. As in the 2 × 2 crossover example, we want to pool information across periods, taking account of the correlation among repeated responses for each individual. To do so, we use a marginal model where the primary covariates are defined as follows:

$$x_1(x_2) = \begin{cases} 1 & \text{period } 2(3), \\ 0 & \text{otherwise,} \end{cases} \qquad x_3(x_4) = \begin{cases} 1 & \text{treatment B(C)}, \\ 0 & \text{otherwise,} \end{cases}$$

$$x_5(x_6) = \begin{cases} 1 & \text{the previous assignment is B(C)}, \\ 0 & \text{otherwise.} \end{cases}$$

We first examine the carry-over effect by fitting a model

$$\begin{aligned} \operatorname{logit} \Pr(Y_{ij} = 1) = \beta_0 &+ \beta_1 x_{ij1} + \beta_2 x_{ij2} + \beta_3 x_{ij3} \\ &+ \beta_4 x_{ij4} + \beta_5 x_{ij5} + \beta_6 x_{ij6}, \end{aligned} \qquad (8.3.1)$$

for $j = 1, 2, 3$ and $i = 1, \ldots, 86$. We considered two different models for the association: that the marginal odds ratios were constant for all three pairs of times (Model 1); and that they took three distinct values (Model 2). The inferences for $\boldsymbol{\beta}$ did not change materially as we changed the assumption about the association.

Results for Models 1 and 2 reported in Table 8.4 suggest that there is moderate evidence of a carry-over effect for the high dose analgesic treatment. The odds of dysmenorrhoea relief in periods 2 or 3 are reduced by a

Table 8.4. Coefficients and (standard errors) from logistic regression analyses using GEE for the 3 × 3 crossover trial on primary dysmenorrhoea. Models were fitted using the alternating logistic regression implementation of GEE.

	Model			
Variable	1	2	3	4
Intercept	−1.08	−1.10	−1.21	−1.19
	(0.32)	(0.32)	(0.42)	(0.42)
$\text{Period}_2(x_1)$	0.42	0.38	0.96	0.88
	(0.41)	(0.41)	(0.72)	(0.72)
$\text{Period}_3(x_2)$	0.59	0.55	0.56	0.53
	(0.46)	(0.45)	(0.79)	(0.80)
$\text{Treatment}_\text{B}(x_3)$	2.09	2.09	2.74	2.66
	(0.42)	(0.42)	(0.69)	(0.67)
$\text{Treatment}_\text{C}(x_4)$	2.07	2.12	2.00	2.01
	(0.42)	(0.42)	(0.57)	(0.57)
$\text{Carryover}_\text{B}(x_5)$	−0.15	−0.091	−0.32	−0.34
	(0.51)	(0.50)	(0.55)	(0.55)
$\text{Carryover}_\text{C}(x_6)$	−0.92	−0.86	−0.86	−0.81
	(0.44)	(0.43)	(0.49)	(0.49)
$x_1 \cdot x_3$			−1.55	−1.42
			(0.87)	(0.84)
$x_1 \cdot x_4$			−0.052	0.006
			(0.89)	(0.90)
$x_2 \cdot x_3$			−0.39	−0.33
			(0.92)	(0.89)
$x_2 \cdot x_4$			0.42	0.44
			(0.91)	(0.92)
$\log \gamma_{12}$	−0.22	−0.96	−0.19	−0.87
	(0.38)	(0.62)	(0.35)	(0.90)
$\log \gamma_{13}$	−0.22	0.11	−0.19	0.18
	(0.38)	(0.72)	(0.35)	(0.75)
$\log \gamma_{23}$	−0.22	0.29	−0.19	0.20
	(0.38)	(0.70)	(0.35)	(0.68)

factor of 60% ($0.6 = 1 - \exp(-0.919)$) among patients who received treatment C in the previous period rather than A, irrespective of the current treatment assignment.

We next examine the data for possible treatment-by-period interactions by adding $x_1 \cdot x_3, x_1 \cdot x_4, x_2 \cdot x_3$ and $x_2 \cdot x_4$ to the previous model. It appears, as shown for models 3 and 4 of Table 8.4, that the assumption that treatment effects are constant over time is adequate. We therefore return to the first model, and conclude that the odds of dysmenorrhoea relief for the group receiving the low (high) dose of analgesic is $\exp(2.03) = 7.6$ ($\exp(2.07) = 7.9$) times higher than when using the placebo and that the two doses of analgesic have similar effects.

Jones and Kenward (1987) use canonical parameters in a log-linear model to analyse three-period crossover trials. For these data, they used a model in which $\text{logit}\,\Pr(Y_{ij} \mid Y_{ik}, k \neq j, \boldsymbol{x}_{ij})$ is a linear function of the other responses, $Y_{ik}, k \neq j$, and of the covariates defined above. This model found little evidence of carry-over effects. The lack of statistical significance in their analysis is likely due to the fact that the variables x_5 and x_6 were modelled simultaneously with Y_{ij-1}. When there are treatment effects, as is the case here, the carry-over effects of variables x_5 and x_6 will be partly attributed to Y_{ij-1}, which has also been affected by the treatment during the last period. By conditioning on the prior outcome, we attribute some of the effect of the last-period treatment to the last-period outcome. By the analogous argument, the estimated treatment effects will also be smaller in the conditional model as applied by Jones and Kenward (1987). The conceptual difficulties in conditioning on other outcomes with longitudinal and other studies that generate correlated data have been addressed in more detail by Liang *et al.* (1992).

Example 8.3. A conventional randomized trial

In clinical trials pre–post designs are common in practice. Here, the primary response variables of each patient are measured prior to and after the randomization has taken place. To illustrate how marginal models may be applied to this design for binary responses, we consider the schizophrenia trial described in Example 1.7 in which the response variable, Positive and negative symptom noting scale (PANSS), is dichotomized as one if PANSS ≥ 80 and 0 otherwise.

Figure 8.1 shows the estimated prevalence in two groups (1: risperidone of 6 mg; 0: haloperidol) at baseline and at 1, 2, 4, 6, and 8 weeks after randomization. There is a clear trend of decline in risk for having PANSS $\geq$ 80 for both groups. A scientific question of interest is whether the apparent difference in trend between the two groups is clinically meaningful. To formulate this objective statistically, we consider the following marginal model for the binary response Y_{ij}:

$$\text{logit}\,\Pr(Y_{ij} = 1) = \beta_0 + \beta_1 x_{i1} + \beta_2 x_{ij2} + \beta_3 x_{i1} \cdot x_{ij2},$$

for $j = 0, 1, \ldots, 5$ and $i = 1, \ldots, m$, where $m = 170$, the number of subjects included in this analysis. Here x_{i1} is the treatment status defined earlier

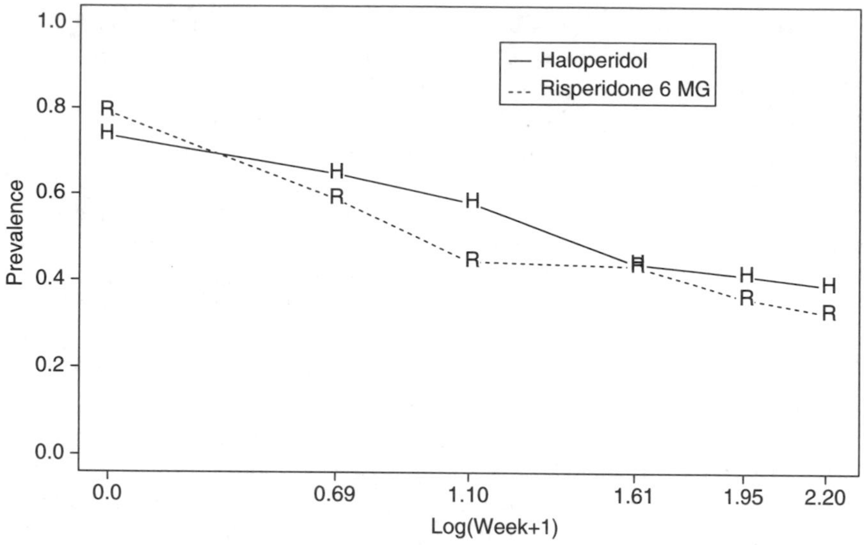

Fig. 8.1. Prevalence of PANSS $\geq$ 80 as a function of time (in weeks) from randomization estimated separately for risperidone (6 mg) and haloperidol group.

and $x_{ij2} = \log(t_j + 1)$, where t_j is time in weeks from randomization. Thus, for example, $x_{i02} = \log 1 = 0$ and $x_{i52} = \log 6$. We have applied the logarithmic transformation to the t_j's to capture the empirical phenomenon, as shown in Fig. 8.1, of greater rate of decline in earlier weeks. The primary coefficient of interest is β_3 which describes the difference, in logit scale, in change of prevalence over time between two treated groups. With up to six observations per subject in the span of eight weeks, it is of interest to explore the pattern of within-subject association to insure that such an association is properly acknowledged in GEE. Figure 8.2 shows, for each one of the groups, the plots of the estimated log-odds ratio relating two binary responses from the same subject versus the lag time. It is evident that the degree of within-subject association, as measured by log-odds ratio, decreases as the time between visits increases. Such a pattern, which appears to be linear, is similar between the two treatment groups. To capture this empirical phenomenon, we consider for $j < k = 0, 1, \ldots, 5$,

$$\log \text{OR}(Y_{ij}, Y_{ik}) = \alpha_0 + \alpha_1 \, | \, x_{ij2} - x_{ik2} \, | \, .$$

The results based upon the GEE analysis are presented in Table 8.5. They suggest that for patients in the haloperidol group, the prevalence of having

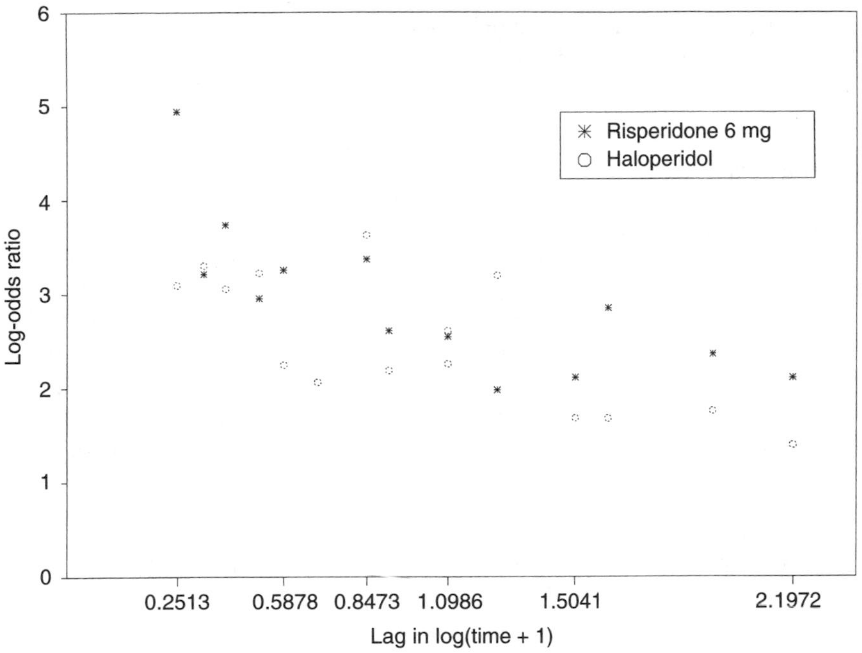

Fig. 8.2. Estimated log-odds ratio versus lag time, in log scale, for risperidone (6 mg) and haloperidol.

PANSS ≥ 80 decreases significantly ($\hat{\beta}_2 = -0.445 \pm 0.131$) at the rate of 26% ($0.26 = 1 - 2^{-0.455}$) per week at baseline and less drastically at the rate of 8% ($0.08 = 1 - (6/5)^{-0.445}$) per week at week four. The decline of prevalence for patients receiving risperidone of 6 mg is more pronounced at the rate of 43% ($0.43 = 1 - 2^{-0.445-0.371}$) per week at baseline and 14% at week four. The difference between the two groups in prevalence change over time is statistically significant at the 0.05 level (Z-statistic $= -0.371/0.185 = -2.01$). The results from the statistical modelling are consistent with the empirical finding in Fig. 8.2 that the log-odds ratio measuring the degree of within-subject association decreases as the lag time increases. Thus the odds ratio for repeated observations measured at baseline and at week one is estimated as $23.63 = \exp(3.803 - 0.924 \cdot \log 2)$ but drops to $6.56 = \exp(3.803 - 0.924 \cdot \log 8)$ if the second observation was measured at week eight. Finally, the finding concerning the treatment effect as captured by β_3 appears to be stable as long as the within-subject association is properly modelled; see results from Models 1–3 of Table 8.5. However, if the within-subject association is ignored, results for β_3 under Model 4 are very different, both quantitatively and qualitatively, than the rest. It is important to point out that in this trial, more that 50% of

Table 8.5. Marginal model coefficients (standard errors) from GEE for the pre-post trial on schizophrenia.

	Model			
Variable	1	2	3	4
Logistic regression				
Intercept	0.976	0.965	0.974	1.060
	(0.222)	(0.221)	(0.222)	(0.225)
Treatment (x_1)	0.110	0.087	0.120	0.005
	(0.315)	(0.313)	(0.315)	(0.320)
Time (x_2)	−0.445	−0.458	−0.449	−0.724
	(0.131)	(0.129)	(0.131)	(0.141)
$x_1 \cdot x_2$	−0.371	−0.351	−0.366	−0.156
	(0.185)	(0.184)	(0.184)	(0.202)
Within-subject association				
Intercept	3.803	2.884	3.605	—
	(0.410)	(0.456)	(0.591)	
lag time (z)	−0.924	—	−0.778	—
	(0.337)		(0.444)	
Treatment (x_1)	—	0.258	0.397	—
		(0.641)	(0.809)	
$x_1 \cdot z$	—	—	−0.302	—
			(0.673)	

the subjects dropped out during the eight week follow-up period and that there is strong evidence that dropout is related to response. The issue of missing data will be addressed in Chapter 13, where we will revisit this example.

Example 8.4. Respiratory infection in Indonesian preschool children

Two hundred and seventy-five preschool children in Indonesia were examined for up to six consecutive quarters for the presence of respiratory infection. This is a subset of a cohort studied by Sommer *et al.* (1984). A primary question of interest is whether the prevalence of respiratory infection is higher among children who suffer xerophthalmia, an ocular manifestation of chronic vitamin A deficiency. Also of interest is the change in the prevalence of respiratory infection with age. It is worth noting that either question can be addressed using both cross-sectional and longitudinal data. In what follows, we will look specifically at the ageing question.

Table 8.6. Prevalence of respiratory infection and xerophthalmia by visit.

	Visit (season)					
Prevalence (%)	1 (Su*)	2 (A)	3 (W)	4 (S)	5 (Su)	6 (A)
Respiratory infection	12.6	4.6	7.3	3.8	14.9	9.4
Xerophthalmia	3.9	6.1	6.2	5.5	3.1	3.0
No. of children	230	214	177	183	195	201

*Su = Summer; A = Autumn; W = Winter; S = Spring.

The prevalence of respiratory infection in six consecutive quarters, as shown in Table 8.6, reveals a possible seasonal trend with a summer maximum. The prevalence of xerophthalmia also indicates some seasonality, with a maximum in winter.

We begin our analysis by considering only data from the first visit. The results are summarized in Table 8.7. Model 1 in Table 8.7 is a logistic regression of respiratory infection on xerophthalmia and age (centred at 36 months), adjusting for gender and height for age as a percentage of the United States National Center for Health Statistics standard. The results suggest a strong cross-sectional age effect on the prevalence of respiratory infection. The effect is non-linear on the logit scale, as the quadratic term for age is statistically significant and negative in sign. As shown in Fig. 8.3, the cross-sectional analysis suggests that the prevalence of respiratory infection increases from age 12 months and reaches its peak at 20 months before starting to decline. If we now include the data from all six visits (Model 2 in Table 8.7), this concave relationship is preserved qualitatively, as shown in Fig. 8.3. We note that an annual sine and cosine have been included in Model 2 to adjust for seasonality but that this has very little impact on the age coefficients. The discrepancy among the age coefficients in Models 1 and 2 may be explained by Fig. 8.4 in which the cross-sectional age effects on respiratory infection are displayed graphically for each of six visits. The age coefficients in Model 2 can be interpreted as weighted averages of the cross-sectional age coefficients from each visit.

The association between respiratory infection and xerophthalmia is positive, although not statistically significant at the 5% level. There is limited information about the association with xerophthalmia in this partial data set which includes only 52 events of vitamin A deficiency. See Sommer *et al.* (1984) for an analysis of the complete data set of over 23 000 observations. We now want to distinguish the contributions of cross-sectional and longitudinal information to the estimated relationship of respiratory infection and age. That is, we want to separate differences among sub-populations of

Table 8.7. Logistic regressions of the prevalence of respiratory function on age and xerophthalmia adjusting for gender, season, and height for age. Models 1 and 2 estimate cross-sectional effects; Models 3 and 4 distinguish cross-sectional from longitudinal effects. Models 2–4 are fitted using the alternating logistic regression implementation of GEE.

	Model			
Variable	1	2	3	4
Intercept	−1.47	−2.05	−1.76	−2.21
	(0.36)	(0.21)	(0.25)	(0.32)
Gender	−0.66	−0.49	−0.53	−0.53
	(0.44)	(0.24)	(0.24)	(0.24)
Height for age	−0.11	−0.042	−0.051	−0.048
	(0.041)	(0.023)	(0.025)	(0.024)
Seasonal cosine	—	−0.59	—	−0.54
		(0.17)		(0.21)
Seasonal sine	—	−0.16	—	−0.016
	—	(0.14)	—	(0.18)
Xerophthalmia	0.44	0.50	0.53	0.64
	(1.15)	(0.44)	(0.45)	(0.44)
Age	−0.089	−0.030	—	—
	(0.027)	(0.008)	—	—
Age^2	−0.0026	−0.0010	—	—
	(0.0011)	(0.0004)	—	—
Age at entry	—	—	−0.053	−0.053
	—	—	(0.013)	(0.013)
(Age at entry)^2	—	—	−0.0013	−0.0013
	—	—	(0.0005)	(0.0005)
Follow-up time	—	—	−0.19	−0.082
	—	—	(0.071)	(0.099)
(Follow-up)^2	—	—	0.013	0.007
	—	—	(0.004)	(0.007)
$\log(\gamma)$		0.49	0.46	0.49
		(0.27)	(0.26)	(0.26)

children at different ages at a fixed time (cross-sectional) from changes in children over time (longitudinal). To do so, we first decompose the variable age_{ij}, the age of the ith child at the jth visit, where $j = 1, \ldots, 6$, as the sum

$$\text{age}_{i1} + (\text{age}_{ij} - \text{age}_{i1}).$$

If we allow separate regression coefficients β_C and β_L for age_{i1} and $\text{age}_{ij} - \text{age}_{i1}$, respectively, the regression coefficient β_L describes the change of

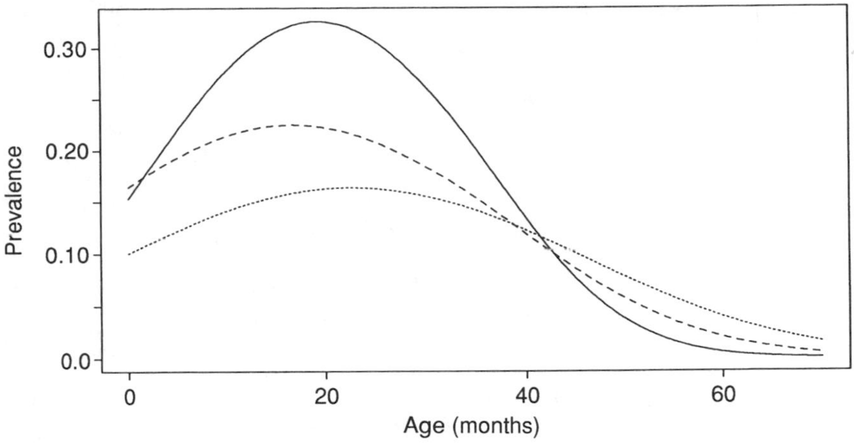

Fig. 8.3. Prevalence of respiratory infection as a function of age for three different models. – – – – –: Model 1; ......: Model 2; – – –: Model 3.

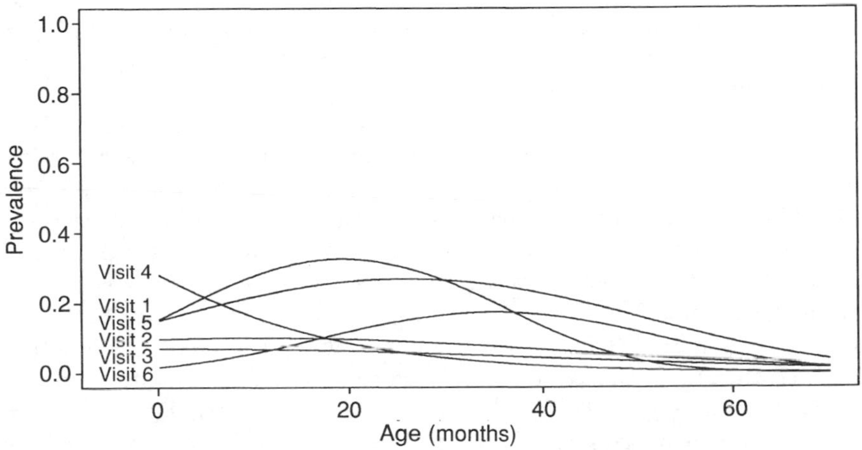

Fig. 8.4. Prevalence of respiratory infection as a function of age estimated separately for each of the six visits.

the risk of respiratory infection as the children grow older. The parameter β_C describes the age effect which would be estimated from purely cross-sectional data. The reader is referred to a more detailed discussion on this distinction in Sections 1.2 and 2.2. Note that the distinction between β_C and β_L defined for linear models holds only approximately for logistic and other non-linear models.

Results for Model 3 in Table 8.7 provide a different picture of how the risk of respiratory infection may be associated with age. The cross-sectional

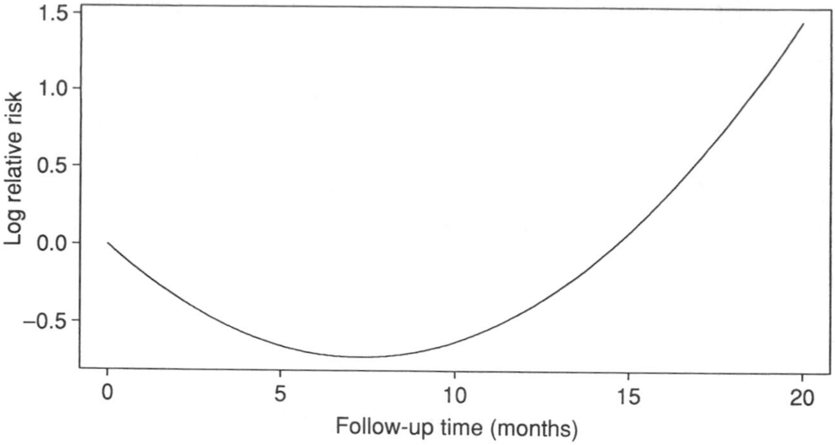

Fig. 8.5. The logarithm of the risk of respiratory infection as a function of follow-up time relative to the risk at an individual's first visit.

parameters suggest that the risk of respiratory infection climbs steadily in the first 20 months of life before declining; see Fig. 8.3. The longitudinal age parameters suggest otherwise. The risk of respiratory infection declines in the first 7 to 8 months of follow-up before rising later in life; see Fig. 8.5. This pattern is consistent even if we subdivide the study population into five cohorts according to the age at entry, namely, 0–12, 13–24, 25–36, 37–48, and 49 months or older. This pattern of a convex relationship between age and the risk of respiratory infection appears to coincide with the pattern of seasonality noted earlier. To determine whether seasonality is responsible, we add the annual harmonic in Model 4. The results are shown in the last column of Table 8.6. In fact, the longitudinal age parameters are now all insignificant. It makes sense that we can learn little about the effects of ageing from data collected over 18 months if we restrict our attention to longitudinal information. This is especially true in the presence of a substantial seasonal signal. On the other hand, much can be learned by comparing children of different ages so long as we can assume that there are no cohort effects, which would confound the inferences about age effects.

8.4 Counted responses

8.4.1 *Parametric modelling for count data*

Count data are increasingly common in the biological sciences. Examples include the number of panic attacks occurring during a six-month interval after receiving treatment for mental illness; the number of sexual partners in a three-month period recorded in an HIV prevention programme, and the number of infant deaths per month before and after introduction of a prenatal care programme. Traditionally, the Poisson distribution has been the most commonly used model for count data. It has the form

$$\Pr(Y = y) = \mu^y e^{-\mu}/y!, \quad y = 0, 1, 2, \dots .$$

The Poisson distribution is completely specified by the parameter μ, which is both the mean and the variance of the distribution, that is, $\mu = \mathrm{E}(Y) = \mathrm{Var}(Y)$. Unfortunately, the Poisson assumption that the mean and variance are equal is often inconsistent with empirical evidence.

To illustrate the problem, consider the seizure data in Table 1.5, which represent the number of epileptic seizures in each of four two-week intervals, for treatment and control groups with a total of 59 individuals. Table 8.8 gives the ratio of the sample variances to the means of the counts for each treatment-by-visit combination. A high degree of extra-Poisson variation is evident as the variance-to-mean ratios range from 7 to 39, whereas ratios of one correspond to the Poisson model. A commonly used model for *over-dispersed* count data, where the variance exceeds the mean, is the negative-binomial distribution. Here, we assume that given a rate μ_i, the Y_{ij} are independent Poisson variates with mean and variance equal to μ_i. The over-dispersion arises because the μ_i are assumed to vary across subjects according to a gamma distribution with mean μ and variance $\phi\mu^2$. Then, the marginal distribution of Y_{ij} has mean μ and variance $\mu + \phi\mu^2$ which exceeds the Poisson variance when $\phi > 0$. The negative binomial and other *random-effects* models for count data are discussed in more detail in Chapter 9.

In the regression context, we want to relate the counted response to explanatory variables. The most common assumption is

$$\log \mathrm{E}(Y_{ij}) = \boldsymbol{x}_{ij}'\boldsymbol{\beta}, \tag{8.4.1}$$

so that $\boldsymbol{\beta}$ describes the change in the log of the population-average count per unit change in x. If β_1 is the coefficient associated with the treatment assignment variable in the seizure data of Example 1.6, then $\exp(\beta_1)$ represents the ratio of average seizure rates, measured as the number of seizures

Table 8.8. Variance-to-mean ratios for the epileptic seizure data.

	Visit			
Treatment	1	2	3	4
Treated	38.7	16.8	23.8	18.8
Placebo	10.8	7.5	24.5	7.3

per two-week period, for the treated patients compared to that among the control patients. A negative value of β_1 is evidence that the treatment is effective relative to the placebo in controlling the seizure rate.

To account for the over-dispersion which is not prescribed by the Poisson distribution, one can assume instead that

$$\mathrm{Var}(Y_{ij}) = \phi_{ij}\mathrm{E}(Y_{ij}), \tag{8.4.2}$$

with $\phi_{ij} > 1$. To control the number of over-dispersion parameters, a regression model for the ϕ_{ij} is needed. For this, we can assume $\phi_{ij} = \phi(\boldsymbol{\alpha}_1)$, where α_1 is a vector of q_1 parameters. A simple version of $\phi(\boldsymbol{\alpha}_1)$ would be $\phi_{ij} = \phi_1$ if treated and ϕ_2 if control. Alternatively, we may allow a different ϕ at different time points, constant across subjects.

Until now, we have assumed that the interval lengths, t_{ij}, during which the events are observed, are the same for each subject, and for each visit. This is appropriate for the seizure data where the intervals after treatment are all two weeks. A special problem may emerge if the observations are collected at irregular times and Y_{ij} represents the number of events between successive visits. This problem, however, can be easily corrected by decomposing the marginal mean, $\mu_{ij} = \mathrm{E}(Y_{ij})$, into the product of t_{ij}, the known observation period, and λ_{ij}, an unknown parameter representing the rate of the counting process per unit time. The log-linear model (8.4.1) can then be applied to λ_{ij}, that is,

$$\log \lambda_{ij} = \boldsymbol{x}'_{ij}\boldsymbol{\beta},$$

so that a regression coefficient in $\boldsymbol{\beta}$ is a logarithm of the ratio of rates per unit interval of time. We note that

$$\log \mathrm{E}(Y_{ij}) = \log t_{ij} + \boldsymbol{x}'_{ij}\boldsymbol{\beta}.$$

This equation shows that we can take account of different interval lengths by introducing an *offset*, $\log t_{ij}$, into the log-linear model as explained in more detail by McCullagh and Nelder (1989).

Thus far, we have ignored parametric models for the correlation among repeated observations on a unit. The most natural models involve random effects, which will be discussed in Chapter 9. Taking a marginal approach, we can specify a parametric model for the correlation coefficient $\rho = \rho(\boldsymbol{\alpha}_2)$, where $\boldsymbol{\alpha}_2$ is a q_2-vector of parameters. As with binary responses, the ranges of correlations for pairs of counts are restricted by their means. Sensible models in addition to random effects models for the association among counts need further development.

8.4.2 *Generalized estimating equation approach*

We have suggested the use of $\boldsymbol{S}_{\boldsymbol{\beta}}$ in (8.2.4) to estimate the regression coefficient $\boldsymbol{\beta}$ for binary responses. The same estimating function can be used here, except that $\boldsymbol{S_\beta}$ depends not only on $\boldsymbol{\beta}$ and $\boldsymbol{\alpha}_2$, but also on $\boldsymbol{\alpha}_1$ because of the need to account for over-dispersion. Let $\boldsymbol{\alpha} = (\boldsymbol{\alpha}_1, \boldsymbol{\alpha}_2)$ be a vector of $q = q_1 + q_2$ parameters. We can now solve simultaneously the equations $\boldsymbol{S_\beta} = 0$ and

$$\boldsymbol{S}_\alpha(\boldsymbol{\beta}, \boldsymbol{\alpha}) = \sum_{i=1}^{m} \left(\frac{\partial \boldsymbol{\eta}_i}{\partial \boldsymbol{\alpha}}\right)' (\boldsymbol{W}_i - \boldsymbol{\eta}_i) = 0,$$

where $R_{ij} = \{Y_{ij} - \mu_{ij}\}/\{v(\mu_{ij})\}^{1/2}$, $\boldsymbol{W}_i' = (R_{i1}R_{i2}, \ldots, R_{in_i-1}R_{in_i}, R_{i1}^2, \ldots, R_{in_n}^2)$ and $\boldsymbol{\eta}_i = \mathrm{E}(\boldsymbol{W}_i)$.

There are two minor discrepancies between this procedure and the one suggested in Section 8.2.3. Firstly, the n_i squared terms of the R_{ij}'s have been added to $\boldsymbol{W}_i$ to estimate the overdispersion parameters, $\boldsymbol{\phi} = \boldsymbol{\phi}(\boldsymbol{\alpha}_1)$. Secondly, the diagonal matrix $\boldsymbol{H}_i$ used in (8.2.5) is set to be the identity matrix, so that $(\boldsymbol{S_\beta}, \boldsymbol{S_\alpha})$ depends on $\boldsymbol{\beta}$ and $\boldsymbol{\alpha}$ only. For binary data, $\mathrm{Cov}(Y_{ij}, Y_{ik})$ for $j \neq k$ is completely specified by (8.2.1) and (8.2.3), and no additional parameters are introduced. However, this is not the case for count data. By forcing $\boldsymbol{H}_i$ to be the identity matrix we potentially lose efficiency in estimating $\boldsymbol{\alpha}$. Our experience has suggested that this loss of efficiency has very little impact on the $\boldsymbol{\beta}$ estimation. Using $\boldsymbol{H}_i = \boldsymbol{I}$ avoids estimating additional higher-order parameters, and this reduces sampling variation.

Example 8.5. Epileptic seizures

We now revisit the seizure count data set considered briefly in Section 8.4.1. Fifty-nine epileptics suffering from partial seizures were randomized to receive either the anti-epileptic drug progabide ($m_1 = 31$) or a placebo ($m_2 = 28$). Patients from the two groups appear to be comparable in terms of baseline age (in years) and eight-week baseline seizure counts as shown in Table 8.9. The main objective of this study was to determine whether progabide reduces the rate of seizures.

Table 8.10 gives the mean seizure rates per two weeks stratified by treatment group and time (baseline versus visits 1–4). Overall, there is very

Table 8.9. Summary statistics for the epileptic seizure data.

Group	Age	Baseline seizure counts in 8 weeks
Treatment	27.7 ± 1.19	31.6 ± 5.03
Placebo	29.0 ± 1.13	30.8 ± 4.93

Table 8.10. Averaged seizure rates (per two weeks) by treatment and visit.

Treatment	Visit	Seizure rate
Progabide	Baseline	7.90
		(6.91)*
	1–4	7.96
		(5.71)*
Placebo	Baseline	7.70
	1–4	8.60
Cross-product ratio		0.90**
		(0.74)*

*Summary statistics when patient #207 is deleted.
**0.90 = (7.96/7.90)/(8.60/7.70).

little change in two-week seizure counts for the treated group (7.96/7.90 = 101%) and a small increase in the placebo group (8.60/7.70 = 112%). The treatment effect, measured by the cross-product ratio, is reported in the last row of Table 8.10. Patient number 207 appears to be very unusual. They had an extremely high seizure count (151 in eight weeks) at baseline and their count doubled after treatment to 302 seizures in eight weeks. If their data are set aside, the cross-product ratio drops from 0.90 to 0.74, giving some indication of a treatment benefit.

For more formal inference we now use a log-linear regression fitted by the GEE method as described in Sections 8.4.1 and 8.4.2. To estimate the overall treatment effect, we use the following model:

$$\log \mathrm{E}(Y_{ij}) = \log t_{ij} + \beta_0 + \beta_1 x_{ij1} + \beta_2 x_{i2} + \beta_3 x_{ij1} \cdot x_{i2},$$
$$j = 0, 1, 2, 3, 4, \quad i = 1, \ldots, 59. \tag{8.4.3}$$

Here, $t_{ij} = 8$ if $j = 0$ and $t_{ij} = 2$ if $j = 1, 2, 3, 4$. The $\log t_{ij}$ term is needed to account for different observation periods. The covariates are defined as

$$x_{ij1} = \begin{cases} 1 & \text{if visit } 1, 2, 3 \text{ or } 4, \\ 0 & \text{if baseline,} \end{cases} \qquad x_{i2} = \begin{cases} 1 & \text{if progabide,} \\ 0 & \text{if placebo.} \end{cases}$$

The variable x_{i2} is included in the model to allow different distributions of baseline seizure counts between the treated and placebo groups. The parameter $\exp(\beta_1)$ is the ratio of the average seizure rate after treatment to before treatment for the placebo group. The coefficient of interest, β_3, represents the difference in the logarithm of the post- to pre-treatment

Table 8.11. Log-linear regression coefficients and robust standard errors (in parentheses) for analysis of seizure rates. The model in (8.4.3) was fitted using GEE assuming exchangeable correlation, with and without patient number 207 who had unusual pre- and post-randomization seizure counts.

Variable	Complete data	Patient 207 deleted
Intercept	1.35	1.35
	(0.16)	(0.16)
Time (x_1)	0.11	0.11
	(0.12)	(0.12)
Treatment (x_2)	0.027	−0.11
	(0.22)	(0.19)
$x_1 \cdot x_2$	−0.10	−0.30
	(0.21)	(0.17)
Over-dispersion parameter	19.4	10.4
Correlation coefficient	0.78	0.60

ratio between the progabide and placebo groups. A negative coefficient corresponds to a greater reduction (or smaller increase) in the seizure counts for the progabide group.

The results given in Table 8.11 suggest that, overall, there is very little difference between the treatment and placebo groups in the change of seizure counts before and after the randomization ($\hat{\beta}_3 = -0.10 \pm 0.21$) if patient number 207 is included. If this patient is set aside, there is modest evidence that progabide is favoured over the placebo. Note also that different conclusions would be drawn if the strong over-dispersion ($\hat{\phi} = 19.44$) was ignored since the standardized test statistic, $Z = \hat{\beta}_3/\sqrt{\{\text{Var}(\hat{\beta}_3)\}}$ would have been inflated by $(19.4)^{1/2} = 4.4$, and would be statistically significant at the 5% level.

8.5 Sample size calculations revisited

In Section 2.4 we presented sample size formulas for longitudinal studies with continuous and binary responses. The focus was on the simple two-group comparison with equal sizes for both groups. In clinical trials, patients may be randomized to three or more groups with varying numbers of subjects participating. Furthermore, it is important in observational studies that major confounding effects be adequately adjusted through, for example, regression modelling, and that such an adjustment be appropriately acknowledged when calculating the sample size needed. In this section, we outline a general approach for sample size calculations with longitudinal observations addressing the limitations mentioned above. The approach was developed by Liu and Liang (1997) who extended the earlier work by Self and Mauritsen (1988) for independent observations. In general, unlike in Section 2.4, no closed form expressions for sample size are available.

We assume that the scientific objective can be formulated through a marginal model. Specifically, we assume that

$$h(\mu_{ij}) = \boldsymbol{x}_{ij}'\boldsymbol{\beta} + \boldsymbol{z}_{ij}'\boldsymbol{\lambda},$$

where $\boldsymbol{\beta}$, a $p \times 1$ vector, representing parameters of interest and $\boldsymbol{\lambda}$, a $q \times 1$ vector, is introduced to allow adjustment for other effects. The hypothesis of interest is then H_0: $\boldsymbol{\beta} = \boldsymbol{\beta}_0$, a pre-specified value for $\boldsymbol{\beta}$. Thus, in conventional clinical trials where patients are assigned to one of three treated groups of different dosage levels or to the placebo group, $\boldsymbol{x}_{ij}$ would represent $p = 3$, dummy variables indicating treatment status, with the placebo as the reference group. In cross-over trials with two treatments (A versus B), p would be equal to 1 with

$$(x_{i1}, x_{i2}) = \begin{cases} (1,0) & \text{if subject receives Treatment A followed by B,} \\ (0,1) & \text{if subject receives Treatment B followed by A.} \end{cases}$$

In observational studies where confounding adjustment is critical, $\boldsymbol{z}_{ij}$ would represent q major confounding variables measured at the jth visit whereas $\boldsymbol{x}_{ij}$ would represent dummy variables for different exposure levels of interest such as maternal smoking status.

To test the null hypothesis that $\boldsymbol{\beta} = \boldsymbol{\beta}_0$, we consider the following GEE test statistic

$$T = \boldsymbol{S}_{\boldsymbol{\beta}}'(\boldsymbol{\beta}_0, \hat{\boldsymbol{\lambda}}_0, \boldsymbol{\alpha})\mathbf{B}_0^{-1}\boldsymbol{S}_{\boldsymbol{\beta}}(\boldsymbol{\beta}_0, \hat{\boldsymbol{\lambda}}_0, \boldsymbol{\alpha}),$$

where

$$\boldsymbol{S}_{\boldsymbol{\beta}}(\boldsymbol{\beta}_0, \hat{\boldsymbol{\lambda}}_0, \boldsymbol{\alpha}) = \sum_{i=1}^{m} \left(\frac{\partial \boldsymbol{\mu}_i(\boldsymbol{\beta}_0, \hat{\boldsymbol{\lambda}}_0)}{\partial \boldsymbol{\beta}} \right)' V_i^{-1}(\boldsymbol{\beta}_0, \hat{\boldsymbol{\lambda}}_0, \boldsymbol{\alpha})(\boldsymbol{y}_i - \boldsymbol{\mu}_i(\boldsymbol{\beta}_0, \hat{\boldsymbol{\lambda}}_0)),$$

$$\mathbf{B}_0 = \text{Cov}\{\boldsymbol{S}_{\boldsymbol{\beta}}(\boldsymbol{\beta}_0, \hat{\boldsymbol{\lambda}}_0, \boldsymbol{\alpha})\}, \quad V_i = \text{Cov}(\boldsymbol{Y}_i; \boldsymbol{\beta}, \boldsymbol{\lambda}, \boldsymbol{\alpha}),$$

and $\hat{\boldsymbol{\lambda}}_0$ is an estimator of $\boldsymbol{\lambda}$ under H_0 obtained by solving

$$\sum_{i=1}^{m} \left(\frac{\partial \boldsymbol{\mu}_i(\boldsymbol{\beta}_0, \boldsymbol{\lambda})}{\partial \boldsymbol{\lambda}} \right)' V_i^{-1}(\boldsymbol{\beta}_0, \boldsymbol{\lambda}, \boldsymbol{\alpha})(\boldsymbol{y}_i - \boldsymbol{\mu}_i(\boldsymbol{\beta}_0, \boldsymbol{\lambda})) = 0.$$

Under H_0, T converges as $m \to \infty$ to a χ_p^2 distribution whereas under H_1, $\boldsymbol{\beta} = \boldsymbol{\beta}_1$ and $\boldsymbol{\lambda} = \boldsymbol{\lambda}_1$, T follows a non-central chi-square distribution asymptotically with the non-centrality parameter

$$\nu = \boldsymbol{\zeta}'\mathbf{B}_1^{-1}\boldsymbol{\zeta}. \tag{8.5.1}$$

Here, $\boldsymbol{\zeta} = \mathrm{E}_{H_1}(\boldsymbol{S}_{\boldsymbol{\beta}}(\boldsymbol{\beta}_0, \boldsymbol{\lambda}_0, \boldsymbol{\alpha}))$ and $\mathbf{B}_1 = \mathrm{Cov}_{H_1}(\boldsymbol{S}_{\boldsymbol{\beta}}, \boldsymbol{\lambda}_0, \boldsymbol{\alpha})$; see Liu and Liang (1997) for detailed expressions. In particular, $\boldsymbol{\zeta}$ involves the calculation of $\boldsymbol{\mu}_i' - \boldsymbol{\mu}_i^*$, where $\mu_{ij}' = h(\boldsymbol{x}_{ij}'\boldsymbol{\beta}_1 + \boldsymbol{z}_{ij}'\boldsymbol{\lambda}_1)$, $\mu_{ij}^* = h(\boldsymbol{x}_{ij}'\boldsymbol{\beta}_0 + \boldsymbol{z}_{ij}'\boldsymbol{\lambda}_0^*)$ and λ_0^* denotes the estimate of λ which is obtained when H_1 is true but we assume H_0, that is we fix $\beta = \beta_0$.

To complete the process, we further assume that $n_i = n$ and that the covariates $\{(\boldsymbol{x}_{ij}, \boldsymbol{z}_{ij}), j = 1, \ldots, n\}$ are discrete with L distinct values. Thus, in conventional clinical trials with $p + 1$ treatments as mentioned earlier, $x_{ij} = x_i$ and $z_{ij} \equiv 1$, hence $L = p + 1$. In this setting, both $\boldsymbol{\zeta}$ and $\mathbf{B}_1$ in (8.5.1) have expressions of the form $\boldsymbol{\zeta} = m\tilde{\boldsymbol{\zeta}}$ and $\mathbf{B}_1 = m\tilde{\mathbf{B}}_1$, where $\tilde{\boldsymbol{\zeta}}$ and $\tilde{\mathbf{B}}_1$ involves combinations weighted according to probabilities associated with each of L distinct values that the covariates take. We can then obtain an explicit expression for the necessary sample size, m, as

$$m = \nu \Big/ \left(\tilde{\boldsymbol{\zeta}}\tilde{\mathbf{B}}_1^{-1}\tilde{\boldsymbol{\zeta}}\right), \tag{8.5.2}$$

where ν is derived from a non-central chi-squared distribution in accordance with the specified types I and II errors.

Through simulations, Liu and Liang (1997) found that the sample size calculations outline above lead to an excellent agreement between the simulated power and the pre-specified power. As expected, the sample size formula in (8.5.2) coincides with that in Section 2.4 for the special cases considered therein.

8.6 Further reading

This chapter has discussed the fitting of marginal models to discrete longitudinal data. We have emphasized the problem of describing the relationship between the marginal expectation of the response and covariates at each visit. In contrast to Chapter 5, we have given very little attention to the mechanisms by which the within-subject association may have arisen. Readers interested in this issue are referred to Zeger *et al.* (1988) and Thall and Vail (1990).

The use of GEE to estimate regression coefficients specified by marginal models has been studied extensively over the last fifteen years. For more detailed treatments, see Liang and Zeger (1986), Zeger and Liang (1986),

Prentice (1988), Zhao and Prentice (1990), Thall and Vail (1990), Liang *et al.* (1992), and Fitzmaurice and Laird (1993).

It is not uncommon in biomedical studies to encounter response variables which are categorical with more than two categories. A typical example is when the response measures the severity of injury. Regression models for polytomous responses, ordinal or nominal, are available. See, for example, McCullagh (1980) and Anderson (1984). Extensions of GEE to this situation can be found in Stram *et al.* (1988), Liang *et al.* (1992) and Heagerty and Zeger (1996).

Extensions of GEE for discrete survival outcomes is presented in TenHave and Uttal (1994), Guo and Lin (1994), Shih (1998), Clayton (1992) and Heagerty and Zeger (2000).

Readers are referred to the book by Jones and Kenward (1989) for the use of crossover designs in clinical trials. For the more common pre-post designs, there is extensive literature on how the response variable measured at baseline might best be utilized. See, for example, Stanek (1988), Laird and Wang (1990), Frison and Pocock (1992, 1997) and Liang and Zeger (2000) and the references therein.

9

Random effects models

9.1 Introduction

Chapter 8 has dealt with marginal models whose regression parameters have population average interpretations. In this chapter we consider random effects models in which the regression coefficients measure the more direct influence of explanatory variables on the responses for heterogeneous individuals. Linear models with random effects were discussed in Section 5.2 in the context of a general framework for parametric modelling of correlation in longitudinal data. The use of random effects in the generalized linear model (GLM) family was introduced in Section 7.2 where the coefficients were contrasted with those from marginal and transition models. In Chapter 7, we used the notation $\boldsymbol{\beta}, \boldsymbol{\beta}^*$, and $\boldsymbol{\beta}^{**}$ to distinguish marginal, random effects and transition coefficients, respectively. For the remainder of the book, we will use $\boldsymbol{\beta}$ for any regression coefficients as long as the type of model is clear from the context.

As discussed in Section 7.2, the basic premise of the random effects model is that there is natural heterogeneity among subjects in a subset of the regression coefficients, for example in the intercepts. Using the GLM framework, we assume that conditional on unobservable variables $\boldsymbol{U}_i$, we have independent responses from a distribution in the exponential family (see Appendix A, equation (A.5.1)) such that

$$h\{\mathrm{E}(Y_{ij} \mid \boldsymbol{U}_i)\} = \boldsymbol{x}_{ij}'\boldsymbol{\beta} + \boldsymbol{d}_{ij}'\boldsymbol{U}_i. \tag{9.1.1}$$

Here, h is the link function and $\boldsymbol{x}_{ij}$ and $\boldsymbol{d}_{ij}$ are covariate vectors of length p and q, respectively.

To illustrate briefly, consider the 2×2 crossover trial data in Example 8.1 and suppose that a person's response follows the logistic model

$$\text{logit } \Pr(Y_{ij} = 1 \mid U_i) = \beta_0 + U_i + \beta_1 x_{ij}, \tag{9.1.2}$$

where x_{ij} indicates whether the person received placebo ($x = 0$) or drug ($x = 1$). This model states that each person on placebo has their own probability of a normal response ($Y = 1$) given by

$$P(Y_i = 1) = \exp(\beta_0 + U_i)/\{1 + \exp(\beta_0 + U_i)\}.$$

It further states that a person's odds of a normal response are multiplied by $\exp(\beta_1)$ when taking the drug, regardless of the initial risk.

Another simple case is when $\boldsymbol{x}_{ij} = \boldsymbol{d}_{ij}$ so that each individual can be thought to have their own regression coefficients $\boldsymbol{\beta} + \boldsymbol{U}_i$. With a large number of observations for a subject, we could estimate their individual coefficients from $\boldsymbol{y}_i$. But in practice, we have limited data and must borrow strength across subjects to make inferences about either $\boldsymbol{\beta}$ or the $\boldsymbol{U}_i$. This is accomplished by assuming that the $\boldsymbol{U}_i$ are independent realizations from a distribution.

There are two distinct approaches to inference about random effects models. The first is appropriate when we are interested in a particular subset of regression coefficients, none of which are assumed to vary across subjects. For example, suppose we want to estimate the drug effect in the crossover trial and believe that only the intercept, not the drug effect, varies across individuals. Here, we can treat the $\boldsymbol{U}_i$ as nuisance effects and condition them out of the problem. That is, we can attempt to use only that part of the data which does not contain information about the $\boldsymbol{U}_i$ when making inference about particular coefficients. The second approach is appropriate when the subject-specific coefficients are themselves of interest or when conditioning away the information about the random effects discards too much information about an important regression coefficient. Here, we operate as if the $\boldsymbol{U}_i$ are an independent sample from some distribution and estimate both the fixed effects, $\boldsymbol{\beta}$, and the random effects, $\boldsymbol{U}_i$, under this working model.

In random intercept models, the choice between these two approaches relates to the distinction between cross-sectional and longitudinal information discussed in Sections 1.1 and 1.4, and illustrated in Fig. 1.1. With the conditional likelihood approach, we use only longitudinal information, that is, comparisons within subjects, to estimate $\boldsymbol{\beta}$. When we assume that the $\boldsymbol{U}_i$ follow a distribution, we combine both longitudinal and cross-sectional information. The relative weight given to each source is determined by the variability among the $\boldsymbol{U}_i$. When there is large variability across subjects, the analysis should weight the longitudinal information more heavily since comparisons within a subject are likely to be more precise than comparisons among subjects.

Note that a fundamental assumption of the random effects model is that the $\boldsymbol{U}_i$ are independent of the explanatory variables. If this assumption is incorrect in the random intercept case, the conditional analysis will still give a consistent estimate of $\boldsymbol{\beta}$. The random effects analysis will not. Econometricians (e.g. Hausman, 1978) have developed what they call *specification tests* to check the random effects assumption. The model for longitudinal data in Section 1.4, which includes both cross-sectional and longitudinal parameters, is one way to allow random intercepts to depend on explanatory variables.

The remainder of the chapter is organized as follows. Section 9.2 discusses estimation of $\boldsymbol{\beta}$ in the random effects GLM using both conditional and full maximum likelihood. The latter is computationally expensive to implement in general, and we shall review an approximate method which works reasonably well for estimation of $\boldsymbol{\beta}$ in certain situations. Chapter 11 discusses some recent developments for full likelihood-based approaches which improve on the approximate methods described here. We consider logistic models for binary data in Section 9.3 and Poisson regression models for count data in Section 9.4.

9.2 Estimation for generalized linear mixed models

In the random effects GLM we assume:

(1) the conditional distribution of Y_{ij} given $\boldsymbol{U}_i$ follows a distribution from the exponential family with density $f(y_{ij} \mid \boldsymbol{U}_i; \boldsymbol{\beta})$;

(2) given $\boldsymbol{U}_i$, the repeated measurements, $Y_{i1}, \ldots, Y_{n_i}$, are independent;

(3) the $\boldsymbol{U}_i$ are independent and identically distributed with density function $f(\boldsymbol{U}_i; G)$.

Let $\boldsymbol{U} = (\boldsymbol{U}_1, \ldots, \boldsymbol{U}_m)$. In the subsection below on conditional likelihood, we will treat the random effects as if they were fixed parameters to be removed from the problem, so that we need not rely on the third assumption above. In the subsection on maximum likelihood estimation, we will treat $\boldsymbol{U}$ as a set of unobserved variables which we then integrate out of the likelihood, adopting the assumption that the random effects distribution is Gaussian with mean zero and variance matrix G.

9.2.1 *Conditional likelihood*

In this subsection, we review conditional maximum likelihood estimation for $\boldsymbol{\beta}$. McCullagh and Nelder (1989, Section 7.2) present a more general treatment for GLMs. The main idea is to treat the random effects, $\boldsymbol{U}_i$, as a set of nuisance parameters and to estimate $\boldsymbol{\beta}$ using the conditional likelihood of the data given the sufficient statistics for the $\boldsymbol{U}_i$.

Treating $\boldsymbol{U}$ as fixed, the likelihood function for $\boldsymbol{\beta}$ and $\boldsymbol{U}$ is

$$\prod_{i=1}^{m}\prod_{j=1}^{n_i} f(y_{ij} \mid \boldsymbol{\beta}, \boldsymbol{U}_i) \propto \prod_{i=1}^{m}\prod_{j=1}^{n_i} \exp\{\theta_{ij} y_{ij} - \psi(\theta_{ij})\}, \tag{9.2.1}$$

where $\theta_{ij} = \theta_{ij}(\boldsymbol{\beta}, \boldsymbol{U})$. To simplify the discussion, we restrict attention to canonical link functions (McCullagh and Nelder, 1989, p. 32) for which $\theta_{ij} = \boldsymbol{x}_{ij}'\boldsymbol{\beta} + \boldsymbol{d}_{ij}'\boldsymbol{U}_i$. Then the likelihood above can be written as

$$\exp\left\{\boldsymbol{\beta}'\sum_{i,j}\boldsymbol{x}_{ij}y_{ij} + \sum_i \boldsymbol{U}_i'\sum_j \boldsymbol{d}_{ij}y_{ij} - \sum_{i,j}\psi(\theta_{ij})\right\}. \tag{9.2.2}$$

Hence, the sufficient statistics for $\boldsymbol{\beta}$ and $\boldsymbol{U}_i$ are $\sum_{i,j}\boldsymbol{x}_{ij}y_{ij}$ and $\sum_j \boldsymbol{d}_{ij}y_{ij}$ respectively, and $\sum_j \boldsymbol{d}_{ij}y_{ij}$ is sufficient for $\boldsymbol{U}_i$ for fixed $\boldsymbol{\beta}$.

The conditional likelihood is proportional to the conditional distribution of the data given the sufficient statistics for the $\boldsymbol{U}_i$. The contribution from subject i has the form

$$\begin{aligned} f\left(\boldsymbol{y}_i \mid \sum_j \boldsymbol{d}_{ij}y_{ij} = \boldsymbol{b}_i; \boldsymbol{\beta}\right) &= \frac{f(\boldsymbol{y}_i; \boldsymbol{\beta}, \boldsymbol{U}_i)}{f\left(\sum_j \boldsymbol{d}_{ij}y_{ij} = \boldsymbol{b}_i; \boldsymbol{\beta}, \boldsymbol{U}_i\right)} \\ &= \frac{f\left(\sum_j \boldsymbol{x}_{ij}y_{ij} = \boldsymbol{a}_i, \sum_j \boldsymbol{d}_{ij}y_{ij} = \boldsymbol{b}_i; \boldsymbol{\beta}, \boldsymbol{U}_i\right)}{f\left(\sum_j \boldsymbol{d}_{ij}y_{ij} = \boldsymbol{b}_i; \boldsymbol{\beta}, \boldsymbol{U}_i\right)}. \end{aligned} \tag{9.2.3}$$

For a discrete GLM this expression can be written as

$$\frac{\sum_{R_{i1}} \exp(\boldsymbol{\beta}'\boldsymbol{a}_i + \boldsymbol{U}_i'\boldsymbol{b}_i)}{\sum_{R_{i2}} \exp\left(\boldsymbol{\beta}'\sum_j \boldsymbol{x}_{ij}y_{ij} + \boldsymbol{U}_i'\boldsymbol{b}_i\right)},$$

where R_{i1} is the set of possible values for $\boldsymbol{y}_i$ such that $\sum_j \boldsymbol{x}_{ij}y_{ij} = \boldsymbol{a}_i$ and $\sum_j \boldsymbol{d}_{ij}y_{ij} = \boldsymbol{b}_i$, and R_{i2} is the set of values for $\boldsymbol{y}_i$ such that $\sum_j \boldsymbol{d}_{ij}y_{ij} = \boldsymbol{b}_i$. The conditional likelihood for $\boldsymbol{\beta}$ given the data for all m individuals simplifies to

$$\prod_{i=1}^{m} \frac{\sum_{R_{i1}} \exp(\boldsymbol{\beta}'\boldsymbol{a}_i)}{\sum_{R_{i2}} \exp\left(\boldsymbol{\beta}'\sum_{j=1}^{n_i} \boldsymbol{x}_{ij}y_{ij}\right)}. \tag{9.2.4}$$

For simple cases such as the random intercept model, the conditional likelihood is reasonably easy to maximize (Breslow and Day, 1980). Random intercept models for binary and count data are considered in more detail below.

9.2.2 *Maximum likelihood estimation*

Here, we will treat the $\boldsymbol{U}_i$ as a sample of independent unobservable variables from a random effects distribution. Qualitatively, this assumption implies that we can learn about one individual's coefficients by understanding the variability in coefficients across the population. When there is little variability, we should rely on the population average coefficients to estimate those for an individual. When there is substantial variation, we must rely more heavily on the data from each individual in estimating their own coefficients. This idea was illustrated in Section 5.5, where our objective was to estimate an individual subject's CD4 trajectory.

The likelihood function for the unknown parameter $\boldsymbol{\delta}$, which is defined to include both $\boldsymbol{\beta}$ and the elements of G, is

$$L(\boldsymbol{\delta}; \boldsymbol{y}) = \prod_{i=1}^{m} \int \prod_{j=1}^{n_i} f(y_{ij} \mid \boldsymbol{U}_i; \boldsymbol{\beta}) f(\boldsymbol{U}_i; G)\, \mathrm{d}\boldsymbol{U}_i. \tag{9.2.5}$$

This is just the marginal distribution of $\boldsymbol{Y}$ obtained by integrating the joint distribution of $\boldsymbol{Y}$ and $\boldsymbol{U}$ with respect to $\boldsymbol{U}$. In some special cases such as the Gaussian linear model (Chapters 4–6), the integral above has a closed form, but for most non-Gaussian models, numerical methods are required for its evaluation.

To find the maximum likelihood estimate, we can solve the score equations obtained by setting to zero the derivative with respect to $\boldsymbol{\delta}$ of the log likelihood. If we imagine that the 'complete' data for an individual comprise $(\boldsymbol{y}_i, \boldsymbol{U}_i)$ and if we restrict attention for the moment to canonical link functions, then the *complete data* score function for $\boldsymbol{\beta}$ has a particularly simple form

$$\boldsymbol{S}_{\boldsymbol{\beta}}(\boldsymbol{\delta} \mid \boldsymbol{y}, \boldsymbol{U}) = \sum_{i=1}^{m} \sum_{j=1}^{n_i} \boldsymbol{x}_{ij} \{y_{ij} - \mu_{ij}(\boldsymbol{U}_i)\} = 0, \tag{9.2.6}$$

where $\mu_{ij}(\boldsymbol{U}_i) = \mathrm{E}(y_{ij} \mid \boldsymbol{U}_i) = h^{-1}(\boldsymbol{x}'_{ij}\boldsymbol{\beta} + \boldsymbol{d}'_{ij}\boldsymbol{U}_i)$. The observed data score equations are obtained by taking the expectation of the complete data equations with respect to the conditional distribution of the unobserved random effects given the data. That is, we define the observed data score functions, $\boldsymbol{S}_{\boldsymbol{\beta}}(\boldsymbol{\delta} \mid \boldsymbol{y})$, as the expectations of the complete data score functions, $\boldsymbol{S}_{\boldsymbol{\beta}}(\boldsymbol{\delta} \mid \boldsymbol{y}, \boldsymbol{U})$, with respect to the conditional distribution of $\boldsymbol{U}$ given $\boldsymbol{y}$. This gives,

$$\boldsymbol{S}_{\boldsymbol{\beta}}(\boldsymbol{\delta} \mid \boldsymbol{y}) = \sum_{i=1}^{m} \sum_{j=1}^{n_i} \boldsymbol{x}_{ij} [y_{ij} - \mathrm{E}\{\mu_{ij}(\boldsymbol{U}_i) \mid \boldsymbol{y}_i\}] = 0. \tag{9.2.7}$$

The score equations for G can similarly be obtained as

$$\boldsymbol{S}_G(\boldsymbol{\delta} \mid \boldsymbol{y}) = \frac{1}{2} G^{-1} \left\{ \sum_{i=1}^{m} \mathrm{E}(\boldsymbol{U}_i \boldsymbol{U}'_i \mid \boldsymbol{y}_i) \right\} G^{-1} - \frac{m}{2} G^{-1} = 0. \tag{9.2.8}$$

To solve for the maximum likelihood estimate of $\boldsymbol{\delta}$, a common strategy is to use the EM algorithm (Dempster *et al.*, 1977). This algorithm iterates between an E-step, which involves evaluating the expectations in the score equations above using the current values of the parameters, and an M-step, in which we solve the score equations to give updated parameter estimates.

The dimension of the integration involved in the conditional expectations is q, the dimension of $\boldsymbol{U}_i$. When q is one or two, numerical integration techniques can be implemented reasonably easily (e.g. Crouch and Spiegelman, 1990). For higher dimensional problems, Monte Carlo integration methods can be used. See, for example, the application of Gibbs sampling in Zeger and Karim (1991).

An alternative strategy is to approximate the score equations in such a way that the integrations can be avoided. This approach has been used by Stiratelli *et al.* (1984) for logistic models with Gaussian random effects, Karim (1991), Schall (1991), and Breslow and Clayton (1993) for random effects GLMs, and Lindstrom and Bates (1990) for non-linear regression models with Gaussian random effects and errors. The central idea is to use conditional modes rather than conditional means in the score equation for $\boldsymbol{\beta}$. This is equivalent to approximating the conditional distribution of $\boldsymbol{U}_i$ given $\boldsymbol{y}_i$ by a Gaussian distribution with the same mode and curvature. By using modes rather than means, we replace the integration with an optimization that can be incorporated into the M-step.

To specify the algorithm more completely, let $v_{ij} = \mathrm{Var}(y_{ij} \mid \boldsymbol{U}_i)$ and $Q_i = \mathrm{diag}\{v_{ij}h'(\mu_{ij})^2\}$. Let $\boldsymbol{z}_i$ be the surrogate response defined to have elements $z_{ij} = h(\mu_{ij}) + (y_{ij} - \mu_{ij})h'(\mu_{ij})$, $j = 1, \ldots, n_i$ and define the $n_i \times n_i$ matrix $V_i = Q_i + D_i G D_i'$, where D_i is the $n_i \times q$ matrix whose jth row is $\boldsymbol{d}_{ij}$. For a fixed G, updated values of $\boldsymbol{\beta}$ and $\boldsymbol{U}$ are obtained by iteratively solving

$$\hat{\boldsymbol{\beta}} = \left(\sum_{i=1}^{m} X_i' V_i^{-1} X_i\right)^{-1} \sum_{i=1}^{m} X_i' V_i^{-1} \boldsymbol{z}_i \tag{9.2.9}$$

and

$$\hat{\boldsymbol{U}}_i = G D_i V_i^{-1}(\boldsymbol{z}_i - X_i \boldsymbol{\beta}).$$

These equations are an application of Harville's (1977) method for linear random effects models to a linearized version of the possibly non-linear estimating equations in the GLM extension.

To estimate G, note that the score equation (9.2.8) implies that

$$\hat{G} = m^{-1} \sum_{i=1}^{m} \mathrm{E}(\boldsymbol{U}_i \boldsymbol{U}_i' \mid \boldsymbol{y}_i) \tag{9.2.10}$$

$$= m^{-1} \sum_{i=1}^{m} \mathrm{E}(\boldsymbol{U}_i \mid \boldsymbol{y}_i)\mathrm{E}(\boldsymbol{U}_i \mid \boldsymbol{y}_i)' + m^{-1} \sum_{i=1}^{m} \mathrm{Var}(\boldsymbol{U}_i \mid \boldsymbol{y}_i). \tag{9.2.11}$$

The quantity $\hat{\boldsymbol{U}}_i$ is an estimate of $\mathrm{E}(\boldsymbol{U}_i \mid \boldsymbol{y}_i)$. An estimate of the conditional variance is $(D_i'Q_i^{-1}D_i + G^{-1})^{-1}$. Note that the parameters appear on both sides of equations (9.2.9) and (9.2.10) so that the algorithm proceeds by iteratively updating first the estimates of the regression coefficients and the random effects, and then the variance of the random effects, until the parameter estimates converge. A variety of slightly different algorithms for estimation of G have been proposed. See Breslow and Clayton (1993) for one specific implementation and an evaluation of its performance.

This approximate method gives reasonable estimates of $\boldsymbol{\beta}$ in many problems. The estimates of $\boldsymbol{U}_i$ and G are more sensitive to the Gaussian approximation to the conditional distribution. The approximation breaks down when there are few observations per subject and the GLM is far from the Gaussian. Karim (1991) and Breslow and Clayton (1993) have evaluated this approximate method for some specific random effects GLMs. More recently, Breslow and Lin (1995) and Lin and Breslow (1996) proposed a bias correction method by expanding the approximate likelihood, which they termed penalized quasi-likelihood, at random effects parameters G. They found that bias reduction is satisfactory, especially for large values of G.

9.3 Logistic regression for binary responses

9.3.1 *Conditional likelihood approach*

In this section, we consider the random intercept logistic model for binary data given by

$$\operatorname{logit} \Pr(Y_{ij} = 1 \mid U_i) = \beta_0 + U_i + \boldsymbol{x}_{ij}'\boldsymbol{\beta}. \tag{9.3.1}$$

To simplify the discussion, we will write $\gamma_i = \beta_0 + U_i$ and assume that $\boldsymbol{x}_{ij}$ does not include an intercept term. The joint likelihood function for $\boldsymbol{\beta}$ and the γ_i is proportional to

$$\prod_{i=1}^{m} \exp\left[\gamma_i \sum_{j=1}^{n_i} y_{ij} + \left(\sum_{j=1}^{n_i} y_{ij}\boldsymbol{x}_{ij}'\right)\boldsymbol{\beta} - \sum_{j=1}^{n_i} \log\left\{1 + \exp(\gamma_i + \boldsymbol{x}_{ij}'\boldsymbol{\beta})\right\}\right]. \tag{9.3.2}$$

The conditional likelihood for β given the sufficient statistics for the γ_i has the form

$$\prod_{i=1}^{m} \frac{\exp\left(\sum_{j=1}^{n_i} y_{ij}\boldsymbol{x}_{ij}'\boldsymbol{\beta}\right)}{\sum_{R_i} \exp\left(\sum_{\ell=1}^{y_{i\cdot}} \boldsymbol{x}_{i\ell}'\boldsymbol{\beta}\right)} \tag{9.3.3}$$

where $y_{i\cdot} = \sum_{j=1}^{n_i} y_{ij}$ and the index set R_i contains all the $\binom{n_i}{y_{i\cdot}}$ ways of choosing $y_{i\cdot}$ positive responses out of n_i repeated observations.

Table 9.1. Notation for a 2×2 crossover trial.

Group	$(1,1)$	$(0,1)$	$(1,0)$	$(0,0)$
AB	a_1	b_1	c_1	d_1
BA	a_2	b_2	c_2	d_2

The conditional likelihood above is equivalent to the one derived in stratified case-control studies (Breslow and Day, 1980). In that context, there are m strata; in the ith stratum, there are $y_{i.}$ cases and $n_i - y_{i.}$ controls. This connection is important in that any statistical package suitable for the analysis of the stratified case-control studies can be used to fit a random intercept logistic model to binary longitudinal data with little or no modification.

Example 9.1. The 2×2 crossover trial

Let a, b, c, and d denote the numbers of response pairs for each of the four possible combinations of outcomes in a 2×2 crossover trial, as shown in Table 9.1.

For example, b_1 is the number of subjects in the first group, who received the active treatment (A) followed by placebo (B) with outcomes (1,0), that is with a normal response ($Y = 1$) at the first visit and an abnormal response ($Y = 0$) at the second.

For the logistic model (9.3.1) which includes only the treatment variable x_1, the conditional likelihood (9.2.4) reduces to

$$\left\{\frac{\exp(\beta_1)}{1+\exp(\beta_1)}\right\}^{b_1+b_2}\left\{\frac{1}{1+\exp(\beta_1)}\right\}^{c_1+c_2}.$$

The estimate of β_1 which maximizes this conditional likelihood is

$$\hat{\beta}_1 = \log\{(b_1+b_2)/(c_1+c_2)\}.$$

Its variance can be estimated by $(b_1+b_2)^{-1} + (c_1+c_2)^{-1}$.

If the period effect (x_2) is now added to the model, the conditional likelihood function becomes

$$\frac{\exp\{(\beta_1+\beta_2)b_1\}}{\{1+\exp(\beta_1+\beta_2)\}^{b_1+c_1}}\;\frac{\exp\{(\beta_1-\beta_2)b_2\}}{\{1+\exp(\beta_1-\beta_2)\}^{b_2+c_2}}.$$

The maximum conditional likelihood estimate of β_1 and the corresponding variance estimate are, respectively

$$\hat{\beta}_1 = \frac{1}{2}\log\left(\frac{b_1 b_2}{c_1 c_2}\right), \quad \widehat{\mathrm{Var}}(\hat{\beta}_1) = \frac{1}{4}\left(b_1^{-1} + c_1^{-1} + b_2^{-1} + c_2^{-1}\right).$$

For the 2×2 crossover data on cerebrovascular deficiency, previously discussed as Example 8.1, we have $b_1 = 6$, $c_1 = 0$, $b_2 = 4$, and $c_2 = 2$. For the model including the treatment variable only, the treatment effect, β_1, is estimated as $\log\{(6+4)/(0+2)\} = 1.61$ with estimated standard error 0.77. A similar result is obtained when the period effect is included in the model. The treatment effect is now estimated as $\frac{1}{2}\log\{(6 \times 4)/(0.5 \times 2)\} = 1.59$ with estimated standard error 0.85. Note that we have used the convention of replacing the zero cell with 0.5 in this calculation. Nevertheless, the data indicate that the odds of a normal electrocardiogram for the treated patients are about five times ($5 = \exp(1.6)$) greater than the odds for patients receiving the placebo. This finding from the conditional inference is to be contrasted with the results from fitting a marginal model in Example 8.1 of Section 8.3. For the marginal model, we estimated a roughly two-fold increase in the odds for the treated group. The smaller value from the marginal analysis is consistent with the theoretical inequality stated in Section 7.4.

Example 9.2. The 3×3 crossover trial

Table 9.2 gives the results of fitting a random intercept logistic regression model by conditional likelihood to the crossover data from Example 8.2. The table reports the estimated regression coefficients and their standard errors.

Strong treatment effects are evident after adjusting for period and carryover effects. The chance of dysmenorrhoea relief for a patient is increased by a factor of $\exp(1.98) = 7.3$ if her treatment is switched from placebo to a low dose of analgesic and by a factor of $\exp(1.71) = 5.5$ if treatment is switched from placebo to a high dose.

The principal advantage of the conditional likelihood approach is that we remove the random effects from the likelihood by which we estimate $\boldsymbol{\beta}$, thus avoiding the assumption that they are a sample from a particular probability distribution. The disadvantage is that we rely entirely on within-subject comparisons. So persons with $y_{i.} = n_i$ or $y_{i.} = 0$ provide no information about the regression coefficients. In the 2×2 crossover

Table 9.2. Results for a conditional likelihood analysis of data from a 3×3 crossover trial.

	Treatment		Period		Carryover	
Variable	B	C	2	3	B	C
Coefficient	1.98	1.71	0.69	0.85	−0.14	−1.24
Standard error	(0.45)	(0.41)	(0.56)	(0.58)	(0.60)	(0.65)

trials, this means that $a_1 + d_1 + a_2 + d_2$ pairs are uninformative. In the example considered, this accounts for 82% (55/67) of the subjects under observation. Consequently, standard errors of regression estimates tend to be larger than in a marginal or random effects analysis. For example, the standard error of the regression coefficient for the treatment variable is here 0.91, as opposed to a value of 0.23 obtained from the marginal model. At the extreme, the conditional analysis provides no information about coefficients of explanatory variables which do not vary over time. This can be seen by examining (9.3.3). The product of any time-independent covariate and its coefficient will factor out of the sum in both the numerator and denominator and cancel from the conditional likelihood. This is sensible since we have conditioned away all information about each subject's intercept and thus cannot use estimates which are based entirely upon comparisons across subjects.

We now turn to the situation in which the $\boldsymbol{U}_i$ are treated as an independent sample from a random effects distribution. We begin by reviewing the traditional but simpler random effects models for binary data and then consider the logistic-Gaussian model more specifically.

9.3.2 *Random effects models for binary data*

Historically, the motivation for random effects models has been the observation that the variability among clustered binary responses exceeds what would be expected due to binomial variation alone. Random effects models were introduced to account for this so-called *extra-binomial variation.* The beta-binomial distribution (Skellam, 1948) was one of the earliest. Let $\{Y_{i1}, \ldots, Y_{in_i}\}$ represent the n_i binary responses from cluster i. Here the cluster could be a litter in a teratology experiment, a family or household in a genetic study or an individual in a longitudinal study. The beta-binomial distribution assumes that:

(1) conditional on μ_i, the responses $Y_{i1}, \ldots, Y_{in_i}$ are independent with common probability μ_i;

(2) the μ_i follow a beta distribution with mean μ and variance $\delta\mu(1-\mu)$.

Unconditionally, the total number of positive responses for a cluster, $Y_{i.} = Y_{i1} + \cdots + Y_{in}$, has a beta-binomial distribution with

$$\mathrm{E}(Y_{i.}) = n_i \mu_i$$

and

$$\mathrm{Var}(Y_{i.}) = n_i \mu_i (1-\mu_i)\{1 + (n_i - 1)\delta\}.$$

The over-dispersion parameter δ is the correlation for each pair of binary responses from the same cluster.

The beta-binomial distribution has been used to model the incidence of non-infectious diseases in a household (Griffiths, 1973), the number of malformed foetuses in a litter (Williams, 1975), and the number of chromosomal aberrant cells among repeated samples for an individual (Prentice, 1986). Prentice (1986) points out that the correlation coefficient, δ, need not be positive in the beta-binomial model as previously thought, but that its lower bound is

$$\delta_0 = \max\{-\mu/(n-\mu-1), -(1-\mu)/(n+\mu)\}.$$

The beta-binomial framework can be extended so that a parametric model may be imposed on the cluster-specific means, μ_i. For example, μ_i might be assumed to depend on cluster-level explanatory variables, $\boldsymbol{x}_i$, through a logistic function, $\text{logit}(\mu_i) = \boldsymbol{x}_i'\boldsymbol{\beta}$.

Originally, it was assumed that the beta-binomial distribution required each response from the same cluster to have a common probability, μ_i. In the regression set-up, this required the covariates to be the same for all observations within a cluster, that is, $\boldsymbol{x}_{i1} = \cdots = \boldsymbol{x}_{in_i} = \boldsymbol{x}_i$. However, Rosner (1984) has extended the beta-binomial to allow the covariates to vary within clusters. His model for one cluster is formally equivalent to the following n_i logistic regressions:

$$\begin{aligned} &\text{logit}\Pr(Y_{ij} = 1 \mid y_{i1}, \ldots, y_{ij-1}, y_{ij+1}, \ldots, y_{in_i}, \boldsymbol{x}_{ij}) \\ &\quad = \log\left(\frac{\theta_{i1} + w_{ij}\theta_{i2}}{1-\theta_{i1} + (n_i - 1 - w_{ij})\theta_{i2}}\right) + \boldsymbol{x}_{ij}'\boldsymbol{\beta}^*, \quad j = 1, \ldots, n_i, \quad (9.3.4) \end{aligned}$$

where $w_{ij} = y_{i.} - y_{ij}$, θ_{i1} is an intercept parameter and θ_{i2} characterizes the association between pairs of responses for the same cluster. This clever extension of the beta binomial does have some important limitations. First, its regression coefficients, $\boldsymbol{\beta}^*$, measure the effect of $\boldsymbol{x}_{ij}$ on Y_{ij} which cannot first be explained by the other responses in the cluster. Hence, the effects of cluster-level covariates may often be attributed to the other observations within the cluster, rather than to the covariate itself. This drawback is particularly severe when the cluster sizes vary so that different numbers of other responses are conditioned upon in the different clusters. This is a particular problem for longitudinal studies where the number of observations per person often varies. In addition, in longitudinal studies, it may be awkward to model the probability for the first response as a function of responses which come later in time. See, for example, Jones and Kenward (1987) who consider models for crossover trials.

The logistic model introduced in Section 9.1 adds the random effects on the same scale as the fixed effects. To our knowledge, this approach was first considered in the biostatistical literature by Pierce and Sands (1975) in an unpublished Oregon State University report. They assumed a Gaussian distribution for a univariate random intercept. Since then, the logistic model with Gaussian random effects has been studied extensively, including work by Williams (1982), Stiratelli *et al.* (1984), Anderson and Aitkin (1985), Gilmour *et al.* (1985), Zeger *et al.* (1988), Zeger and Karim (1991), Breslow and Clayton (1993), and Waclawiw and Liang (1993). One exception is Conoway (1990), who used a log–log link and a log–gamma distribution for the random intercepts.

9.3.3 *Examples of logistic models with Gaussian random effects*

The approach to fitting the random effects model within the GLM framework has been covered in Section 9.2. No particular computational simplification arises when we focus on the logistic model with Gaussian random effects. The likelihood function for $\boldsymbol{\beta}$ and G is

$$L(\boldsymbol{\beta}, G; \boldsymbol{y}) = \prod_{i=1}^{m} \int \prod_{j=1}^{n_i} \{\mu_{ij}(\boldsymbol{\beta}, \boldsymbol{U}_i)\}^{y_{ij}} \{1 - \mu_{ij}(\boldsymbol{\beta}, \boldsymbol{U}_i)\}^{1-y_{ij}} f(\boldsymbol{U}_i; G) \mathrm{d}\boldsymbol{U}_i, \tag{9.3.5}$$

where $\mu_{ij}(\boldsymbol{\beta}, \boldsymbol{U}_i) = \mathrm{E}(Y_{ij} \,|\, \boldsymbol{U}_i; \boldsymbol{\beta})$. With the logit link and Gaussian assumption on the $\boldsymbol{U}_i$, this reduces to

$$\prod_{i=1}^{m} \int \exp\left[\boldsymbol{\beta}' \sum_j \boldsymbol{x}_{ij} y_{ij} + \boldsymbol{U}_i' \sum_j \boldsymbol{d}_{ij} y_{ij} - \sum_j \log\{1 + \exp(\boldsymbol{x}_{ij}'\boldsymbol{\beta} + \boldsymbol{d}_{ij}'\boldsymbol{U}_i)\}\right]$$
$$\times (2\pi)^{-1} \,|\, G \,|^{-q/2} \exp(-\boldsymbol{U}_i' G^{-1} \boldsymbol{U}_i / 2) \mathrm{d}\boldsymbol{U}_i,$$

where G is the $q \times q$ variance matrix of each $\boldsymbol{U}_i$. Crouch and Spiegelman (1990) present numerical integration methods tailored to the logistic-Gaussian integral above. Zeger and Karim (1991) have used a Gibbs sampling Monte Carlo algorithm to simulate from a posterior distribution similar to this likelihood function. In the examples below, we use the approximation method by Breslow and Clayton (1993), which has been implemented in SAS (GLIMMIX) to obtain maximum likelihood estimates and their estimated standard errors for count data regression models, and we use numerical integration methods implemented in SAS (NLMIXED) to obtain MLEs for binary response models.

Example 9.1. (continued)

For the 2×2 crossover trial on cerebrovascular deficiency, we assume a logistic regression model with additive effects of treatment, period, and a random intercept $\gamma_i = \beta_0 + U_i$, assumed to follow a Gaussian distribution with variance G. Table 9.3 gives maximum likelihood estimates of $\boldsymbol{\beta}$ and $G^{1/2}$. For comparison, the table also presents regression coefficients obtained by fitting a marginal model.

Table 9.3. Regression estimates and standard errors (in parentheses) of random effects and marginal models fitted to the 2×2 crossover data for cerebrovascular deficiency adapted from Jones and Kenward (1989) and presented in Table 8.1.

	Random effects model	Marginal model	Ratio of random effects to marginal
Intercept	2.2 (1.0)	0.67 (0.29)	3.4
Treatment	1.8 (0.93)	0.57 (0.23)	3.3
Period	−1.0 (0.84)	−0.30 (0.23)	3.3
$G^{1/2}$	5.0 (2.3)	—	

Focusing first on the maximum likelihood estimates, there is clear evidence of substantial heterogeneity among subjects. The standard deviation of the random intercept distribution is estimated to be 5.0 with a standard error of 2.3. By the Gaussian assumption for the intercepts on the logit scale, roughly 95% of subjects would fall within 9.8 logit units of the overall mean. But this range on the logit scale translates into probabilities which range from essentially 0 to 1. Hence, the data suggest that some people have little chance and others very high chance of a normal reading given either treatment. Assuming a constant treatment effect for all persons, the odds of a normal response for a subject are estimated to be $6.0 = \exp(1.8)$ times higher on the active drug than on the placebo.

The last column of Table 9.3 presents the ratios of regression estimates obtained from the random effects model and from the marginal model. The three ratios are all close to $(0.346\hat{G}+1)^{1/2} = 3.1$, the theoretical value discussed in Section 7.4 and in Zeger *et al.* (1988).

Example 9.3. The pre–post trial on schizophrenia

As discussed in Chapter 7, a distinctive feature of random effects models is that natural heterogeneity across subjects is modelled directly through subject-specific parameters. This example serves to illustrate that sometimes random intercepts alone may not sufficiently capture the variation exhibited in the data. Table 9.4 presents results from two random effects models: Model 1 with random intercepts to capture variations in baseline risk among subjects, and Model 2 with random intercepts and slopes, the latter for subject variations in changes of risk over time. As in Section 8.3, we consider three independent variables: treatment status (x_1), time in weeks from baseline (x_2) and their interaction (x_3). For Model 1, the estimate for β_3 is -0.877 ($\widehat{\text{SE}} = 0.349$) suggesting that on average, the rate of change for the risk of having PANSS ≥ 80 is considerably lower for the risperidone group than the haloperidol group. For example, the

Table 9.4. Regression estimates and standard errors (in parentheses) of random effects models for the pre–post trial on schizophrenia.

	Model	
Variable	1	2
Intercept	2.274 (0.236)	2.400 (0.610)
Treatment (x_1)	0.236 (0.690)	0.319 (0.740)
Time (x_2)	−1.037 (0.234)	−1.034 (0.430)
$x_1 \cdot x_2$	−0.877 (0.349)	−1.247 (0.561)
G_{11}	11.066	12.167
G_{12}		0.143
G_{22}		3.532

G_{11} and G_{22} denote the variances of random intercepts and slopes respectively; G_{12} denotes the covariance between random intercepts and slopes.

risk for each patient in the haloperidol group at week 5 reduces by 17% ($0.17 = 1-(6/5)^{-1.037}$) compared to that at week 4. However, for a patient receiving risperidone of 6 mg, their risk at week 5 reduces by as much as 29% ($0.29 = 1 - (6/5)^{-1.037-0.877}$) relative to that at week 4. The estimate ($\hat{G}_{11} = 11.07$) for the variance of random intercepts suggests a strong degree of heterogeneity for baseline risks. When random slopes are added to the model, $\hat{\beta}_3$ increases in magnitude, from -0.877 to -1.247, representing a 42% inflation. This addition of random slopes is justified by the substantial estimate of their variance, $\hat{G}_{22} = 3.532$, as shown in Table 9.4. This extra variation across subjects is also more accurately reflected in the standard error estimates of the $\hat{\beta}$'s in Model 2. For example, the s.e. for $\hat{\beta}_3$ in Model 2 (0.561) is almost twice the size of that for $\hat{\beta}_3$ (0.349) in Model 1.

Example 9.4. Respiratory infection in Indonesian preschool children

Fitting a random effects model to the data from the Indonesian study allows us to address the question of how an individual child's risk for respiratory infection would change if their vitamin A status were to change. This is accomplished by allowing each child to have a distinct intercept which represents their propensity for infection. Table 9.5 gives regression estimates from models analogous to Models 2–4 in Table 8.7. Here, we have accounted for correlation by including random intercepts which are assumed to follow a Gaussian distribution with variance G.

Note that the estimates of the random effects standard deviation are around 0.7, statistically significantly different from zero but smaller than

Table 9.5. Regression estimates and standard errors (in parentheses) of random effects models for the Indonesian study on respiratory infection (Sommer *et al.*, 1984).

	Model		
Variable	1	2	3
Intercept	−2.2	−1.9	−2.4
	(0.24)	(0.30)	(0.37)
Sex	−0.51	−0.56	−0.55
	(0.25)	(0.26)	(0.26)
Height for age	−0.044	−0.052	−0.049
	(0.022)	(0.022)	(0.022)
Seasonal cosine	−0.61	—	−0.56
	(0.17)		(0.22)
Seasonal sine	−0.17	—	−0.019
	(0.17)		(0.22)
Xerophthalmia	0.54	0.57	0.69
	(0.48)	(0.48)	(0.49)
Age	−0.031	—	—
	(0.0079)		
Age^2	−0.0011	—	—
	(0.00040)		
Age at entry	—	−0.054	−0.055
		(0.011)	(0.011)
Age at entry^2	—	−0.0014	−0.0014
		(0.00049)	(0.00050)
Follow-up time	—	−0.20	−0.085
		(0.074)	(0.10)
Follow-up time^2	—	0.014	0.0069
		(0.0048)	(0.0068)
$G^{1/2}$	0.72	0.71	0.72
	(0.23)	(0.24)	(0.24)

in the crossover trial of Example 9.1. Among children with linear predictor equal to the intercept, −2.2, in Model 1 (average age, weight, female, vitamin A sufficient), about 95% would have a probability of infection between 0.03 and 0.31. This still represents considerable heterogeneity in the propensity for infection. The relative odds of infection associated with xerophthalmia (vitamin A deficiency) arc estimated to be exp(0.54) = 1.7 in Model 1 and are not significantly different from 1. The lack of significance of the effect is due to the small number of xerophthalmia cases (52) in this illustrative subset of the original data. Finally, the longitudinal age effect on the risk of respiratory infection seen in Model 2 can be explained, to a large extent, by the seasonal trend as shown by fitting Model 3.

Because there is less heterogeneity among subjects, the regression estimates seen above are similar to the marginal model coefficients in Table 8.7. Again, the ratios of the marginal and random effects coefficients are close to $(0.346\hat{G}+1)^{1/2}$ as discussed in Section 7.4.

9.4 Counted responses

9.4.1 *Conditional likelihood method*

We now consider conditional maximum likelihood estimation of the random intercept log-linear model for count data. Specifically, we assume that conditional on $\gamma_i = \beta_0 + U_i$,

(1) Y_{ij} follows a Poisson distribution such that

$$\log \mathrm{E}(Y_{ij} \mid \gamma_i) = \gamma_i + \boldsymbol{x}'_{ij}\boldsymbol{\beta} + \log(t_{ij}), \quad j = 1, \ldots, n_i;$$

and

(2) $Y_{i1}, \ldots, Y_{in_i}$ are independent.

Under these assumptions, the likelihood function for $\boldsymbol{\beta}$ and $\gamma_1, \ldots, \gamma_m$ is completely specified and is proportional to

$$\prod_{i=1}^{m} \exp\left\{ \gamma_i \sum_{j=1}^{n_i} y_{ij} + \boldsymbol{\beta}' \sum_{j=1}^{n_i} y_{ij}\boldsymbol{x}_{ij} \right.$$
$$\left. + \sum_{j=1}^{n_i} y_{ij} \log(t_{ij}) - \sum_{j=1}^{n_i} t_{ij} \exp(\gamma_i + \boldsymbol{x}'_{ij}\boldsymbol{\beta}) \right\}. \qquad (9.4.1)$$

By conditioning on $y_{i.} = \sum_{j=1}^{n_i} y_{ij}$ as was done in Section 9.2.1, we obtain the following conditional likelihood which depends on $\boldsymbol{\beta}$ only:

$$\prod_{i=1}^{m} \binom{y_{i.}}{y_{i1}, \ldots, y_{in_i}} \prod_{j=1}^{n_i} \left(\frac{t_{ij} e^{\boldsymbol{x}'_{ij}\boldsymbol{\beta}}}{\sum_{\ell=1}^{n_i} t_{i\ell} e^{\boldsymbol{x}'_{i\ell}\boldsymbol{\beta}}} \right)^{y_{ij}}. \qquad (9.4.2)$$

The contribution in (9.4.2) for subject i is a multinomial probability in which

$$\pi_{ij} = t_{ij} \exp(\boldsymbol{x}'_{ij}\boldsymbol{\beta}) \Big/ \sum_{\ell=1}^{n_i} t_{i\ell} \exp(\boldsymbol{x}'_{i\ell}\boldsymbol{\beta})$$

represents the probability that each of the $y_{i.}$ events will fall into 'category j', $j = 1, \ldots, n_i$. We now use the conditional likelihood approach to continue the analysis of the seizure data.

Example 9.5. Epileptic seizures

Returning to Example 8.5, we first consider the model

$$\log \mathrm{E}(Y_{ij} \mid \gamma_i) = \gamma_i + \beta_1 x_{ij1} + \beta_2 x_{ij2} + \beta_3 x_{ij1} x_{ij2} + \log(t_{ij}),$$
$$j = 0, 1, \ldots, 4; \quad i = 1, \ldots, 59,$$

where

$$x_{ij1} = \begin{cases} 1 & \text{if the } i\text{th subject is assigned to the progabide group,} \\ 0 & \text{if the } i\text{th subject is assigned to the placebo group,} \end{cases}$$

$$x_{ij2} = \begin{cases} 1 & \text{if } j = 1, 2, 3, \text{ or } 4, \\ 0 & \text{if } j = 0. \end{cases}$$

Here, γ_i is the expected baseline seizure count for the ith subject, $i = 1, \ldots, 59$. The coefficient β_2 represents the log ratio of the seizure rates post versus pre-randomization for the placebo group. Note that this is assumed to take the same value for each subject. Similarly, $\beta_2 + \beta_3$ represents the log ratio of rates for the treated group so that β_3 is the treatment effect coefficient.

Because $\boldsymbol{x}_{i1} = \boldsymbol{x}_{i2} = \boldsymbol{x}_{i3} = \boldsymbol{x}_{i4}$ and $t_{i0} = 8 = t_{i1} + \cdots + t_{i4}$, the conditional likelihood for $\boldsymbol{\beta}$ reduces to

$$\prod_{i=1}^{28} \binom{y_{i\cdot}}{y_{i0}} \left(\frac{\exp(\beta_2)}{1+\exp(\beta_2)}\right)^{y_{i\cdot}-y_{i0}} \left(\frac{1}{1+\exp(\beta_2)}\right)^{y_{i0}}$$
$$\times \prod_{i=29}^{59} \binom{y_{i\cdot}}{y_{i0}} \left(\frac{\exp(\beta_2+\beta_3)}{1+\exp(\beta_2+\beta_3)}\right)^{y_{i\cdot}-y_{i0}} \left(\frac{1}{1+\exp(\beta_2+\beta_3)}\right)^{y_{i0}}.$$

Thus, the conditional likelihood reduces to a comparison of two sets of binomial observations with 'sample sizes' 28 and 31. In the placebo group, each subject contributes a statistic $y_{i0}/y_{i\cdot}$ for estimating the parameter $\pi_1 = 1/\{1+\exp(\beta_2)\}$, which is the common probability that an individual's seizure occurred before rather than after the randomization. Similarly, the common probability in the progabide group is $\pi_2 = 1/\{1+\exp(\beta_2+\beta_3)\}$. Thus, a negative value for β_3 indicates that a relatively larger fraction of the total seizures in the treatment group occurred before rather than after randomization as compared to the placebo group. In other words, a negative β_3 indicates that the treatment is effective.

Table 9.6 gives the conditional maximum likelihood estimates of β_2 and β_3 and their standard errors. With the full data set, there is modest evidence that progabide is more effective than the placebo in reducing the occurrence of seizures ($\hat{\beta}_3 = -0.10 \pm 0.065$). With possible outlier

Table 9.6. Results of conditional likelihood analysis (coefficient ± standard error) of seizure data.

	Complete data	Patient# 207 deleted
β_2	0.11 ± 0.047	0.11 ± 0.047
β_3	-0.10 ± 0.065	-0.30 ± 0.070
Pearson's χ^2	289.9	227.1

patient number 207 deleted, a stronger treatment effect is suggested, ($\hat{\beta}_3 = -0.30 \pm 0.070$). However, the calculation of the Pearson χ^2 statistic

$$\sum_{i=1}^{28} \frac{(y_{i0} - y_{i.}\hat{\pi}_1)^2}{y_{i.}\hat{\pi}_1(1-\hat{\pi}_1)} + \sum_{i=29}^{59} \frac{(y_{i0} - y_{i.}\hat{\pi}_2)^2}{y_{i.}\hat{\pi}_2(1-\hat{\pi}_2)},$$

where $\hat{\pi}_1 = 1/\{1+\exp(\hat{\beta}_2)\}$ and $\hat{\pi}_2 = 1/\{1+\exp(\hat{\beta}_2+\hat{\beta}_3)\}$, also reveals that the fitted model is grossly inadequate. For example, with 57 degrees of freedom in the full data, the fitted model is rejected at the 0.01 level. The same conclusion is reached when the outlying individual is set aside. An important implication of this observation is that the estimated standard errors for the elements of $\hat{\boldsymbol{\beta}}$ may be too small. This may be due to the inadequacy of the assumption that the change in seizure rate is common to everyone within a treatment group.

One way to address this possibility is to introduce a random effect U_{i2} for the pre–post explanatory variable x_2. However, the conditional likelihood method would no longer be appropriate since all relevant information about β_3 will be conditioned away. We must instead use the random effects approach which is the topic of the following sub-section.

9.4.2 *Random effects models for counts*

The Poisson distribution has a long tradition as a model for count data, but in biomedical applications it is rarely the case that $\text{Var}(Y) = \text{E}(Y)$ as is implied by the Poisson assumption. Typically, the variance exceeds the mean (Breslow, 1984). As discussed in Section 9.3.2 for binomial data, this over-dispersion can be explained by assuming that there is natural heterogeneity among the expected responses across observations. If the means are assumed to follow a gamma distribution, the marginal distribution of the counts is the *negative binomial* distribution. Specifically, this distribution arises from the assumptions that

(1) conditional on μ_i, the response variable Y_{ij} has a Poisson distribution with mean μ_i;

(2) the μ_i are independent gamma random variables with mean μ and variance $\phi\mu^2$.

Then, the unconditional distribution of Y_{ij} is negative binomial with

$$\mathrm{E}(Y_{ij}) = \mu \quad \text{and} \quad \mathrm{Var}(Y_{ij}) = \mu + \phi\mu^2. \tag{9.4.3}$$

The use of the negative binomial model dates back at least to the work of Greenwood and Yule (1920) who modelled over-dispersed accident counts.

The simplest extension of the negative binomial model is to assume that the μ_i depend on covariates $\boldsymbol{x}_i$ through some parametric function. The most common is the log-linear model for which

$$\log(\mu_i) = \boldsymbol{x}_i'\boldsymbol{\beta}. \tag{9.4.4}$$

One important limitation of this model for application to longitudinal data is that the explanatory variables in the regression above do not vary within subjects. Morton (1987) proposed a solution to this problem. In the longitudinal context, if we once again let $Y_{i1}, \ldots, Y_{in_i}$ denote the counted responses from the ith subject, Morton (1987) assumed that

(1) conditional on an independent unobserved variable ϵ_i, $\mathrm{E}(Y_{ij} \mid \epsilon_i) = \exp(\boldsymbol{x}_{ij}'\boldsymbol{\beta})\epsilon_i$, $j = 1, \ldots, n_i$;
(2) $\mathrm{Var}(Y_{ij} \mid \epsilon_i) = \phi\mathrm{E}(Y_{ij} \mid \epsilon_i)$;
(3) $\mathrm{E}(\epsilon_i) = 1$ and $\mathrm{Var}(\epsilon_i) = \sigma^2$.

Note that assumptions (1), (2), and (3) imply that $\mathrm{E}(Y_{ij}) = \exp(\boldsymbol{x}_{ij}'\boldsymbol{\beta}) = \mu_{ij}$ and $\mathrm{Var}(Y_{ij}) = \phi\mu_{ij} + \sigma^2\mu_{ij}^2$. Morton (1987) extended this approach to include more complicated nesting structures as well. He used a quasi-likelihood estimation approach, which is similar to GEE, for estimating $\boldsymbol{\beta}, \phi$, and σ^2. An attractive feature of this model is that it is not necessary to specify the complete distribution of ϵ_i, only its first two moments.

The model that is the focus of the remainder of this chapter adds the random effects on the same scale as the fixed effects as follows:

(1′) $\log \mathrm{E}(Y_{ij} \mid \boldsymbol{U}_i) = \boldsymbol{x}_{ij}'\boldsymbol{\beta} + \boldsymbol{d}_{ij}'\boldsymbol{U}_i$;

(2′) given $\boldsymbol{U}_i$, the responses $Y_{i1}, \ldots, Y_{in_i}$ are independent Poisson variables with mean $\mathrm{E}(Y_{ij} \mid U_i)$;

(3′) the $\boldsymbol{U}_i$ are independent realizations from a distribution with density function $f(\boldsymbol{U}_i; G)$.

This second approach allows the contribution of the random effects to vary within a subject, that is, $\boldsymbol{d}_{ij}$ need not be constant for a given i. If this flexibility is needed, the second approach is to be preferred. In fact, the expression (1) is readily seen as a special case of (1′) with $d_{ij} = 1$ and $\boldsymbol{U}_i = \log(\epsilon_i)$. On the other hand, in order to make inferences about

$\boldsymbol{\beta}$ and G, one needs to specify a distribution for the $\boldsymbol{U}_i$. The following sub-section illustrates the use of Poisson regression with Gaussian random effects by re-analysing the seizure data.

9.4.3 *Poisson–Gaussian random effects models*

Example 9.5. (continued)

In this section we fit two models to the progabide data which differ only on how the random effects are incorporated. Model 1 is a log-linear model with a random intercept. In Model 2, we add a second random effect for the pre/post-treatment indicator (x_2) so that

$$\log \mathrm{E}(Y_{ij} \mid \boldsymbol{U}_i) = \beta_0 + \beta_1 x_{ij1} + \beta_2 x_{ij2} + \beta_3 x_{ij1} x_{ij2} + U_{i1} + x_{ij2} U_{i2} + \log(t_{ij}),$$

where $\boldsymbol{U}_i = (U_{i1}, U_{i2})$ is assumed to follow a Gaussian distribution with mean (0,0) and variance matrix G with elements

$$\begin{pmatrix} G_{11} & G_{12} \\ G_{21} & G_{22} \end{pmatrix}.$$

The inclusion of U_{i2} allows us to address the concern raised at the end of Section 9.4.1, that there might be heterogeneity among subjects in the ratio of the expected seizure counts before and after the randomization. The degree of heterogeneity can be measured by the magnitude of G_{22}, the variance of U_{i2}. Both models were fitted using the approximate maximum likelihood algorithm outlined in Section 9.2.2.

Table 9.7 presents results from fitting Models 1 and 2, with and without patient number 207. As expected, the results from Model 1 are in close agreement with those from the conditional approach given in Section 9.4.1. However, this model is refuted by the statistical significance of G_{22}, which in Model 2 using the complete data we estimate to be 0.24 with standard error 0.062.

Focusing on the results for Model 2 fitted to the complete data, subjects in the placebo group have expected seizure rates after treatment which are estimated to be roughly the same as before treatment ($\exp(\hat{\beta}_2) = \exp(0.002) = 1.002$). For the progabide group, the seizure rates are reduced after treatment by about 27% ($1 - \exp(0.002 - 0.31) = 0.27$). Hence, the treatment seems to have a modest effect: the estimated effect is $\hat{\beta}_3 = -0.31$ with a standard error of 0.15. Finally, if we set aside for the moment patient number 207, who had unusually high seizure rates, then the evidence that progabide is effective is somewhat stronger, with $\hat{\beta}_3 = -0.34 \pm 0.15$. The analysis without patient 207 is only exploratory, and is carried out in order to understand this patient's influence on the overall results. Patient number 207 has been identified because of unusual seizure counts and perhaps has special medical problems.

Table 9.7. Estimates and standard errors (in parentheses) for random effects Poisson regression models fitted to the progabide data with and without patient number 207.

	Model 1		Model 2	
Variable	Complete data	Without 207	Complete data	Without 207
Intercept	1.0	1.0	1.1	1.1
	(0.15)	(0.14)	(0.14)	(0.13)
Treatment	−0.023	−0.009	0.050	−0.029
	(0.20)	(0.19)	(0.18)	(0.19)
Time	0.11	0.11	0.002	0.010
	(0.047)	(0.047)	(0.11)	(0.11)
Treatment-	−0.10	−0.30	−0.31	−0.34
by-time	(0.065)	(0.070)	(0.15)	(0.15)
G_{11}	0.62	0.53	0.51	0.46
	(0.12)	(0.10)	(0.10)	(0.10)
G_{12}	—	—	0.054	0.014
			(0.056)	(0.053)
G_{22}	—	—	0.24	0.22
			(0.062)	(0.059)

9.5 Further reading

Throughout this chapter, we have used the Gaussian distribution as a convenient model for the random effects. When the regression coefficients are of primary interest, the specific form of the random effects distribution is less important. However, when the random effects are themselves the focus, as in the CD4 + example in Chapter 5, inferences are more dependent on the assumptions about their distribution. Lange and Ryan (1989) suggest a graphical way to test the Gaussian assumption when the response variables are continuous. When the response variables are discrete, the same task becomes more difficult. Davidian and Gallant (1992) have recently developed a non-parametric approach to estimating the random effects distribution with non-linear models.

The statistical literature on random effects GLMs has grown enormously in the last decade. Key papers in the biostatistics literature include: Laird and Ware (1982); Stiratelli *et al.* (1984); Gilmour *et al.* (1985); Schall (1990); Zeger and Karim (1991); Waclawiw and Liang (1993); Solomon and Cox (1992); Breslow and Clayton (1993); Drum and McCullagh (1993); Breslow and Lin (1995) and Lin and Breslow (1996). These papers also provide useful additional references.

10
Transition models

This chapter considers extensions of generalized linear models (GLMs) for describing the conditional distribution of each response y_{ij} as an explicit function of past responses $y_{ij-1}, \ldots, y_{i1}$ and covariates x_{ij}. We will focus on the case where the observation times t_{ij} are equally spaced. To simplify notation, we denote the history for subject i at visit j by $\mathcal{H}_{ij} = \{y_{ik},\ k = 1, \ldots, j-1\}$. As above, we will continue to condition on the past and present values of the covariates without explicitly listing them.

The most useful transition models are Markov chains for which the conditional distribution of y_{ij} given $\mathcal{H}_{ij}$ depends only on the q prior observations $y_{ij-1}, \ldots, y_{ij-q}$. The integer q is referred to as the model *order*. Sections 10.1 and 10.2 provide a general treatment of Markov GLMs and fitting procedures. Section 10.3 deals with categorical data. Section 10.4 briefly discusses models for counted responses which are in an earlier stage of development than the corresponding models for categorical data.

10.1 General

As discussed in Section 7.3, a transition model specifies a GLM for the conditional distribution of Y_{ij} given the past responses, $\mathcal{H}_{ij}$. The form of the conditional GLM is

$$f(y_{ij} \mid \mathcal{H}_{ij}) = \exp\{[y_{ij}\theta_{ij} - \psi(\theta_{ij})]/\phi + c(y_{ij}, \phi)\}, \qquad (10.1.1)$$

for known functions $\psi(\theta_{ij})$ and $c(y_{ij}, \phi)$. The conditional mean and variance are

$$\mu_{ij}^{\mathrm{C}} = \mathrm{E}(Y_{ij} \mid \mathcal{H}_{ij}) = \psi'(\theta_{ij}) \quad \text{and} \quad v_{ij}^{\mathrm{C}} = \mathrm{Var}(Y_{ij} \mid \mathcal{H}_{ij}) = \psi''(\theta_{ij})\phi.$$

We will consider transition models where the conditional mean and variance satisfy the equations

$$h(\mu_{ij}^{\mathrm{C}}) = \boldsymbol{x_{ij}}'\boldsymbol{\beta} + \sum_{r=1}^{s} f_r(\mathcal{H}_{ij}; \boldsymbol{\alpha}),$$

for suitable functions $f_r(\cdot)$, and

$$v_{ij}^{\mathrm{C}} = v(\mu_{ij}^{\mathrm{C}})\phi, \tag{10.1.2}$$

where h and v are known link and variance functions determined from the specific form of the density function above. Appendix A.5 gives additional details on GLMs.

In words, the transition model expresses the conditional mean μ_{ij}^{C} as a function of both the covariates $\boldsymbol{x_{ij}}$ and of the past responses $y_{ij-1}, \ldots, y_{ij-q}$. Past responses or functions thereof are simply treated as additional explanatory variables. We assume that the past affects the present through the sum of s terms, each of which may depend on the q prior values. The following examples with different link functions illustrate the range of transition models which are available.

Linear link – a linear regression with autoregressive errors for Gaussian data (Tsay, 1984) is a Markov model. It has the form

$$Y_{ij} = \boldsymbol{x_{ij}}'\boldsymbol{\beta} + \sum_{r=1}^{q} \alpha_r (Y_{ij-r} - \boldsymbol{x}'_{ij-r}\boldsymbol{\beta}) + Z_{ij},$$

where the Z_{ij} are independent, mean-zero, Gaussian innovations. This is a transition model with $h(\mu_{ij}^{\mathrm{C}}) = \mu_{ij}^{\mathrm{C}}$, $v(\mu_{ij}^{\mathrm{C}}) = 1$, and $f_r = \alpha_r(y_{ij-r} - \boldsymbol{x_{ij-r}}'\boldsymbol{\beta})$. Note that the present observation, Y_{ij}, is a linear function of $\boldsymbol{x_{ij}}$ and of the earlier deviations $Y_{ij-r} - \boldsymbol{x}'_{ij-r}\boldsymbol{\beta}$, $r = 1, \ldots, q$.

Logit link – an example of a logistic regression model for binary responses that comprises a first-order Markov chain (Cox, 1970; Korn and Whittemore, 1979; Zeger *et al.*, 1985) is

$$\text{logit } \Pr(Y_{ij} = 1 \,|\, \mathcal{H}_{ij}) = \boldsymbol{x_{ij}}'\boldsymbol{\beta} + \alpha y_{ij-1},$$

previously given as equation (7.3.1). Here

$$h(\mu_{ij}^{\mathrm{C}}) = \text{logit}(\mu_{ij}^{\mathrm{C}}) = \log\left(\frac{\mu_{ij}^{\mathrm{C}}}{1 - \mu_{ij}^{\mathrm{C}}}\right), \quad v(\mu_{ij}^{\mathrm{C}}) = \mu_{ij}^{\mathrm{C}}(1 - \mu_{ij}^{\mathrm{C}})$$

and

$$f_r(\mathcal{H}_{ij}, \alpha) = \alpha_r y_{ij-r}, \quad s = q = 1.$$

A simple extension to a model of order q has the form

$$\text{logit } \Pr(Y_{ij} = 1 \,|\, \mathcal{H}_{ij}) = \boldsymbol{x_{ij}}'\boldsymbol{\beta}_q + \sum_{r=1}^{q} \alpha_r y_{ij-r}.$$

The notation $\boldsymbol{\beta}_q$ indicates that the value and interpretation of the regression coefficients changes with the Markov order, q.

Log-link – with count data we can assume a log-linear model where Y_{ij} given $\mathcal{H}_{ij}$ follows a Poisson distribution. Zeger and Qaqish (1988) discussed a first-order Markov chain with $f_1 = \alpha\{\log(y^*_{ij-1}) - \boldsymbol{x_{ij-1}}'\boldsymbol{\beta}\}$, where $y^*_{ij} = \max(y_{ij}, d), 0 < d < 1$. This leads to

$$\mu^{\mathrm{C}}_{ij} = \mathrm{E}(Y_{ij} \mid \mathcal{H}_{ij}) = \exp(\boldsymbol{x_{ij}}'\boldsymbol{\beta}) \left(\frac{y^*_{ij-1}}{\exp(\boldsymbol{x}'_{ij-1}\boldsymbol{\beta})} \right)^{\alpha}.$$

The constant d prevents $y_{ij-1} = 0$ from being an absorbing state whereby $y_{ij-1} = 0$ forces all future responses to be 0. Note when $\alpha > 0$, we have an increased expectation, μ^{C}_{ij}, when the previous outcome, y_{ij-1}, exceeds $\exp(\boldsymbol{x}'_{ij-1}\boldsymbol{\beta})$. When $\alpha < 0$, a higher value at t_{ij-1} causes a lower value at t_{ij}.

Within the linear regression model, the transition model can be formulated with $f_r = \alpha_r(y_{ij-r} - \boldsymbol{x_{ij-1}}'\boldsymbol{\beta})$ so that $\mathrm{E}(Y_{ij}) = \boldsymbol{x_{ij}}'\boldsymbol{\beta}$ whatever the value of q. In the logistic and log-linear cases, it is difficult to formulate models in such a way that $\boldsymbol{\beta}$ has the same meaning for different assumptions about the time dependence. When $\boldsymbol{\beta}$ is the scientific focus, the careful data analyst should examine the sensitivity of the substantive findings to the choice of time-dependence model. This issue is discussed below by way of example.

Section 7.5 briefly discussed the method of conditional maximum likelihood for fitting the simplest logistic transition model. We now consider estimation in more detail.

10.2 Fitting transition models

As indicated in (7.5.3), in a first-order Markov model the contribution to the likelihood for the ith subject can be written as

$$L_i(y_{i1}, \ldots, y_{in_i}) = f(y_{i1}) \prod_{j=2}^{n_i} f(y_{ij} \mid \mathcal{H}_{ij}).$$

In a Markov model of order q, the conditional distribution of Y_{ij} is

$$f(y_{ij} \mid \mathcal{H}_{ij}) = f(y_{ij} \mid y_{ij-1}, \ldots, y_{ij-q}),$$

so that the likelihood contribution for the ith subject becomes

$$f(y_{i1}, \ldots, y_{iq}) \prod_{j=q+1}^{n_i} f(y_{ij} \mid y_{ij-1}, \ldots, y_{ij-q}).$$

The GLM (10.1.1) specifies only the conditional distribution $f(y_{ij} \mid \mathcal{H}_{ij})$; the likelihood of the first q observation $f(y_{i1}, \ldots, y_{iq})$ is not specified directly.

In the linear model we assume that Y_{ij} given $\mathcal{H}_{ij}$ follows a Gaussian distribution. If $Y_{i1}, \ldots, Y_{iq}$ are also multivariate Gaussian and the covariance structure for the Y_{ij} is weakly stationary, the marginal distribution $f(y_{ij}, \ldots, y_{iq})$ can be fully determined from the conditional distribution model without additional unknown parameters. Hence, full maximum likelihood estimation can be used to fit Gaussian autoregressive models. See Tsay (1984) and references therein for details.

In the logistic and log-linear cases, $f(y_{i1}, \ldots, y_{iq})$ is not determined from the GLM assumption about the conditional model, and the full likelihood is unavailable. An alternative is to estimate $\boldsymbol{\beta}$ and $\boldsymbol{\alpha}$ by maximizing the conditional likelihood

$$\prod_{i=1}^{m} f(y_{iq+1}, \ldots, y_{in_i} \mid y_{i1}, \ldots, y_{iq}) = \prod_{i=1}^{m} \prod_{j=q+1}^{n_i} f(y_{ij} \mid \mathcal{H}_{ij}). \tag{10.2.1}$$

When maximizing (10.2.1) there are two distinct cases to consider. In the first, $f_r(\mathcal{H}_{ij}; \boldsymbol{\alpha}, \boldsymbol{\beta}) = \alpha_r f_r(\mathcal{H}_{ij})$ so that $h(\mu_{ij}^{\mathrm{C}}) = \boldsymbol{x_{ij}}'\boldsymbol{\beta} + \sum_{r=1}^{s} \alpha_r f_r(\mathcal{H}_{ij})$. Here, $h(\mu_{ij}^{\mathrm{C}})$ is a linear function of both $\boldsymbol{\beta}$ and $\boldsymbol{\alpha} = (\alpha_1, \ldots, \alpha_s)$ so that estimation proceeds as in GLMs for independent data. We simply regress Y_{ij} on the $(p+s)$-dimensional vector of extended explanatory variables $(\boldsymbol{x_{ij}}, f_1(\mathcal{H}_{ij}), \ldots, f_s(\mathcal{H}_{ij}))$.

The second case occurs when the functions of past responses include both $\boldsymbol{\alpha}$ and $\boldsymbol{\beta}$. Examples are the linear and log-linear models discussed above. To derive an estimation algorithm for this case, note that the derivative of the log conditional likelihood or conditional score function has the form

$$\boldsymbol{S}^{\mathrm{C}}(\boldsymbol{\delta}) = \sum_{i=1}^{m} \sum_{j=q+1}^{n_i} \frac{\partial \mu_{ij}^{\mathrm{C}}}{\partial \boldsymbol{\delta}} {v_{ij}^{\mathrm{c}}}^{-1} (y_{ij} - \mu_{ij}^{\mathrm{C}}) = 0, \tag{10.2.2}$$

where $\boldsymbol{\delta} = (\boldsymbol{\beta}, \boldsymbol{\alpha})$. This equation is the conditional analogue of the GLM score equation discussed in Appendix A.5. The derivative $\partial \mu_{ij}/\partial \boldsymbol{\delta}$ is analogous to $\boldsymbol{x_{ij}}$ but it can depend on $\boldsymbol{\alpha}$ and $\boldsymbol{\beta}$. We can still formulate the estimation procedure as an iterative weighted least squares as follows. Let $\boldsymbol{Y_i}$ be the $(n_i - q)$-vector of responses for $j = q+1, \ldots, n_i$ and $\boldsymbol{\mu}_{ij}^{\mathrm{C}}$ its expectation given $\mathcal{H}_{ij}$. Let $\boldsymbol{X}_i^*$ be an $(n_i - q) \times (p+s)$ matrix with kth row $\partial \mu_{iq+k}/\partial \boldsymbol{\delta}$ and $\boldsymbol{W_i} = \mathrm{diag}(1/v_{ik+q}^{\mathrm{C}},\ k = 1, \ldots, n_i - q)$ an $(n_i - q) \times (n_i - q)$ diagonal weighting matrix. Finally, let $\boldsymbol{Z_i} = \boldsymbol{X_i^*}\hat{\boldsymbol{\delta}} + (\boldsymbol{Y_i} - \hat{\boldsymbol{\mu}}_i^{\mathrm{C}})$. Then, an updated $\hat{\boldsymbol{\delta}}$ can be obtained by iteratively regressing $\boldsymbol{Z}$ on $\boldsymbol{X}^*$ using weights $\boldsymbol{W}$.

When the correct model is assumed for the conditional mean and variance, the solution $\hat{\boldsymbol{\delta}}$ of (10.2.2) asymptotically, as m goes to infinity, follows a Gaussian distribution with mean equal to the true value, $\boldsymbol{\delta}$, and

$(p+s) \times (p+s)$ variance matrix

$$V_{\hat{\boldsymbol{\delta}}} = \left(\sum_{i=1}^{m} X_i^{*\prime} W_i X_i^* \right)^{1}. \tag{10.2.3}$$

The variance $V_{\hat{\boldsymbol{\delta}}}$ depends on $\boldsymbol{\beta}$ and $\boldsymbol{\alpha}$. A consistent estimate, $\hat{V}_{\hat{\boldsymbol{\delta}}}$, is obtained by replacing $\boldsymbol{\beta}$ and $\boldsymbol{\alpha}$ by their estimates $\hat{\boldsymbol{\beta}}$ and $\hat{\boldsymbol{\alpha}}$. Hence a 95% confidence interval for β_1 is $\hat{\beta}_1 \pm 2\sqrt{\hat{V}_{\hat{\boldsymbol{\delta}}_{11}}}$, where $\hat{V}_{\hat{\boldsymbol{\delta}}_{11}}$ is the element in the first row and column of $\hat{V}_{\hat{\boldsymbol{\delta}}}$.

If the conditional mean is correctly specified and the conditional variance is not, we can still obtain consistent inferences about $\boldsymbol{\delta}$ by using the robust variance from equation (A.6.1) in Appendix A, which here takes the form

$$V_{\mathrm{R}} = \left(\sum_{i=1}^{m} X_i^{*\prime} W_i X_i^* \right)^{-1} \left(\sum_{i=1}^{m} X_i^{*\prime} W_i V_i W_i X_i^* \right) \left(\sum_{i=1}^{m} X_i^{*\prime} W_i X_i^* \right)^{-1}. \tag{10.2.4}$$

A consistent estimate $\hat{V}_{\mathrm{R}}$ is obtained by replacing $V_i = \mathrm{Var}(\boldsymbol{Y_i} \mid \mathcal{H}_i)$ in the equation above by its estimate, $(\boldsymbol{Y_i} - \hat{\boldsymbol{\mu}}_{\boldsymbol{i}}{}^{\mathrm{C}})(\boldsymbol{Y_i} - \hat{\boldsymbol{\mu}}_{\boldsymbol{i}}{}^{\mathrm{C}})'$.

Interestingly, use of the robust variance will often give consistent confidence intervals for $\hat{\boldsymbol{\delta}}$ even when the Markov assumption is violated. However, in that situation, the interpretation of $\hat{\boldsymbol{\delta}}$ is questionable since $\mu_{ij}^{\mathrm{C}}(\hat{\boldsymbol{\delta}})$ is not the conditional mean of Y_{ij} given $\mathcal{H}_{ij}$.

10.3 Transition models for categorical data

This section discusses Markov chain regression models for categorical responses observed at equally spaced intervals. We begin with logistic models for binary responses and then briefly consider extensions to multinominal and ordered categorical outcomes.

As discussed in Section 7.3, a first-order binary Markov chain is characterized by the transition matrix

$$\begin{pmatrix} \pi_{00} & \pi_{01} \\ \pi_{10} & \pi_{11} \end{pmatrix},$$

where $\pi_{ab} = \Pr(Y_{ij} = b \mid Y_{ij-1} = a)$, $a, b = 0, 1$. For example, π_{01} is the probability that $Y_{ij} = 1$ when the previous response is $Y_{ij-1} = 0$. Note that each row of a transition matrix sums to one since $\Pr(Y_{ij} = 0 \mid Y_{ij-1} = a) + \Pr(Y_{ij} = 1 \mid Y_{ij-1} = a) = 1$. As its name implies, the transition matrix records the probabilities of making each of the possible transitions from one visit to the next.

In the regression setting, we model the transition probabilities as functions of covariates $x_{ij} = (1, x_{ij1}, x_{ij2}, \ldots, x_{ijp})$. A very general model uses a separate logistic regression for $\Pr(Y_{ij} = 1 \mid Y_{ij-1} = y_{ij})$, $y_{ij} = 0, 1$. That is, we assume that

$$\text{logit} \Pr(Y_{ij} = 1 \mid Y_{ij-1} = 0) = \boldsymbol{x}'_{ij}\boldsymbol{\beta}_0$$

and

$$\text{logit} \Pr(Y_{ij} = 1 \mid Y_{ij-1} = 1) = \boldsymbol{x}'_{ij}\boldsymbol{\beta}_1,$$

where $\boldsymbol{\beta}_0$ and $\boldsymbol{\beta}_1$ may differ. In words, this model assumes that the effects of explanatory variables will differ depending on the previous response. A more concise form for the same model is

$$\text{logit} \Pr(Y_{ij} = 1 \mid Y_{ij-1} = y_{ij-1}) = \boldsymbol{x}'_{ij}\boldsymbol{\beta}_0 + y_{ij-1}\boldsymbol{x}'_{ij}\boldsymbol{\alpha}, \qquad (10.3.1)$$

so that $\boldsymbol{\beta}_1 = \boldsymbol{\beta}_0 + \boldsymbol{\alpha}$. Equation (10.3.1) expresses the two regressions as a single logistic model which includes as predictors the previous response y_{ij-1} as well as the interaction of y_{ij-1} and the explanatory variables. An advantage of the form in (10.3.1) is that we can now easily test whether simpler models fit the data equally well. For example, we can test whether $\boldsymbol{\alpha} = (\alpha_0, 0)$ so that in (10.3.1) $y_{ij-1}\boldsymbol{x_{ij}}'\alpha = \alpha_0 Y_{ij-1}$. This assumption implies that the covariates have the same effect on the response probability whether $y_{ij-1} = 0$ or $y_{ij-1} = 1$.

Alternately, we can test whether a more limited subset of $\boldsymbol{\alpha}$ is zero indicating that the associated covariates can be dropped from the model. Each of these alternatives is nested within the saturated model so that standard statistical methods for nested models can be applied.

In many problems, a higher order Markov chain may be needed. The second-order model has transition matrix

		Y_{ij}	
Y_{ij-2}	Y_{ij-1}	0	1
0	0	π_{000}	π_{001}
0	1	π_{010}	π_{011}
1	0	π_{100}	π_{101}
1	1	π_{110}	π_{111}

Here, $\pi_{abc} = \Pr(Y_{ij} = c \mid Y_{ij-2} = a, Y_{ij-1} = b)$; for example π_{011} is the probability that $Y_{ij} = 1$ given $Y_{ij-2} = 0$ and $Y_{ij-1} = 1$. By analogy with the regression models for a first-order chain, we could now fit four separate logistic regressions, one for each of the four possible histories (Y_{ij-2}, Y_{ij-1}), namely $(0,0)$, $(0,1)$, $(1,0)$, and $(1,1)$ with regression coefficients $\boldsymbol{\beta}_{00}$, $\boldsymbol{\beta}_{01}$, $\boldsymbol{\beta}_{10}$, and $\boldsymbol{\beta}_{11}$, respectively. But it is again more convenient to write a single equation as follows

$$\begin{aligned}&\text{logit } \Pr(Y_{ij}=1 \mid Y_{ij-2}=y_{ij-2}, Y_{ij-1}=y_{ij-1})\\ &\quad = \boldsymbol{x}_{ij}'\boldsymbol{\beta} + y_{ij-1}\boldsymbol{x}_{ij}'\boldsymbol{\alpha}_1 + y_{ij-2}\boldsymbol{x}_{ij}'\boldsymbol{\alpha}_2 + y_{ij-1}y_{ij-2}\boldsymbol{x}_{ij}'\boldsymbol{\alpha}_3. \qquad (10.3.2)\end{aligned}$$

By plugging in the different values for y_{ij-2} and y_{ij-1}, we obtain $\boldsymbol{\beta}_{00}=\boldsymbol{\beta}$; $\boldsymbol{\beta}_{01}=\boldsymbol{\beta}+\boldsymbol{\alpha}_1$; $\boldsymbol{\beta}_{10}=\boldsymbol{\beta}+\boldsymbol{\alpha}_2$; and $\boldsymbol{\beta}_{11}=\boldsymbol{\beta}+\boldsymbol{\alpha}_1+\boldsymbol{\alpha}_2+\boldsymbol{\alpha}_3$. We would again hope that a more parsimonious model fits the data equally well so that many of the components of the $\boldsymbol{\alpha}_i$ would be zero.

An important special case of (10.3.2) occurs when there are no interactions between the past responses, y_{ij-1} and y_{ij-2}, and the explanatory variables, that is, when all elements of the $\boldsymbol{\alpha}_i$ are zero except the intercept term. In this case, the previous responses affect the probability of a positive outcome but the effects of the explanatory variables are the same regardless of the history. Even in this situation, we must still choose between Markov models of different order. For example, we might start with a third-order model which can be written in the form

$$\begin{aligned}&\text{logit } \Pr(Y_{ij}=1 \mid Y_{ij-3}=y_{ij-3}, Y_{ij-2}=y_{ij-2}, Y_{ij-1}=y_{ij-1})\\ &\quad = \boldsymbol{x}_{ij}'\boldsymbol{\beta} + \alpha_1 y_{ij-1} + \alpha_2 y_{ij-2} + \alpha_3 y_{ij-3} + \alpha_4 y_{ij-1}y_{ij-2}\\ &\qquad + \alpha_5 y_{ij-1}y_{ij-3} + \alpha_6 y_{ij-2}y_{ij-3} + \alpha_7 y_{ij-1}y_{ij-2}y_{ij-3}. \qquad (10.3.3)\end{aligned}$$

A second-order model can be used if the data are consistent with $\alpha_3=\alpha_5=\alpha_6=\alpha_7=0$; a first-order model is implied if $\alpha_j=0$ for $j=2,\ldots,7$. As with any regression coefficients, the interpretation and value of $\boldsymbol{\beta}$ in (10.3.3) depends on the other explanatory variables in the model, in particular on which previous responses are included. When inferences about $\boldsymbol{\beta}$ are the scientific focus, it is essential to check their sensitivity to the assumed order of the Markov regression model.

As discussed in Section 10.2, when the Markov model is correctly specified, the transition events are uncorrelated so that ordinary logistic regression can be used to estimate regression coefficients and their standard errors. However, there may be circumstances when we choose to model $\Pr(Y_{ij} \mid Y_{ij-1},\ldots,Y_{ij-q})$ even though it does not equal $\Pr(Y_{ij} \mid \mathcal{H}_{ij})$. For example, suppose there is heterogeneity across people in the transition matrix due to unobserved factors, so that a reasonable model is

$$\Pr(Y_{ij}=1 \mid Y_{ij-1}=y_{ij-1}, U_i) = (\beta_0 + U_i) + \boldsymbol{x}_{ij}'\boldsymbol{\beta} + \alpha y_{ij-1},$$

where $U_i \sim N(0,\sigma^2)$. We may still wish to estimate the population-averaged transition matrix, $\Pr(Y_{ij} \mid Y_{ij-1}=y_{ij-1})$. But here the random intercept U_i makes the transitions for a person correlated. Correct inferences about the population-averaged coefficients can be drawn using the GEE approach described in Section 7.5.

10.3.1 *Indonesian children's study example*

We illustrate the Markov models for binary longitudinal data with the respiratory disease data from our subset of 1200 records from the Indonesian Children's Health Study. Ignoring dependence on covariates for the moment, the observed first-order transitions are as presented in Table 10.1.

The table gives the number and frequency of transitions from the infection state at one visit to the next. These rates estimate the transition probabilities $\Pr(Y_{ij} \mid Y_{ij-1})$. Note that there are 855 transitions among the 1200 observations, since for example we did not observe the child's status prior to visit one. For children who did not have respiratory disease at the prior visit ($Y_{ij-1} = 0$), the frequency of respiratory infection was 7.7%. Among children who did have infection at the prior visit, the proportion was 13.5%, or 1.76 times as high.

An important question is whether vitamin A deficiency, as indicated by the presence of the ocular disease xerophthalmia, is associated with a higher prevalence of respiratory infection. Sommer *et al.* (1984) have demonstrated this relationship in an analysis of the entire Indonesian data set which includes over 20 000 records on 3500 children. In our subset, we can form the cross-tabulation shown in Table 10.2 of xerophthalmia and respiratory infection at a given visit, using the 855 observations in Table 10.1.

Table 10.1. Number (frequency) of transitions from respiratory disease status Y_{ij-1} at visit $j-1$ to disease status Y_{ij} at visit j for Indonesian Children's Health Study data.

	Y_{ij}		
Y_{ij-1}	0	1	
0	721 (0.923)	60 (0.077)	781 (1.0)
1	64 (0.865)	10 (0.135)	74 (1.0)
			855

Table 10.2. Cross-tabulation of respiratory disease Y_{ij} against xerophthalmia status x_{ij} for Indonesian children's health study data from visits 2 to 6.

	Y_{ij}		
x_{ij}	0	1	
0	748	65	813
	(0.920)	(0.080)	(1.0)
1	37	5	42
	(0.881)	(0.119)	(1.0)
			855

Table 10.3. Cross-tabulation of current respiratory disease status Y_{ij} against xerophthalmia x_{ij} and previous respiratory disease status Y_{ij-1} for the Indonesian children's study data from visits 2 to 7.

	Y_{ij}			Y_{ij}		
x_{ij}	0	1		0	1	
0	688	56	744	60	9	69
	(0.925)	(0.075)	(1.0)	(0.870)	(0.130)	(1.0)
1	33	4	37	4	1	5
	(0.892)	(0.108)	(1.0)	(0.800)	(0.200)	(1.0)
			781			74
	$Y_{ij-1} = 0$			$Y_{ij-1} = 1$		

The frequency of respiratory infection is $1.49 = 0.119/0.080$ times as high among children who are vitamin A deficient. But there is clearly correlation among repeated respiratory disease outcomes for a given child. We can control for this dependence by examining the effect of vitamin A deficiency separately for transitions starting with $Y_{ij-1} = 0$ or $Y_{ij-1} = 1$ as in Table 10.3. Among children free of infection at the prior visit, the frequency of respiratory disease is $1.44 = 0.108/0.075$ times as high if the child has xerophthalmia. Among those who suffered infection at the prior visit, the xerophthalmia relative risk is $1.54 = 0.200/0.130$. Hence, the xerophthalmia effect is similar for $Y_{ij-1} = 0$ or $Y_{ij-1} = 1$ even though Y_{ij-1} is a strong predictor of Y_{ij}.

This exploratory analysis suggests a model

$$\text{logit Pr}(Y_{ij} = 1 \mid Y_{ij-1} = y_{ij-1}) = \boldsymbol{x}'_{ij}\boldsymbol{\beta} + \alpha y_{ij-1}.$$

Table 10.4 presents logistic regression results for that model and a number of others. For each set of predictor variables, the table reports the

Table 10.4. Logistic regression coefficients, standard errors (within round parentheses), and robust standard errors (within square parentheses) for several models fitted to the 855 respiratory disease transitions in the Indonesian children's health study data.

	Model				
Variable	1	2	3	4	5
Intercept	−2.44	−2.51	−2.51	−2.85	−2.81
	(0.13)	(0.14)	(0.14)	(0.19)	(0.18)
	[0.14]	[0.14]	[0.14]	[0.18]	[0.17]
Current	0.44	0.40	0.42	0.79	0.78
xerophthalmia	(0.50)	(0.55)	(0.50)	(0.58)	(0.52)
(1 = yes; 0 = no)	[0.54]	[0.51]	[0.53]	[0.49]	[0.53]
Age − 36				−0.024	−0.023
(months)				(0.0077)	(0.0073)
				[0.0070]	[0.0065]
Season				1.23	1.11
(1 = 2nd qtr;				(0.29)	(0.28)
0 = other)				[0.29]	[0.27]
Y_{ij-1}		0.61	0.62	0.82	0.62
		(0.39)	(0.37)	(0.47)	(0.38)
		[0.41]	[0.39]	[0.44]	[0.40]
Y_{ij-1} by		0.11		−0.11	
xerophthalmia		(1.3)		(1.4)	
		[1.1]		[1.1]	
Y_{ij-1} by age				0.00063	
				(0.029)	
				(0.024]	
Y_{ij-1} by season				−1.24	
				(1.2)	
				[1.1]	

regression coefficient, the standard error from (10.2.3) reported by ordinary logistic regression procedures, and the robust standard error defined by (10.2.4).

The first model predicts the risk of infection using only xerophthalmia status and should reproduce Table 10.2. The frequency of infection among children without xerophthalmia in Table 10.2 is 8.0% which equals $\exp(-2.44)/\{1+\exp(-2.44)\}$, where -2.44 is the intercept for Model 1 in Table 10.4. The log odds ratio calculated from Table 10.2 is

$$\log\{(0.119/0.881)/(0.080/0.920)\} = 0.44,$$

which is the coefficient for xerophthalmia in Model 1 of Table 10.4. The advantage of the logistic regression formulation is that standard errors are readily calculated.

Model 2 allows the association between xerophthalmia and respiratory disease to differ among children with respiratory disease at the prior visit and reproduces the transition rates from Table 10.3. For children without infection at the prior visit ($Y_{ij-1} = 0$), the log odds ratio for xerophthalmia calculated from Table 10.3 is $\log\{(0.108/0.892)/(0.075/0.925)\} = 0.40$, which equals the coefficient for current xerophthalmia in Model 2. The log odds ratio for children with infection at the prior visit is $0.40 + 0.11 = 0.51$, the sum of the xerophthalmia effect and the xerophthalmia-by-previous-infection interaction.

A comparison of Tables 10.2 and 10.3 indicates that the association of xerophthalmia and respiratory infection is similar for children who did and did not have respiratory infection at the previous visit. This is confirmed by the xerophthalmia-by-previous-infection interaction term in Model 2 which is 0.11 with approximate, robust 95% confidence interval (−2.1, 2.3). In Model 3, the interaction has been dropped.

If the first-order Markov assumption is valid, that is, if $\Pr(Y_{ij} \mid \mathcal{H}_{ij}) = \Pr(Y_{ij} \mid Y_{ij-1})$, then the standard errors estimated by ordinary logistic regression are valid. The robust standard errors have valid coverage in large samples even when the Markov assumption is incorrect. Hence a simple check of the sensitivity of inferences about a particular coefficient to the Markov assumption is whether the ordinary and robust standard errors are similar. They are similar for both coefficients in Model 1.

Models 1, 2, and 3 illustrate the use of logistic regression to fit simple Markov chains. The strength of this formulation is the ease of adding additional predictors to the model. This is illustrated in Models 4 and 5, where the child's age and a binary indicator of season (1 = 2nd quarter; 0 = other) have been added. In Model 4, we fit all interactions with Y_{ij-1} which is the same as fitting separate logistic regressions for the cases $Y_{ij-1} = 0$ and 1. None of the interactions with prior infection are important so they are dropped in Model 5.

Having controlled for age, season, and respiratory infection at the prior visit in Model 5, there is mild evidence in these data for an association between xerophthalmia and respiratory infection; the xerophthalmia coefficient is 0.78 with robust standard error 0.53. As with any regression, it is important to check the sensitivity of the scientific findings to choice of model. With transition models, we must check whether the regression inferences about $\boldsymbol{\beta}$ change with the model for the time dependence. To illustrate, we add Y_{ij-2} as a predictor to Model 5. Because we are using two prior visits as predictors, only data from visits 3 through 7 are relevant giving a total of 591 transitions. Interestingly, the inclusion of Y_{ij-2} reduces the influence of season and Y_{ij-1}, and increases the xerophthalmia coefficient to 1.73. Controlling for respiratory infection at the two prior visits nearly doubles the xerophthalmia coefficient. This example demonstrates an essential feature of transition models: explanatory variables (e.g. xerophthalmia) and previous responses are treated symmetrically as predictors of the current response. Hence, as the time-dependence model changes, so might inferences about the explanatory variables. Even when the time dependence is not of primary scientific interest, the sensitivity of the regression inferences must be checked by fitting a variety of time-dependence models.

10.3.2 *Ordered categorical data*

The ideas underlying logistic regression models for binary responses carry over to outcomes with more than two categories. In this sub-section, we consider models for ordered categorical data, and then briefly discuss nominal response models. The books by McCullagh and Nelder (1989, Chapter 5) and Agresti (1990, Chapter 9) provide expanded discussions for the case of independent observations. Agresti (1999) provides an overview of methods for both independent and clustered ordinal data.

To formulate a transition model for ordered categorical data, let Y_{ij} indicate a response variable which can take C ordered categorical values, labelled $0, 1, \ldots, C-1$. An example of ordered data is a rating of health status as: poor, fair, good, or excellent. While the outcomes are ordered, any numerical scale that might be assigned would be arbitrary.

The first-order transition matrix for Y_{ij} is defined by $\pi_{ab} = \Pr(Y_{ij} = b \mid Y_{ij-1} = a)$ for $a, b = 0, 1, \ldots, C-1$. As with binary data ($C = 2$), a saturated model of the transition matrix can be obtained by fitting a separate regression for each of the C possible values of Y_{ij-1}. That is, we model $\Pr(Y_{ij} = b \mid Y_{ij-1} = a)$ separately for each $a = 0, 1, \ldots, C-1$. With ordered categorical outcomes, we can use a *proportional odds* model (Snell, 1964 and McCullagh, 1980) which we now briefly review.

Since the response categories for ordinal data are usually arbitrary, we would like a regression model whose coefficients have the same interpretation when we combine or split categories. This is achieved by working with the cumulative probabilities $\Pr(Y \leq a)$ rather than the cell probabilities, $\Pr(Y = a)$. Given the cumulative probabilities, we can derive the cell probabilities since $\Pr(Y \leq a) = \Pr(Y \leq a-1) + \Pr(Y = a),\ a = 1, \ldots, C$.

The proportional odds model for independent observations has the form

$$\operatorname{logit} \Pr(Y \leq a) = \log \frac{\Pr(Y \leq a)}{\Pr(Y > a)} = \theta_a + \boldsymbol{x}'\boldsymbol{\beta},$$

where $a = 0, 1, \ldots, C-2$. Here and for the remainder of this section, we write the model intercepts as θ_a and do not include an intercept term in $\boldsymbol{x}$. Taking $\boldsymbol{x} = 0$, we see that $\Pr(Y \leq a) = \mathrm{e}^{-\theta_a}/(1+\mathrm{e}^{-\theta_a})$. Since $\Pr(Y \leq a)$ is a non-decreasing function of a, we have $\theta_0 \leq \theta_1 \leq \cdots \leq \theta_{C-2}$. If $\theta_a = \theta_{a+1}$, then $\Pr(Y \leq a) = \Pr(Y \leq a+1)$ and categories a and $a+1$ can therefore be collapsed.

The regression parameters $\boldsymbol{\beta}$ have log odds ratio interpretations, since

$$\frac{\Pr(Y \leq a \,|\, \boldsymbol{x}_1)/\Pr(Y > a \,|\, \boldsymbol{x}_1)}{\Pr(Y \leq a \,|\, \boldsymbol{x}_2)/\Pr(Y > a \,|\, \boldsymbol{x}_2)} = \exp\{(\boldsymbol{x}_1 - \boldsymbol{x}_2)'\boldsymbol{\beta}\}.$$

Following Clayton (1992), it is convenient to introduce the vector of variables $Y^* = (Y_0^*, Y_1^*, \ldots, Y_{C-2}^*)$ defined by $Y_a^* = 1$, if $Y \leq a$ and 0 otherwise. If $C = 3, Y^* = (Y_0^*, Y_1^*)$ takes values as shown in Table 10.5. The proportional odds model is simply a logistic regression for the Y_a^*, since

$$\log \frac{\Pr(Y \leq a)}{\Pr(Y > a)} = \operatorname{logit} \Pr(Y_a^* = 1) = \theta_a + \boldsymbol{x}'\boldsymbol{\beta}, \quad a = 0, 1, \ldots, C-2.$$

Here, each Y_a^* is allowed to have a different intercept but the proportional odds model requires that covariates have the same effect on each Y_a^*.

Our first application of the proportional odds model to a Markov chain for ordered categorical responses is the saturated first-order model without covariates. The transition matrix is $\pi_{ab} = \Pr(Y_{ij} = b \,|\, Y_{ij-1} = a)$, $a = 0, 1, \ldots, C-1$. We model the cumulative probabilities,

Table 10.5. Definition of Y^* variables for proportional odds modelling of ordered categorical data.

Y	0	1	2
Y_0^*	1	0	0
Y_1^*	1	1	0

$\Pr(Y_{ij} \le b \,|\, Y_{ij-1} = a) = \pi_{a0} + \pi_{a1} + \cdots + \pi_{ab}$, assuming that

$$\log \frac{\Pr(Y_{ij} \le b \,|\, Y_{ij-1} = a)}{\Pr(Y_{ij} > b \,|\, Y_{ij-1} = a)} = \theta_{ab} \tag{10.3.4}$$

for $a = 0, 1, \ldots, C-1$ and $b = 0, 1, \ldots, C-2$. Now, suppose that covariates $\boldsymbol{x}_{ij}$ have a different effect on Y_{ij} for each previous state Y_{ij-1}. The model can be written as

$$\log \frac{\Pr(Y_{ij} \le b \,|\, Y_{ij-1} = a)}{\Pr(Y_{ij} > b \,|\, Y_{ij-1} = a)} = \theta_{ab} + \boldsymbol{x_{ij}}'\boldsymbol{\beta_a} \tag{10.3.5}$$

for $a = 0, \ldots, C-1$; $b = 0, \ldots, C-2$. As with binary responses, we can rewrite (10.3.5) as a single (although somewhat complicated) regression equation using the interactions between $\boldsymbol{x_{ij}}$ and the vector of derived variables $\boldsymbol{y}^*_{ij-1} = (y^*_{ij-1,0}, \ldots, y^*_{ij-1,C-2})$

$$\log \frac{\Pr(Y_{ij} \le b \,|\, \boldsymbol{Y}^*_{ij-1} = \boldsymbol{y}^*_{ij-1})}{\Pr(Y_{ij} > b \,|\, \boldsymbol{Y}^*_{ij-1} = \boldsymbol{y}^*_{ij-1})}$$

$$= \theta_b + \sum_{\ell=0}^{C-2} \alpha_{\ell b} y^*_{ij-1\ell} + \boldsymbol{x}'_{ij}\left(\boldsymbol{\beta} + \sum_{\ell=0}^{C-2} \gamma_\ell y^*_{ij-1\ell}\right). \tag{10.3.6}$$

Comparing (10.3.5) and (10.3.6), we see that $\theta_{C-1b} - \theta_b$ and $\alpha_{ab} - \theta_{ab} - \theta_{a+1b}$, $a = 0, 1, \ldots, C-2$; $b = 0, 1, \ldots, C-2$. Similary, $\boldsymbol{\beta}_{C-1} = \boldsymbol{\beta}$ and $\gamma_a = \boldsymbol{\beta}_a - \boldsymbol{\beta}_{a+1}$, $a = 0, 1, \ldots, C-2$.

With this formulation, we can test whether or not the effect of $\boldsymbol{x}_{ij}$ on Y_{ij} is the same for adjacent categories of Y_{ij-1} by testing whether $\gamma_a = 0$. A simple special case of (10.3.6) is to assume that $\gamma_0 = \gamma_1 = \cdots = \gamma_{C-2} = 0$ so the covariates $\boldsymbol{x}_{ij}$ have the same effect on Y_{ij} regardless of Y_{ij-1}. As with binary data we can fit models with different subsets of the interactions between $\boldsymbol{y}^*_{ij-1}$ and $\boldsymbol{x}_{ij}$.

The transition ordinal regression model can be estimated using conditional maximum likelihood, that is, by conditioning on the first observation, Y_{i1}, for each person. Standard algorithms for fitting proportional odds models (McCullagh, 1980) can be used by adding the derived variables $\boldsymbol{y}^*_{ij-1}$ and their interactions with $\boldsymbol{x}_{ij}$ as additional covariates. As an alternative, Clayton (1992) has proposed using GEE to fit simultaneously logistic regressions to $Y^*_{ij0}, \ldots, Y^*_{ijC-2}$, again with $\boldsymbol{y}^*_{ij-1}$ and its interactions with $\boldsymbol{x}_{ij}$ as covariates. For the examples studied by Clayton, the GEE estimates were almost fully efficient.

When the categorical response does not have a natural ordering, we must model the transition probabilities, $\pi_{ab} = \Pr(Y_{ij} = b \,|\, Y_{ij-1} = a)$, $a, b = 0, 1, \ldots, C-1$. McCullagh and Nelder (1989) and Agresti (1990) discuss a variety of logistic model formulations for independent responses.

As we have demonstrated for binary and ordered categorical responses, these can be extended to transition models by using indicator variables for the previous state and their interactions with covariates as additional explanatory variables.

10.4 Log-linear transition models for count data

In this section, we consider extensions of the log-linear model in which the conditional distribution of y_{ij} given the past $\mathcal{H}_{ij}$ is Poisson with conditional expectation that depends both on past outcomes $y_{i1}, \ldots, y_{ij-1}$ and on explanatory variables $\boldsymbol{x}_{ij}$. We begin by reviewing three possible models for the conditional mean μ_{ij}^{C}. In each case, we restrict our attention to a first-order Markov chain.

1. $\mu_{ij}^{\mathrm{C}} = \exp(\boldsymbol{x}_{ij}'\boldsymbol{\beta})\{1 + \exp(-\alpha_0 - \alpha_1 y_{ij-1})\}$, $\alpha_0, \alpha_1 > 0$. In this model, suggested by Wong (1986), $\boldsymbol{\beta}$ represents the influence of the explanatory variables when the previous response takes the value $y_{ij-1} = 0$. When $y_{ij-1} > 0$, the conditional expectation is decreased from its maximum value, $\exp(\boldsymbol{x}_{ij}'\boldsymbol{\beta})\{1+\exp(-\alpha_0)\}$, by an amount that depends on α_1. Hence, this model only allows a negative association between the prior and current responses. For a given α_0, the degree of negative correlation increases as α_1 increases. Note that the conditional expectation must vary between $\exp(\boldsymbol{x}_{ij}'\boldsymbol{\beta})$ and twice this value, as a consequence of the constraints on α_0 and α_1.
2. $\mu_{ij}^{\mathrm{C}} = \exp(\boldsymbol{x}_{ij}'\boldsymbol{\beta}+\alpha y_{ij-1})$. This model appears sensible by analogy with the logistic model (7.3.1). But it has limited application for count data because when $\alpha > 0$, the conditional expectation grows as an exponential function of time. In fact, when $\exp(\boldsymbol{x}_{ij}'\boldsymbol{\beta}) = \mu$, corresponding to no dependence on covariates, this assumption leads to a stationary process only when $\alpha < 0$. Hence, the model can describe negative association but not positive association without growing exponentially over time. This is a time series analogue of the *auto-Poisson* process discussed for data on a two-dimensional lattice by Besag (1974).
3. $\mu_{ij}^{\mathrm{C}} = \exp[\boldsymbol{x}_{ij}'\boldsymbol{\beta}+\alpha\{\log(y_{ij-1}^*)-\boldsymbol{x}_{ij-1}'\boldsymbol{\beta}\}]$, *where* $y_{ij-1}^* = \max(y_{ij-1}, d)$ *and* $0 < d < 1$. This is the model introduced by Zeger and Qaqish (1988) and briefly discussed in Section 10.1. When $\alpha = 0$, it reduces to an ordinary log-linear model. When $\alpha < 0$, a prior response greater than its expectation decreases the expectation for the current response and there is negative correlation between y_{ij-1} and y_{ij}. When $\alpha > 0$, there is positive correlation.

For the remainder of this section, we focus on the third Poisson transition model above. It can arise through a simple physical mechanism called a size-dependent branching process. Suppose that $\exp(\boldsymbol{x}_{ij}'\boldsymbol{\beta}) = \mu$.

Suppressing the index i for the moment, let y_j represent the number of individuals in a population at generation j. Let $Z_k(y_{j-1})$ be the number of offspring for person k in generation $j-1$. Then for $y_{j-1} > 0$, the total size of the jth generation is

$$y_j = \sum_{k=1}^{y_{j-1}} Z_k(y_{j-1}).$$

If $y_{j-1} = 0$, we assume that the population is restarted with Z_0 individuals. Now, if we asssume that the random variables Z_k are independent Poisson with expectation $(\mu/y^*_{j-1})^{1-\alpha}$, then the population size will follow the transition model with $\mu^{\mathrm{C}}_j = \mu(y^*_{j-1}/\mu)^\alpha$. The assumption about the number of offspring per person represents a crowding effect. When the population is large, each individual tends to decrease their number of offspring. This leads to a stationary process.

Figure 10.1 displays five realizations of this transition model for different values of α. When $\alpha < 0$, the sample paths oscillate back and forth about their long-term average level since a large outcome at one time decreases the conditional expectation of the next response. When $\alpha > 0$, the process meanders, staying below the long-term average for extended periods. Notice that the sample paths have sharper peaks and broader valleys. This pattern is in contrast to Gaussian autoregressive sample paths for which the peaks and valleys have the same shape. In the Poisson model, the conditional variance equals the conditional mean. When by chance we get a large observation, the conditional mean and variance of the next value are both large; that is, the process becomes unstable and quickly falls towards the long-term average. After a small outcome, the conditional mean and variance are small, so the process tends to be more stable. Hence, there are broader valleys and sharper peaks.

To illustrate the application of this transition model for counts, we have fitted it to the seizure data. *A priori*, there is clear evidence that this model is not appropriate for this data set. The correlations among repeated seizure counts for each person do not decay as the time between observations increases. For example, the correlations of the square root transformed seizure number at the first post-treatment period with those at the second, third, and fourth periods are 0.76, 0.70, and 0.78, respectively. The Markov model implies that these should decrease as an approximately exponential function of lag. Nevertheless, we might fit the first-order model if our goal was simply to predict the seizure rate in the next interval, given only the rate in the previous interval. Because there is only a single observation prior to randomization, we have assumed that the pre-randomization means are the same for the two treatment groups. Letting $d = 0.3$, we estimate the treatment effect (treatment-by-time interaction in Tables 8.11 and 9.6) to be -0.10, with a model-based standard error of 0.083. This standard error

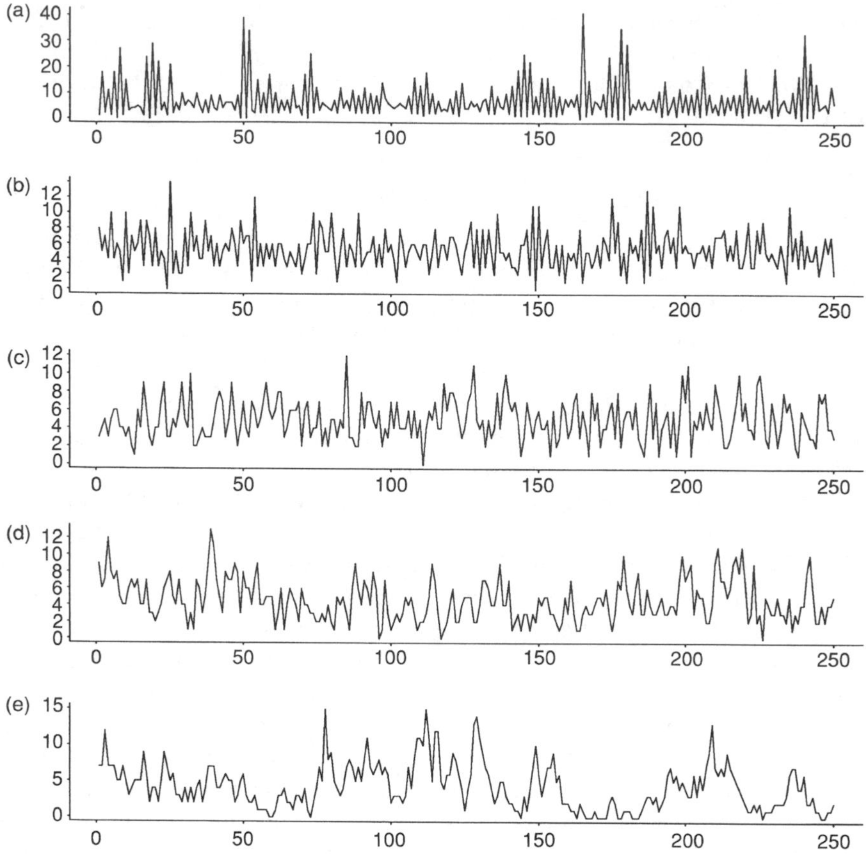

Fig. 10.1. Realizations of the Markov–Poisson time series model: (a) $\alpha = -0.8$; (b) $\alpha = -0.4$; (c) $\alpha = 0.0$; (d) $\alpha = 0.4$; (e) $\alpha = 0.8$.

is not valid because the model does not accurately capture the actual correlation structure in the data. We have also estimated a robust standard error which is 0.30, much larger than 0.083, reflecting the fact that the correlation does not decay as expected for the transition model. The estimate of treatment effect is not sensitive to the constant d; it varies between -0.096 and -0.107 as d ranges from 0.1 to 1.0. The estimate of α for $d = 0.3$ is 0.79 and also is not very sensitive to the value of c.

10.5 Further reading

Markov models have been studied by probabilists and mathematical statisticians for several decades. Feller (1968) and Billingsley (1961) are seminal texts. But there has been little theoretical study of Markov regression models except for the linear model (e.g. Tsay, 1984). This is partly because it is difficult to derive marginal distributions when the conditional distribution is assumed to follow a GLM regression.

Regression models for binary Markov chains are in common use. Examples of applications can be found in Korn and Whittemore (1979), Stern and Coe (1984), and Zeger *et al.* (1985). The reader is referred to papers by Wong (1986), and Zeger and Qaqish (1988) for methods applicable to count data. There has also been very interesting work on Bayesian Markov regression models with measurement error. See, for example, the discussion paper by West *et al.* (1985) and the volume by Spall (1988).

11
Likelihood-based methods for categorical data

11.1 Introduction

In a study of the natural history of schizophrenia, first-episode patients had disease symptoms recorded monthly for up to 10 years following initial hospitalization (Thara *et al.*, 1994). In studies of the health effects of air pollution, asthmatic children recorded the presence or absence of wheezing each day for approximately 60 days (Yu *et al.*, 2000). To determine whether maternal employment correlates with paediatric care utilization and both maternal stress and childhood illness, daily measurements of maternal stress (yes, no) and childhood illness (yes, no) were recorded for 28 consecutive days (Alexander and Markowitz, 1986). Lunn, *et al.* (2001) analyse ordinal allergic severity scores collected daily for 3 months on subjects assigned either to placebo or to one of three doses of active drug. In each of these examples the primary scientific question pertains to the association between specific covariates and a high-dimensional categorical response vector. 'Group-by-time' regression methods that characterize differences over time in the expected outcome among patient subgroups can be used for each of these examples. Although several analysis options exist for discrete longitudinal data, there are few likelihood-based methods that can accommodate such increasingly common long discrete series.

Likelihood-based analysis of longitudinal data remains attractive since a properly specified model leads to efficient estimation, and to valid summaries under missing at random (MAR) drop-out mechanisms as discussed in Chapter 13. A likelihood approach can be used to construct profile likelihood curves for key parameters, to compare nested models using likelihood ratio tests, and to compare non-nested models by considering penalized criteria such as AIC or BIC. However, to be used successfully we need to correctly specify the model form and this requires both tailored exploratory methods to characterize means and covariances, and methods for model checking. Finally, the sensitivity of likelihood-based methods to the underlying model assumptions needs to be understood so that important forms of model violation can be checked in practice.

In Chapter 8 we discussed marginal models and overviewed early approaches to provide likelihood-based inference specifically for binary response data. In Chapter 9 we discussed generalized linear mixed models (GLMMs) and commented on both approximate maximum likelihood and Bayesian estimation options. In Chapter 10 we discussed transition models and the use of the conditional likelihood for inference. The goal of this chapter is to provide a more detailed overview of current choices for likelihood-based analysis of categorical response data. We focus on the common and particularly challenging case of binary response data.

11.1.1 *Notation and definitions*

In this section we distinguish between *conditional* and *marginal* regression coefficients. We define the marginal mean as the average response conditional on the covariates for subject i, $\boldsymbol{X}_i = (\boldsymbol{x}_{i1}, \ldots, \boldsymbol{x}_{in_i})$: $\mu_{ij}^{\mathrm{M}} = \mathrm{E}(Y_{ij} \mid \boldsymbol{X}_i)$. A marginal generalized linear regression model links the marginal mean to covariates using a marginal regression parameter, $\boldsymbol{\beta}^{\mathrm{M}}$: $h(\mu_{ij}^{\mathrm{M}}) = \boldsymbol{x}_{ij}'\boldsymbol{\beta}^{\mathrm{M}}$. In contrast, we define a conditional mean as the average response conditional on the covariates $\boldsymbol{X}_i$ and additional variables $\boldsymbol{A}_{ij}$: $\mu_{ij}^{\mathrm{C}} = \mathrm{E}(Y_{ij} \mid \boldsymbol{X}_i, \boldsymbol{A}_{ij})$. A conditional generalized linear regression model links the conditional mean to both covariates and $\boldsymbol{A}_{ij}$ using a conditional regression parameter, $\boldsymbol{\beta}^{\mathrm{C}}$, and additional parameters, $\boldsymbol{\gamma}$: $h(\mu_{ij}^{\mathrm{C}}) = \boldsymbol{x}_{ij}'\boldsymbol{\beta}^{\mathrm{C}} + \boldsymbol{\gamma}'\boldsymbol{A}_{ij}$. We introduce this additional notation to help highlight some of the differences between marginal regression models discussed in Chapters 7 and 8, and random effects models discussed in Chapter 9, where $\boldsymbol{A}_{ij}$ represents the unobserved latent variable $\boldsymbol{U}_i$, and transition models discussed in Chapter 10, where $\boldsymbol{A}_{ij}$ represents functions of the response history, $\mathcal{H}_{ij}$. In this chapter we show how a correspondence between conditional models and their induced margins can be exploited to obtain likelihood-based inference for either conditional regression models or marginal regression models.

11.2 Generalized linear mixed models

Recall from Section 9.1 that a GLMM structures multiple sources of measured and unmeasured variation using a single model equation:

$$h\{\mathrm{E}(Y_{ij} \mid \boldsymbol{X}_i, \boldsymbol{U}_i)\} = \boldsymbol{x}_{ij}'\boldsymbol{\beta}^{\mathrm{C}} + \boldsymbol{d}_{ij}'\boldsymbol{U}_i,$$

where $\boldsymbol{x}_{ij}$ represents measured covariates, and $\boldsymbol{U}_i$ represents unmeasured random effects. For longitudinal data there are three central generalized linear mixed models:

$$h\{\mathrm{E}(Y_{ij} \mid \boldsymbol{X}_i, \boldsymbol{U}_i)\} = \boldsymbol{x}'_{ij}\boldsymbol{\beta}^{\mathrm{C}} + U_{i0}, \tag{11.2.1}$$

$$h\{\mathrm{E}(Y_{ij} \mid \boldsymbol{X}_i, \boldsymbol{U}_i)\} = \boldsymbol{x}'_{ij}\boldsymbol{\beta}^{\mathrm{C}} + U_{i0} + U_{i1} \cdot t_{ij}, \tag{11.2.2}$$

$$h\{\mathrm{E}(Y_{ij} \mid \boldsymbol{X}_i, \boldsymbol{U}_i)\} = \boldsymbol{x}'_{ij}\boldsymbol{\beta}^{\mathrm{C}} + U_{ij}, \tag{11.2.3}$$

$$\mathrm{cov}(U_{ij}, U_{ik}) = \sigma^2 \rho^{|t_{ij}-t_{ik}|}. \tag{11.2.4}$$

In the first model, (11.2.1), correlation among observations collected on an individual are attributable to a subject-specific 'level', or random intercept. These data assume that there is no additional aspect of time that enters into the dependence model. In (11.2.2) we assume that each subject has an individual 'trend', or follows a random linear trajectory (on the scale of the linear predictor). For binary data this model assumes that $\mu_{ij}^{\mathrm{C}} = h^{-1}(\boldsymbol{x}'_{ij}\boldsymbol{\beta}^{\mathrm{C}} + U_{i0} + U_{i1} \cdot t_{ij})$ which approaches 0 or 1 as $t_{ij} \to \infty$. Finally, (11.2.3) assumes only 'serial' correlation implying that observations close together in time are more highly correlated than observations far removed in time. Figure 11.1 displays simulated data, $Y_{ij} = 0$ or 1, generated from each of these models for $j = 1, 2, \ldots, 25$ time points. The first column of plots shows data for 10 subject generated using random intercepts, while the second column uses random lines, and the third column uses a latent autoregressive process to induce dependence. Even though these data are generated under fairly strong and different random effects parameters ($\mathrm{var}(U_{i0}) = 1.5^2$ for random intercepts, $\mathrm{var}(U_{i0}) = 0.2^2$ for random slopes, and $\mathrm{cov}(U_{ij}, U_{ik}) = 2.5^2 \cdot 0.9^{|j-k|}$ for random autoregressive process), there are only subtle aspects of the data that distinguish the models. First, the latent random lines model in the second column shows subjects in rows 2 and 6 (from the top) that appear to change over time from all 0's to all 1's, and the subject in row 5 switches from all 1's early to all 0's late. This pattern is expected from random lines since $\mu_{ij}^{\mathrm{C}} \to 0$ or 1 as j increases. The data generated using autoregressive random effects exhibit more alternating runs of 0's or 1's than the random intercept data, reflecting the serial association. Finally, these data suggest the challenge that binary data present – detectable differences in the underlying dependence structure may only be weakly apparent even with long categorical series.

In Section 9.2.2 we introduced approximate maximum likelihood methods, referred to as penalized quasi-likelihood (PQL) that are based on a Laplace approximation to the marginal likelihood. For count data and binomial data PQL can work surprisingly well. However, Breslow and Clayton (1993) also demonstrate that PQL approximations yield potentially severely biased estimates of both variance components and regression parameters when used for binary response data. Further research has been directed at removing the bias of PQL by employing higher order Laplace approximations (Breslow and Lin, 1995; Lin and Breslow, 1996; Goldstein

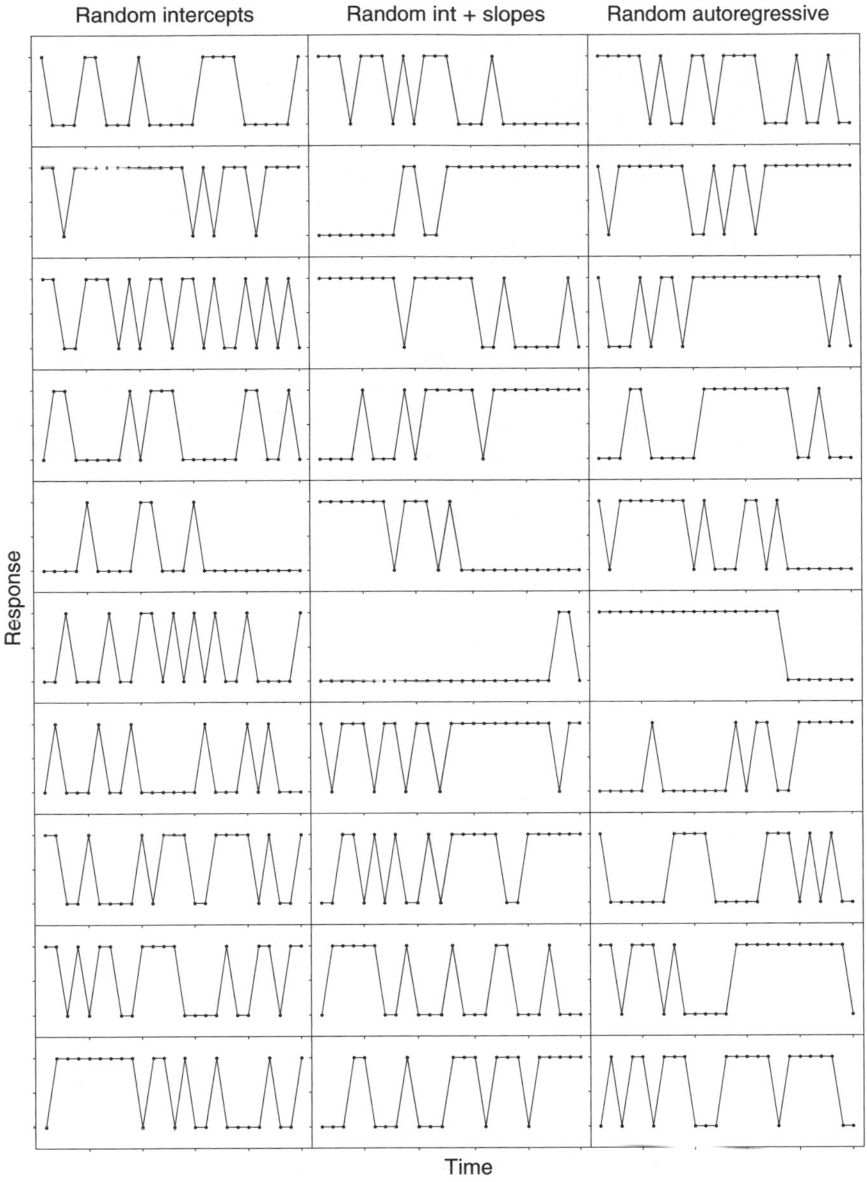

Fig. 11.1. Binary data simulated under GLMMs: Random intercepts $\equiv$ logit $\mathrm{E}(Y_{ij} \mid \boldsymbol{X}_i, U_{i0}) = \beta^{\mathrm{C}} + U_{i0}$; Random intercepts and slopes $\equiv$ logit $\mathrm{E}(Y_{ij} \mid \boldsymbol{X}_i, \boldsymbol{U}_i) = \beta^{\mathrm{C}} + U_{i0} + U_{i1} \cdot j$; Random autoregressive $\equiv$ logit $\mathrm{E}(Y_{ij} \mid \boldsymbol{X}_i, \boldsymbol{U}_i) = \beta^{\mathrm{C}} + U_{ij}$ where $\mathrm{cov}(U_{ij}, U_{ik}) = G\rho^{|j-k|}$.

and Rasbash, 1996). The singular advantage of approximate methods is their computational ease relative to alternative numerical methods which focus on directly maximizing the likelihood function using either quadrature methods or Monte Carlo methods. We review numerical maximum likelihood (ML) approaches in Section 11.2.1. Modern Bayesian computing algorithms have greatly expanded the model forms that can be considered for analysis. In Section 11.2.2 we discuss Markov Chain Monte Carlo (MCMC) analysis for GLMMs.

11.2.1 *Maximum likelihood algorithms*

For low-dimensional random effects standard numerical integration methods can be used to evaluate the likelihood, solve score equations, and compute model-based information matrices. Gauss–Hermite quadrature uses a fixed set of K ordinates and weights $(z_k, w_k)_{k=1}^K$ to approximate the likelihood function. Consider a single scalar random effect $U_i \sim \mathcal{N}(0, G)$ and the likelihood given by equation (9.2.5):

$$
\begin{aligned}
L(\boldsymbol{\delta}, \boldsymbol{Y}) &= \prod_{i=1}^{m} \int \left[\prod_{j=1}^{n_i} f(y_{ij} \mid \boldsymbol{X}_i, U_i; \boldsymbol{\beta}^{\mathrm{C}}) \right] \cdot f(U_i; G)\, \mathrm{d}U_i \\
&= \prod_{i=1}^{m} \int \left[\exp\left\{ \sum_{j=1}^{n_i} \log f(y_{ij} \mid \boldsymbol{X}_i, U_i; \boldsymbol{\beta}^{\mathrm{C}}) \right\} \right] \cdot G^{-1/2} \phi(U_i / G^{1/2})\, \mathrm{d}U_i \\
&\approx \prod_{i=1}^{m} \sum_{k=1}^{K} w_k \cdot \left[\exp\left\{ \sum_{j=1}^{n_i} \log f(y_{ij} \mid \boldsymbol{X}_i, U_i = G^{1/2} z_k; \boldsymbol{\beta}^{\mathrm{C}}) \right\} \right].
\end{aligned}
$$

Monahan and Stefanski (1992) discuss alternatives to Gauss–Hermite and show that the maximal error for Gauss–Hermite quadrature is increasing as the variance of the random effects increases. Specifically, let $M(\eta, \sigma) = \int \mathrm{expit}(\eta + \sigma \cdot z)\phi(z)\mathrm{d}z$, where $\mathrm{expit}(x) = \exp(x)/[1 + \exp(x)]$, and $\phi(z)$ is the standard normal density function. The function $M(\eta, \sigma)$ represents the marginal mean induced by a GLMM where $\mathrm{logit}(\mu^{\mathrm{C}}) = \eta + U$, $U \sim \mathcal{N}(0, \sigma^2)$. Let $\hat{M}(\eta, \sigma) = \sum_{k=1}^{K} w_k \cdot \mathrm{expit}(\eta + \sigma \cdot z_k)$, the approximation to $M(\eta, \sigma)$ using Gauss–Hermite quadrature with K nodes. For $K = 20$, Monahan and Stephanski (1992) show that $\sup_\eta \mid M(\eta, \sigma = 2) - \hat{M}(\eta, \sigma = 2) \mid \approx 10^{-6}$ while $\sup_\eta \mid M(\eta, \sigma = 4) - \hat{M}(\eta, \sigma = 4) \mid \approx 10^{-3}$. Crouch and Spiegelman (1990) also discuss conditions under which 20-point Gaussian quadrature begins to fail.

Adaptive Gaussian quadrature is an alternative numerical integration technique that centres the Gaussian approximation to the likelihood at the posterior mode of the random effects. To derive the adaptive quadrature we begin with the likelihood given above and then consider an arbitrary linear transformation for the placement of the quadrature points:

$$
\begin{aligned}
L(\boldsymbol{\delta}, \boldsymbol{y}) \\
&= \prod_{i=1}^{m} \int \left[\exp\left\{ \sum_{j=1}^{n_i} \log f(y_{ij} \mid \boldsymbol{X}_i, U_i = u; \boldsymbol{\beta}^{\mathrm{C}}) \right\} \right] \cdot G^{-1/2} \phi(u/G^{1/2}) \, \mathrm{d}u \\
&= \prod_{i=1}^{m} \int \left[\exp\left\{ \sum_{j=1}^{n_i} \log f(y_{ij} \mid \boldsymbol{X}_i, U_i = u; \boldsymbol{\beta}^{\mathrm{C}}) \right\} G^{-1/2} \right. \\
&\qquad \left. \times \frac{\phi(u/G^{1/2})}{\phi([u-a]/b)} \right] \cdot \phi([u-a]/b) \, \mathrm{d}u \\
&= \prod_{i=1}^{m} \int \left[\exp\left\{ \sum_{j=1}^{n_i} \log f(y_{ij} \mid \boldsymbol{X}_i, U_i = (a + b \cdot z); \boldsymbol{\beta}^{\mathrm{C}}) \right\} G^{-1/2} \right. \\
&\qquad \left. \times \frac{\phi([a + b \cdot z]/G^{1/2})}{\phi(z)} \cdot \frac{1}{b} \right] \cdot \phi(z) \, \mathrm{d}z \\
&\approx \prod_{i=1}^{m} \sum_{k=1}^{K} w_k \cdot \left[\exp\left\{ \sum_{j=1}^{n_i} \log f(y_{ij} \mid \boldsymbol{X}_i, U_i = (a + b \cdot z_k); \boldsymbol{\beta}^{\mathrm{C}}) \right\} G^{-1/2} \right. \\
&\qquad \left. \times \frac{\phi([a + b \cdot z_k]/G^{1/2})}{\phi(z_k)} \cdot \frac{1}{b} \right].
\end{aligned}
$$

This shows that we can use the Gauss–Hermite quadrature points $(w_k, z_k)_{k=1}^{K}$ after any linear transformation determined by (a, b) as long as the integrand is also modified to contain one additional term (a ratio of normal densities). If the function that we are trying to integrate were of the form $\exp(-\frac{1}{2}(u - a)^2/b^2)$ then evaluation using the linear transformation $a + b \cdot z_k$ would yield an exact result. An adaptive approach uses different values, a_i and b_i for each subject, that provide a quadratic approximation to the ith subject's contribution to the log likelihood, $\sum_j \log f(y_{ij} \mid \boldsymbol{X}_i, U_i; \boldsymbol{\beta}^{\mathrm{C}}) - U_i^2/(2G)$. In Section 9.2.2 we showed that a_i is the posterior mode, $a_i = \hat{U}_i = G D_i V_i^{-1}(\boldsymbol{z}_i - X_i \boldsymbol{\beta}^{\mathrm{C}})$, and b_i is the approximate posterior curvature, $b_i = [\sum_j D'_{ij} V(\mu_{ij}^b) D_{ij} + G^{-1}]^{-1/2}$, where $D_{ij} = \partial \mu_{ij}^b / \partial b$. Liu and Pierce (1994) discuss how this adaptive quadrature is related to higher order Laplace approximation.

Pinheiro and Bates (1995) studied the accuracy of PQL, fixed quadrature, and adaptive quadrature for the non-linear mixed model. Their results suggest that in order to obtain high accuracy with fixed quadrature methods a large number of quadrature points may be necessary (100 or more!), while adaptive quadrature methods proved accurate using 20 points or fewer. Quadrature methods are now implemented in commercial software packages including STATA (fixed quadrature for logistic-normal) and SAS (fixed and adaptive). A key limitation of quadrature methods is that likelihood evaluation requires K^q quadrature points, where q is the dimension of the random effect $\boldsymbol{U}_i$. For q larger than two, the computational burden can become severe. This limitation makes numerical integration using quadrature an excellent choice for random intercept models, for nested random effects, or for random lines, but prohibitive for multidimensional random effect models such as time series or spatial data models.

Monte Carlo ML algorithms have been developed by McCulloch (1997) and Booth and Hobert (2000). Three methods are described and compared in McCulloch (1997): Monte Carlo Expectation-Maximization (MCEM); Monte Carlo Newton–Raphson (MCNR); and Simulated Maximum Likelihood (SML). Hybrid approaches that first use MCEM or MCNR and then switch to SML are advocated. Booth and Hobert (2000) develop adaptations that aim to automate the Monte Carlo ML algorithms and guide the increase in the Monte Carlo sample sizes that is required for the stochastic algorithm to converge. Booth and Hobert (2000) show that efficient estimation can be realized with random intercept models and crossed random effect models, but suggest that the proposed methods may break down when integrals are of high dimension. The advantage of Monte Carlo ML methods is that the approximation error can be made arbitrarily small simply by increasing the size of the Monte Carlo samples. In contrast, to improve accuracy with quadrature methods a new set of nodes and weights, $(z_k, w_k)_{k=1}^K$, must be calculated for a larger value of K.

In summary, fixed, adaptive, and stochastic numerical integration methods have been developed and made commercially accessible for use with GLMMs having low-dimensional random effect distributions. However, none of the numerical ML methods have been made computationally practical for models with random effects distributions with $q > 5$. This aspect makes it impossible to use ML for GLMMs that have serial random effects, such as (11.2.3), greatly limiting application for categorical longitudinal data analysis. Further detail regarding methods for integral approximation can be found in Evans and Swartz (1995).

11.2.2 *Bayesian methods*

Zeger and Karim (1991) discuss use of Gibbs sampling for Bayesian analysis of discrete data using a GLMM. Gibbs sampling is one particular implementation of a wider class of methods for sampling from a posterior distribution known as MCMC. MCMC methods constitute a technical breakthrough for statistical estimation. These methods can handle complex situations with relative ease, allowing inference for fixed effects, random effects, and general functions of fixed and random effects. For example, the autoregressive random effects model (11.2.3) is infeasible to fit using ML methods due to the intractable integrals of dimension n_i that define the marginal likelihood. MCMC can be used fairly easily for this particular problem, as well as for the simpler random intercept and random line models (11.2.1) and (11.2.2). The potential of MCMC has led to an explosion of applications to important and complex modelling scenarios beyond longitudinal data. The books by Gelman *et al.* (1995), Gilks *et al.* (1996), and Carlin and Louis (1996) provide comprehensive introduction and discussion. In this section we provide a brief general overview of the method emphasizing the modelling requirements over the more technical aspects.

A Bayesian approach treats all unknown quantities as random variables and assigns prior probability distributions for the unknown parameters $\boldsymbol{\delta} = (\boldsymbol{\beta}^{\mathrm{C}}, \boldsymbol{G})$ that define the GLMM. Posterior inference is obtained by using the likelihood $L(\boldsymbol{\delta}, \boldsymbol{y})$ to convert prior uncertainty, $\pi(\boldsymbol{\delta})$, into posterior probability statements, $\pi(\boldsymbol{\delta} \mid \boldsymbol{y}) = L(\boldsymbol{y} \mid \boldsymbol{\delta}) \cdot \pi(\boldsymbol{\delta})/f(\boldsymbol{y})$. In the generalized linear mixed model the random effects are also unknown and thus the joint posterior distribution for $\boldsymbol{U} = \mathrm{vec}(\boldsymbol{U}_i)$ and $\boldsymbol{\delta}$ is given by the hierarchical models

$$\pi(\boldsymbol{\delta}, \boldsymbol{U} \mid \boldsymbol{y}) \propto f(\boldsymbol{y} \mid \boldsymbol{U}, \boldsymbol{\delta}) \cdot \ f(\boldsymbol{U} \mid \boldsymbol{\delta}) \cdot \pi(\boldsymbol{\delta}).$$

We note that the marginal posterior distribution for the parameters $\boldsymbol{\delta}$ is obtained by integrating over the random effects $\boldsymbol{U}$,

$$\begin{aligned}\pi(\boldsymbol{\delta} \mid \boldsymbol{y}) &= \int_{\boldsymbol{U}} \pi(\boldsymbol{\delta}, \boldsymbol{U} \mid \boldsymbol{y}) \, \mathrm{d}\boldsymbol{U} \\ &\propto \int_{\boldsymbol{U}} f(\boldsymbol{y} \mid \boldsymbol{U}, \boldsymbol{\delta}) \cdot f(\boldsymbol{U} \mid \boldsymbol{\delta}) \cdot \pi(\boldsymbol{\delta}) \, \mathrm{d}\boldsymbol{U} \\ &\propto L(\boldsymbol{y} \mid \boldsymbol{\delta}) \cdot \pi(\boldsymbol{\delta}),\end{aligned}$$

indicating that the only difference between the maximization of the posterior, $\pi(\boldsymbol{\delta} \mid \boldsymbol{y})$, and the marginal likelihood, $L(\boldsymbol{y} \mid \boldsymbol{\delta})$, is the additional impact of the prior $\pi(\boldsymbol{\delta})$. We review these basic aspects of Bayesian methods for two key reasons. First, it shows that if we can actually solve the harder problem of characterizing the joint posterior $\pi(\boldsymbol{\delta}, \boldsymbol{U} \mid \boldsymbol{y})$ then we can compute the marginal posterior for regression and variance component parameters $\boldsymbol{\delta}$. Second, this shows the well-known result that the posterior distribution closely approximates the likelihood function when weakly informative priors are used.

The MCMC methods can be used to generate samples from the joint posterior $\pi(\boldsymbol{\delta}, \boldsymbol{U} \mid \boldsymbol{y})$. General algorithm details are thoroughly presented elsewhere (Gilks *et al.*, 1996, Carlin and Louis, 1996). The GLMM has a separation of parameters such that $f(\boldsymbol{y} \mid \boldsymbol{U}, \boldsymbol{\delta}) = f(\boldsymbol{y} \mid \boldsymbol{U}, \boldsymbol{\beta}^{\mathrm{C}})$, and $f(\boldsymbol{U} \mid \boldsymbol{\delta}) = f(\boldsymbol{U} \mid \boldsymbol{G})$. These conditional independence relationships allow use of simplified Gibbs steps within MCMC algorithms (Zeger and Karim, 1991). Use of MCMC in practice requires that the samples generated via Markov chains be assessed for convergence to their stationary distribution, and that adequate Monte Carlo sample sizes have been generated to precisely estimate posterior summaries such as means, medians, and standard deviations. Publically available software (BUGS) allows application for models (11.2.1)–(11.2.3) and for more complicated correlated data problems. As with all likelihood-based methods the use of Bayes/MCMC requires careful and thoughtful specification of the data model $f(\boldsymbol{y} \mid \boldsymbol{\delta})$. However, the major contribution of MCMC machinery is that realistically complicated models can now be routinely used in practice, allowing a rich family of correlated data models not previously accessible using direct likelihood methods.

Gelfand and Smith (1990) describe sampling-based approaches for calculation of marginal posterior densities, and Gelfand *et al.* (1990) provide illustration of Bayesian inference based on Gibbs sampling. Zeger and Karim (1991) discuss regression analysis of categorical response data within the GLMM framework, and Albert and Chib (1993), Chib and Greenberg (1998) overview MCMC methods for binary and polytomous data using multivariate probit models. Sun *et al.* (2000) discuss GLMMs where random effects have a serial or spatial correlation structure. Finally, Chib and Carlin (1999) discuss specific computational issues related to the use of MCMC for longitudinal data analysis.

11.3 Marginalized models

The goal of this section is to show that log-linear, random effects, and transition models can be used with multivariate categorical data to either model a conditional regression coefficient as described in Chapters 9 and 10, or as a basis for constructing a correlated data likelihood with a marginal regression structure that is directly modelled.

In marginal regression models, the mean (or first moment) regression parameters represent the change in expected response, such as prevalence with binary outcomes, per unit change in a given predictor without conditioning on the other responses or any latent variables. Correlations among elements of $\boldsymbol{Y}_i$ given $\boldsymbol{X}_i$, even if reasonably attributed to shared unobservable latent variables, or through a dependence on the past outcomes, is accounted for by a separate dependence model. There are several advantages of a direct marginal approach. First, the interpretation of mean parameters, $\boldsymbol{\beta}^{\mathrm{M}}$, is invariant with respect to specification of the dependence model. Two data analysts with the same mean regression but different association models have exactly the same target of estimation, $\boldsymbol{\beta}^{\mathrm{M}}$. In this sense, the mean model is 'separable' from the remainder of the model for the joint distribution. Second, marginal models can be estimated either using semi-parametric methods such as generalized estimating equations (GEE), or using likelihood methods described below.

Often the motivation for adopting a random effects model that conditions on latent variables U_{ij}, or for use of a transition model that conditions on the past outcomes, is simply to account for correlation among repeated measurements. In discussing the role of statistical models, Cox (1990) comments:

> It is important to distinguish the parts of the model that define aspects of subject matter interest, the primary aspects, and the secondary aspects that indicate efficient methods of estimation and assessment of precision. (page 171)

> Especially in empirical models, it is desirable that parameters (e.g. contrasts, regression coefficients and the like) have an interpretation largely independent of the secondary features of the models used. (page 173)

Therefore, if the primary objective of longitudinal analysis is to make inference regarding the mean response as a function of covariates and time, then a marginal mean model may be useful. In this section we describe how the correlation among observations can be characterized by embedding the marginal mean structure within a complete multivariate probability model based on either log-linear, random effects, or transition model dependence assumptions.

Marginalized models separate the model for *systematic variation* (mean) from the model for *random variation* (dependence) when using regression models for longitudinal data. In the first component of a marginalized model a generalized linear model is used for the marginal mean:

$$\text{regression: } h\{\mathrm{E}(Y_{ij} \mid \boldsymbol{X}_i)\} = \boldsymbol{x}_{ij}'\boldsymbol{\beta}^{\mathrm{M}}. \tag{11.3.1}$$

However, the marginal mean only identifies one facet of the complete multivariate distribution for the response $\boldsymbol{Y}_i$. In order to complete model specification we need to characterize the *dependence* among repeated observations. In a marginalized model we specify a second regression to characterize correlation or random variation:

$$\text{dependence: } h\{\mathrm{E}(Y_{ij} \mid \boldsymbol{X}_i, \boldsymbol{A}_{ij})\} = \Delta_{ij}(\boldsymbol{X}_i) + \boldsymbol{\gamma}_{ij}'\boldsymbol{A}_{ij}. \tag{11.3.2}$$

Here we introduce additional variables $\boldsymbol{A}_{ij}$ that are used to structure dependence among the repeated measurements. In general, the link functions in (11.3.1) and (11.3.2) can be different although we usually choose them to be equal so that mean parameters and dependence parameters are on a common scale. One possible choice is $\boldsymbol{A}_{ij} = \{Y_{ik}\colon k \neq j\}$. In this case the parameter $\boldsymbol{\gamma}_{ij}$ indicates how strongly all other response variables, Y_{ik}, predict the current response, Y_{ij}. Although we assume the analysis focus is on the marginal mean given by (11.3.1), specification of the conditional mean in (11.3.2) is useful for describing within-subject correlation and for identifying the joint distribution of $\boldsymbol{Y}_i$. In Section 11.3.2 we describe 'marginalized log-linear models' that are based on (11.3.1) and (11.3.2) using $\boldsymbol{A}_{ij} = \{Y_{ik}\colon k \neq j\}$. Alternatively, we may let $\boldsymbol{A}_{ij} = \boldsymbol{U}_i$, a collection of random effects or latent variables. In this case we also need to describe the population distribution of the random effects. Here γ_{ij} represents variance components that characterize the magnitude of unobserved, or random variation which induces all within-person correlation. In Section 11.3.3 we describe 'marginalized latent variable models' that are based on (11.3.1) and (11.3.2) using $\boldsymbol{A}_{ij} = \boldsymbol{U}_i$. Finally, we may consider $\boldsymbol{A}_{ij} = \{Y_{ik}\colon k < j\} = \mathcal{H}_{ij}$ where (11.3.2) now describes how strongly the past responses predict the current outcome. In Section 11.3.4 we describe 'marginalized transition models' that are based on (11.3.1) and (11.3.2) using $\boldsymbol{A}_{ij} = \mathcal{H}_{ij}$. In this case γ_{ij} characterizes how strongly the past observations predict the current outcome.

In each of these marginalized models the parameter $\Delta_{ij}(\boldsymbol{X}_i)$ represents a function of the marginal means, μ_{ij}^{M}, and dependence parameters, γ_{ij}, such that the conditional model in (11.3.2) is consistent with the marginal mean structure: $\mu_{ij}^{\mathrm{M}} = \mathrm{E}_{\boldsymbol{A}_{ij}}[\mathrm{E}(Y_{ij} \mid \boldsymbol{X}_i, \boldsymbol{A}_{ij})]$. Stated alternatively, when the conditional model in (11.3.2) is averaged over the distribution of $\boldsymbol{A}_{ij}$ the value $\Delta_{ij}(\boldsymbol{X}_i)$ is chosen such that the resulting marginal mean structure is properly induced, $\mu_{ij}^{\mathrm{M}} = \mathrm{E}_{\boldsymbol{A}_{ij}}[h^{-1}\{\Delta_{ij}(\boldsymbol{X}_i) + \gamma_{ij}'\boldsymbol{A}_{ij}\}]$. Likelihood-based estimation methods for marginalized models need to recover $\Delta_{ij}(\boldsymbol{X}_i)$ and evaluate the likelihood function. In each of the following subsections we first review the model assumptions and then overview ML estimation issues.

The structural specification of a marginalized model parallels the components of a generalized linear model for univariate outcomes. McCullagh and Nelder (1989, p. 27) identify a random component that specifies the distribution of the response and therefore determines the likelihood, and a separate systematic component that characterizes the mean response as a function of covariates. Marginalized models for longitudinal data similarly separate the distributional assumptions in (11.3.2) from the regression assumptions in (11.3.1).

11.3.1 *An example using the Gaussian linear model*

Although in this chapter we focus on the use of marginalized models for categorical response data, the model formulation in terms of (11.3.1) and (11.3.2) could equally be adopted for continuous response data. We briefly present the Gaussian version of three marginalized models to derive analytical expressions for $\Delta_{ij}(\boldsymbol{X}_i)$ and to show that each specific pair of models, given in terms of the marginal mean (11.3.1) and a conditional mean (11.3.2), characterizes both the mean and the covariance, and with the assumption of normal errors specifies the multivariate likelihood.

First consider the conditionally specified Gaussian model:

$$\begin{aligned} Y_{ij} \mid Y_{ik}: k \neq j &= \mu_{ij}^{\mathrm{M}} + \sum_{k \neq j} \theta_{ijk}(Y_{ik} - \mu_{ik}^{\mathrm{M}}) + \epsilon_{ij} \\ &= (\mu_{ij}^{\mathrm{M}} - \boldsymbol{\theta}_{ij}' \boldsymbol{\mu}_i^{\mathrm{M}}) + \boldsymbol{\theta}_{ij}' \boldsymbol{Y}_i^* + \epsilon_{ij}, \\ \mathrm{E}(Y_{ij} \mid \boldsymbol{X}_i, \boldsymbol{A}_{ij}) &= \Delta_{ij}(\boldsymbol{X}_i) + \boldsymbol{\theta}_{ij}' \boldsymbol{A}_{ij}, \end{aligned}$$

where $\boldsymbol{\theta}_{ij}$ is the vector $(\theta_{ij1}, \theta_{ij2}, \ldots, \theta_{ijn_i})$ with $\theta_{ijj} = 0$, and $\boldsymbol{A}_{ij} = \boldsymbol{Y}_i^*$, the response vector $\boldsymbol{Y}_i$ with Y_{ij} set to zero. We see that $\Delta_{ij}(\boldsymbol{X}_i) = (\mu_{ij}^{\mathrm{M}} - \boldsymbol{\theta}_{ij}' \boldsymbol{\mu}_i^{\mathrm{M}})$ a function of the marginal mean, $\boldsymbol{\mu}_i^{\mathrm{M}}$, and the dependence parameters $\boldsymbol{\theta}_{ij}$. The covariance of $\boldsymbol{Y}_i$ is $(\boldsymbol{I} - \boldsymbol{\Theta}_i)^{-1}\boldsymbol{R}_i$, where $\boldsymbol{\Theta}_i$ is an $n_i \times n_i$ matrix with rows $\boldsymbol{\theta}_{ij}$, and $\boldsymbol{R}_i$ is a diagonal matrix with diagonal elements equal to $\mathrm{var}(\epsilon_{ij})$. We see that in order to be a valid model we assume $(\boldsymbol{I} - \boldsymbol{\Theta}_i)$ is invertible and require the product $(\boldsymbol{I} - \boldsymbol{\Theta}_i)^{-1}\boldsymbol{R}_i$ to be symmetric, positive definite. Models specified in this fashion are also discussed in the spatial data literature and compared to alternative model specification approaches (see for example Sections 6.3.2 and 6.3.3 of Cressie, 1993).

Next consider an AR(p) formulation:

$$\begin{aligned} Y_{ij} \mid Y_{ik}: k < j &= \mu_{ij}^{\mathrm{M}} + \sum_{k=1}^{p} \gamma_{ij,k}(Y_{ij-k} - \mu_{ij-k}^{\mathrm{M}}) + \epsilon_{ij} \\ &= (\mu_{ij}^{\mathrm{M}} - \boldsymbol{\gamma}_{ij}' \boldsymbol{\mu}_{ij}^*) + \boldsymbol{\gamma}_{ij}' \boldsymbol{H}_{ij-1} + \epsilon_{ij}, \\ \mathrm{E}(Y_{ij} \mid \boldsymbol{X}_i, \boldsymbol{A}_{ij}) &= \Delta_{ij}(\boldsymbol{X}_i) + \boldsymbol{\gamma}_{ij}' \boldsymbol{A}_{ij}, \end{aligned}$$

where $\boldsymbol{\gamma}_{ij}$ is the vector $(\gamma_{ij,1}, \gamma_{ij,2}, \ldots, \gamma_{ij,p})$, $\boldsymbol{\mu}_{ij}^* = (\mu_{ij-1}^{\mathrm{M}}, \mu_{ij-2}^{\mathrm{M}}, \ldots, \mu_{ij-p}^{\mathrm{M}})$, $\boldsymbol{A}_{ij} = \boldsymbol{H}_{ij-1}$, where $\boldsymbol{H}_{ij-1} = (Y_{ij-1}, Y_{ij-2}, \ldots, Y_{ij-p})$. Again we obtain $\Delta_{ij}(\boldsymbol{X}_i) = (\mu_{ij}^{\mathrm{M}} - \boldsymbol{\gamma}_{ij}' \boldsymbol{\mu}_{ij}^*)$ a function of the marginal mean, $\boldsymbol{\mu}_i^{\mathrm{M}}$, and the association parameters $\boldsymbol{\gamma}_{ij}$. The covariance of $\boldsymbol{Y}_i$ is $(\boldsymbol{I} - \boldsymbol{\Gamma}_i)^{-1}\boldsymbol{R}_i(\boldsymbol{I} - \boldsymbol{\Gamma}_i')^{-1}$, where $\boldsymbol{\Gamma}_i$ is the $n_i \times n_i$ lower triangular matrix with rows defined by $\boldsymbol{\gamma}_{ij}$. Here we find that any $\boldsymbol{\Gamma}_i$ leads to a positive semi-definite covariance matrix for $\boldsymbol{Y}_i$ ($\boldsymbol{R}_i$ is assumed to be a diagonal matrix with $\mathrm{var}(\epsilon_{ij})$ on the diagonal). Models specified in this fashion are discussed in the time series literature (see for example Chapter 3 of Diggle, 1990).

Finally, the random effects model can be represented as

$$\begin{aligned} Y_{ij} \mid \boldsymbol{U}_i &= \mu_{ij}^{\mathrm{M}} + \boldsymbol{d}_{ij}' \boldsymbol{U}_i + \epsilon_{ij} \\ &= \mu_{ij}^{\mathrm{M}} + \boldsymbol{d}_{ij}' \boldsymbol{G}^{1/2} \boldsymbol{\xi}_i + \epsilon_{ij}, \\ \mathrm{E}(Y_{ij} \mid \boldsymbol{X}_i, \boldsymbol{A}_{ij}) &= \Delta_{ij}(\boldsymbol{X}_i) + \boldsymbol{\alpha}_{ij}' \boldsymbol{A}_{ij}, \end{aligned}$$

where $\boldsymbol{\alpha}'_{ij} = \boldsymbol{d}'_{ij}\boldsymbol{G}^{1/2}$ and $\boldsymbol{A}_{ij} = \boldsymbol{\xi}_i$ for $\boldsymbol{\xi}_i \sim \mathcal{N}(\boldsymbol{0}, \boldsymbol{I})$. Here we simply have $\Delta_{ij}(\boldsymbol{X}_i) = \mu_{ij}^{\mathrm{M}}$, and the induced covariance of $\boldsymbol{Y}_i$ is $\boldsymbol{D}_i\boldsymbol{G}\boldsymbol{D}'_i + \boldsymbol{R}_i$ where $\boldsymbol{d}_{ij}$ is the jth row of $\boldsymbol{D}_i$.

These examples demonstrate that a multivariate normal model can be specified using marginal means, $\mathrm{E}(Y_{ij} \mid \boldsymbol{X}_i) = \mu_{ij}^{\mathrm{M}}$, combined with conditional expectations $\mathrm{E}(Y_{ij} \mid \boldsymbol{X}_i, \boldsymbol{A}_{ij})$, where $\boldsymbol{A}_{ij}$ can either be the remaining response variables $\{Y_{ik} \colon k \neq j\}$, the past response variables, $\{Y_{ik} \colon k < j\}$, or a latent variable, $\boldsymbol{U}_i$.

11.3.2 *Marginalized log-linear models*

Log-linear models (Bishop *et al.*, 1975) have been widely used for the analysis of cross-classified discrete observations. Balanced binary vectors, $(Y_{i1}, Y_{i2}, \ldots, Y_{in})$ for $i = 1, 2, \ldots, m$, can be considered as a cross-classification of the n component responses. As discussed in Section 8.2.2, a log-linear model is constructed directly for the multivariate probabilities

$$\log \Pr_{\boldsymbol{\theta}_i}(Y_{i1}, \ldots, Y_{in}) = \theta_i^{(0)} + \sum_j \theta_{ij}^{(1)} Y_{ij} + \sum_{j<k} \theta_{ijk}^{(2)} Y_{ij} Y_{ik} + \sum_{j<k<l} \theta_{ijkl}^{(3)} Y_{ij} Y_{ik} Y_{il} + \cdots + \theta_i^{(n)} Y_{i1}, \ldots, Y_{in}.$$

Here the canonical parameter vector $\boldsymbol{\theta}_i = (\boldsymbol{\theta}_i^{(1)}, \boldsymbol{\theta}_i^{(2)}, \ldots, \theta_i^{(n)})$ is unconstrained and $\theta_i^{(0)}$ is a normalizing constant. Given covariates, $\boldsymbol{X}_i$, it is possible to allow $\boldsymbol{\theta}_i$ to depend on $\boldsymbol{X}_i$ or to extend the log-linear model to describe $\log P(\boldsymbol{Y}_i, \boldsymbol{X}_i)$ when $\boldsymbol{X}_i$ is also discrete. However, in either case the log-linear model results in complicated functions for the marginal expectations, $\mathrm{E}(Y_{ij} \mid \boldsymbol{X}_i)$, because these are obtained as sums over the response variable joint distribution

$$\mathrm{E}(Y_{ij} \mid \boldsymbol{X}_i) = \sum_{Y_{ik}, k \neq j} \Pr_{\boldsymbol{\theta}_i}(Y_{i1}, Y_{i2}, \ldots, \underline{Y_{ij} = 1, \ldots}, Y_{in} \mid \boldsymbol{X}_i)$$

yielding mixtures of exponential functions of the canonical parameters $\boldsymbol{\theta}_i$. In a log-linear model, the natural (canonical) univariate regressions are for the conditional expectations

$$\begin{aligned} &\operatorname{logit} \mathrm{E}(Y_{ij} \mid Y_{ik} \colon k \neq j) \\ &= \theta_{ij}^{(1)} + \sum_k \theta_{ijk}^{(2)} Y_{ik} + \sum_{k<l} \theta_{ijkl}^{(3)} Y_{ik} Y_{il} + \cdots + \theta_i^{(n)} \prod_{l \neq j} Y_{il}. \end{aligned}$$

Therefore, although log-linear models are well suited for describing multivariate dependencies, or for modelling joint and conditional distributions, they do not directly facilitate multivariate generalized linear regression modelling of the marginal means.

We now consider the formulation of marginalized log-linear models. Fitzmaurice and Laird (1993) 'marginalized' canonical log-linear models to permit likelihood-based regression estimation of the marginal means by transforming the canonical parameter, $\boldsymbol{\theta}_i = (\boldsymbol{\theta}_i^{(1)}, \boldsymbol{\theta}_i^{(2)}, \ldots, \theta_i^{(n)})$ into the mixed parameter, $\boldsymbol{\theta}_i^* = (\boldsymbol{\mu}_i^{\mathrm{M}}, \boldsymbol{\theta}_i^{(2)}, \ldots, \theta_i^{(n)})$, where $\boldsymbol{\mu}_i^{\mathrm{M}} = (\mu_{i1}^{\mathrm{M}}, \mu_{i2}^{\mathrm{M}}, \ldots, \mu_{in}^{\mathrm{M}})$, with $\mu_{ij}^{\mathrm{M}} = \mathrm{E}(Y_{ij} \mid \boldsymbol{X}_i)$. In their approach the underlying log-linear model parameters, $(\boldsymbol{\theta}_i^{(2)}, \ldots, \theta_i^{(n)})$ are used to describe the covariance of the response vector while the average response variable is directly modelled via the marginal mean.

We use the following pair of regression statements to characterize the marginalized log-linear model

$$h\{\mathrm{E}(Y_{ij} \mid \boldsymbol{X}_i)\} = \boldsymbol{x}_{ij}'\boldsymbol{\beta}^{\mathrm{M}}, \tag{11.3.3}$$

$$\operatorname{logit}\{\mathrm{E}(Y_{ij} \mid \boldsymbol{X}_i, Y_{ik}\colon k \neq j)\} = \Delta_{ij}(\boldsymbol{X}_i) + \boldsymbol{\theta}_{ij}'\boldsymbol{W}_{ij}, \tag{11.3.4}$$

where $\boldsymbol{W}_{ij}$ represents Y_{ik}, pairwise products $Y_{ik}Y_{il}$, and higher order products of $\{Y_{ik}\colon k \neq j\}$. The fact that (11.3.3) identifies the joint distribution of $\boldsymbol{Y}_i$ with $\boldsymbol{\theta}_{ij}$ unconstrained parameters subject only to symmetry conditions such as $\theta_{ijk}^{(2)} = \theta_{ikj}^{(2)}$, is known as the Hammersly–Clifford Theorem (Besag, 1974). The term $\Delta_{ij}(\boldsymbol{X}_i)$ is not a free parameter since it is constrained to satisfy the marginal mean model (11.3.3). The parameters for this model are $\boldsymbol{\beta}^{\mathrm{M}}$ and $\{\boldsymbol{\theta}_{ij}\}_{j=1}^{n}$. As with all marginal regression models the mean model (11.3.3) is separated from the dependence model (11.3.4) and the parameter $\boldsymbol{\beta}^{\mathrm{M}}$ retains the same interpretation for any model assumptions used in (11.3.4). The log-linear association parameters in $\boldsymbol{\theta}_{ij}$ indicate how strongly other outcomes, Y_{ik} $k \neq j$, predict Y_{ij}. This model does not exploit time asymmetry and conditions on both past and future outcomes through $\{Y_{ik}\colon k \neq j\}$ in order to characterize dependence.

With regard to estimation, Fitzmaurice and Laird (1993) showed how iterative proportional fitting (Deming and Stephan, 1940) can be used to transform from the mixed parameter $\boldsymbol{\theta}_i^*$ to the canonical parameter $\boldsymbol{\theta}_i$ in order to evaluate the likelihood function. In this approach the 2^n multivariate probability vector $P_{\boldsymbol{\theta}_i}(Y_{i1}, Y_{i2}, \ldots, Y_{in})$ is recovered for each subject. A related use of log-linear models that also permits marginal regression models is presented by Lang and Agresti (1994), Glonek and McCullagh (1995), and Lang *et al.* (1999). Each of these approaches is limited to applications with small or moderate cluster sizes due to computational demands. In addition, the methods of Fitzmaurice and Laird (1993) are effectively limited to balanced data since the canonical association parameters $(\boldsymbol{\theta}_i^{(2)}, \ldots, \theta_i^{(n)})$ must be separately modelled and estimated for each cluster size n_i.

11.3.3 *Marginalized latent variable models*

Heagerty (1999) and Heagerty and Zeger (2000) have discussed how the flexibility of GLMMs for characterizing unobserved heterogeneity can be combined with a marginal regression model. We refer to these models as marginalized latent variable models, or equivalently as marginalized random effects models.

Once again we assume interest in the marginal mean μ_{ij}^{M} and an associated generalized linear model that characterizes systematic variation. We further assume that correlation among observations is induced via unobserved latent variables U_{ij}, and that observations Y_{ij} would be conditionally independent given these random effects. The model can then be expressed through the pair of regressions

$$h\{\mathrm{E}(Y_{ij} \mid \boldsymbol{X}_i)\} = \boldsymbol{x}_{ij}'\boldsymbol{\beta}^{\mathrm{M}}, \tag{11.3.5}$$

$$h\{\mathrm{E}(Y_{ij} \mid \boldsymbol{X}_i, \boldsymbol{U}_i)\} = \Delta_{ij}(\boldsymbol{X}_i) + U_{ij}. \tag{11.3.6}$$

To complete the model specification we assume a distributional model for U_{ij}, $U_{ij} \sim F_{\boldsymbol{\alpha}}$, indexed by a parameter $\boldsymbol{\alpha}$, such as the normal random effects model

$$\boldsymbol{U}_i \sim \mathcal{N}\{\boldsymbol{0}, \boldsymbol{G}(\boldsymbol{\alpha})\}, \tag{11.3.7}$$

where the parameter $\boldsymbol{\alpha}$ represents variance components that determine $\mathrm{cov}(\boldsymbol{U}_i)$. This random effects specification includes random intercepts, $U_{ij} \equiv U_{i0}$, random lines, $U_{ij} \equiv U_{i0} + U_{i1} \cdot t_{ij}$, and autoregressive random effects. Note that if $\boldsymbol{G}^{1/2}\boldsymbol{G}^{1/2} = \boldsymbol{G}(\boldsymbol{\alpha})$ and $\boldsymbol{A}_i$ is multivariate standard normal, then $\boldsymbol{U}_i = \boldsymbol{G}^{1/2}\boldsymbol{A}_i$ and (11.3.6) becomes

$$h\{\mathrm{E}(Y_{ij} \mid \boldsymbol{X}_i, \boldsymbol{A}_i)\} = \Delta_{ij}(\boldsymbol{X}_i) + \boldsymbol{G}^{1/2}\boldsymbol{A}_i,$$

which has the general marginalized model form that we describe in (11.3.2).

The formulation in (11.3.5)–(11.3.7) is an alternative to the classical GLMM (Breslow and Clayton, 1993) which directly parameterizes the conditional mean function, $\Delta_{ij}(\boldsymbol{X}_i) = \boldsymbol{x}_{ij}'\boldsymbol{\beta}^{\mathrm{C}}$. Recall from Chapter 7 that there is a critical distinction between the marginal parameter, $\boldsymbol{\beta}^{\mathrm{M}}$, and the conditional parameter, $\boldsymbol{\beta}^{\mathrm{C}}$. The conditional regression coefficient $\boldsymbol{\beta}^{\mathrm{C}}$ contrasts the expected response for different values of the measured covariates, $\boldsymbol{x}_{ij}$, for equivalent values of the latent variable U_{ij}. The marginal coefficient does not attempt to control for the unobserved U_{ij} when characterizing averages. For example, a marginal gender contrast compares the mean among men to the mean among women, while a conditional gender contrast compares the mean among men with $U_{ij} = U^*$ to the mean among women who also have $U_{ij} = U^*$. Interpretation of $\boldsymbol{\beta}^{\mathrm{C}}$ can be particularly difficult for multilevel models with cluster-level covariates since no direct matching of U_{ij} is observed for these contrasts. See Graubard and Korn (1994) or Heagerty and Zeger (2000) for further discussion.

Figure 11.2 represents the marginalized latent variable model. The inner dashed box indicates that the marginal regression model characterizes the average response conditional only on covariates. The outer dashed box indicates that the complete multivariate model assumes dependence is induced via the latent variables U_{ij}.

The marginalized model in (11.3.5)–(11.3.7) also permits conditional statements via the implicitly defined $\Delta_{ij}(\boldsymbol{X}_i)$, recognizing their dependence on model assumptions. The parameter $\Delta_{ij}(\boldsymbol{X}_i)$ is a function of both the marginal linear predictor $\eta(\boldsymbol{x}_{ij}) = \boldsymbol{x}'_{ij}\boldsymbol{\beta}^{\mathrm{M}}$ and the random effects distribution $F_{\boldsymbol{\alpha}}(U_{ij})$, and is defined as the solution to the integral equation that links the marginal and conditional means

$$\mu_{ij}^{\mathrm{M}} = \mathrm{E}(\mu_{ij}^{\mathrm{C}}), \tag{11.3.8}$$

$$h^{-1}(\boldsymbol{x}'_{ij}\boldsymbol{\beta}^{\mathrm{M}}) = \int h^{-1}\{\Delta_{ij}(\boldsymbol{X}_i) + U_{ij}\} \mathrm{d}F_{\boldsymbol{\alpha}}(U_{ij}). \tag{11.3.9}$$

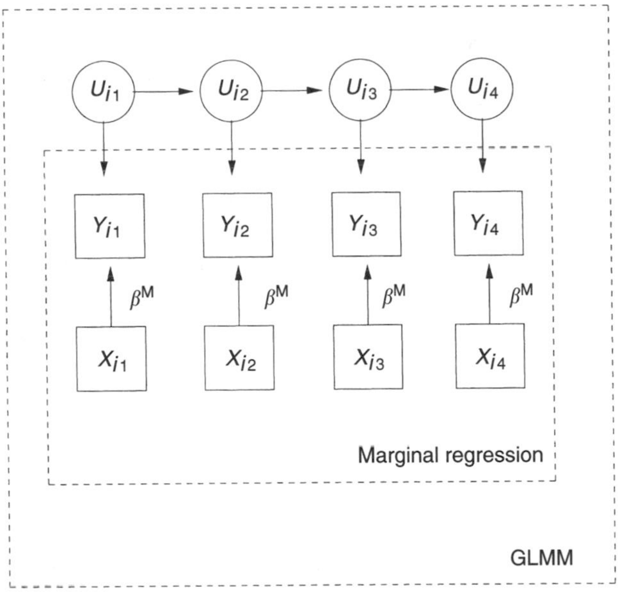

Fig. 11.2. Diagram representing a marginalized latent variable model. The inner dashed box indicates that the model specifies a marginal generalized linear model, $h\{\mathrm{E}(Y_{ij} \mid \boldsymbol{X}_i)\} = \boldsymbol{x}'_{ij}\boldsymbol{\beta}^{\mathrm{M}}$, induced from an underlying GLMM for $\mathrm{E}(Y_{ij} \mid \boldsymbol{X}_i, \boldsymbol{U}_i)$.

We assume that $\text{var}(U_{ij}) = \sigma^2(\boldsymbol{X}_i)$, allowing explicit dependence on covariates $\boldsymbol{X}_i$ since this represents a mixed model formulation, $U_{ij} = U_{i0} + U_{i1} \cdot x_{ij}$, and the case where random intercepts have a different magnitude of variation depending on the value of a cluster-level covariate, $\text{var}(U_{i0} \mid X_i = 0) = \sigma_0^2$, and $\text{var}(U_{i0} \mid X_i = 1) = \sigma_1^2$. In the common case where $U_{ij} \sim \mathcal{N}\{0, \sigma^2(\boldsymbol{X}_i)\}$, we can rewrite $U_{ij} = \sigma(\boldsymbol{X}_{ij}) \cdot \xi$, where $\xi \sim \mathcal{N}(0,1)$ and the integral equation becomes

$$h^{-1}\{\eta(\boldsymbol{x}_{ij})\} = \int h^{-1}\{\Delta_{ij}(\boldsymbol{X}_i) + \sigma(\boldsymbol{X}_i) \cdot \xi\}\phi(\xi)\, \mathrm{d}\xi,$$

where ϕ is the standard normal density function. Given $\eta(\boldsymbol{x}_{ij})$ and $\sigma(\boldsymbol{X}_i)$, the integral equation can be numerically solved for $\Delta_{ij}(\boldsymbol{X}_i)$. See Heagerty (1999) for details of the linkage between $\eta(\boldsymbol{x}_{ij})$ and $\Delta_{ij}(\boldsymbol{X}_i)$ when $h = \text{logit}$.

For certain link function and mixing distribution combinations the transformation between conditional and marginal mean can be obtained analytically. For example, using a probit link function and Gaussian random effects, $U = \sigma(X) \cdot \xi$ for $\xi \sim \mathcal{N}(0,1)$, yields the relationship

$$\Phi\{\eta(X)\} = \mathrm{E}\left[\Phi\{\Delta(X) + \sigma(X) \cdot \xi\}\right] = \Phi\left\{\frac{\Delta(X)}{\sqrt{1 + \sigma^2(X)}}\right\}$$

showing that the marginal linear predictor, $\eta(X)$, is a rescaling of the conditional linear predictor, $\Delta(X)$. If the variance of the latent variable is independent of X, then the marginal and conditional model structures will be the same (i.e. linear, or additive in multiple covariates), however, if $\sigma(X)$ depends on covariates, then the marginal and conditional models will have different functional forms. A key example where heterogeneity or over-dispersion is assumed to depend on covariates is in teratologic applications where the intra-litter correlation is a function of the dose, X (see Prentice, 1986 and Aerts and Claeskens, 1997 for examples using the beta-binomial model). Similarly for count data, Grömping (1996) discusses the relationship between the marginal and conditional mean for a log link with normal mixing distribution, where

$$\begin{aligned}\exp\{\eta(X)\} &= \mathrm{E}[\exp\{\Delta(X) + \sigma(X) \cdot \xi\}] \\ &= \exp\{\Delta(X) + \tfrac{1}{2}\sigma^2(X)\}.\end{aligned}$$

Again, if $\sigma(X) = \sigma_0$, then the marginal and conditional models are nearly equivalent, but if heterogeneity is allowed to depend on covariates, as in mixed effects models, the functional form of the marginal and conditional models will differ. For example, a mixed model that has $\Delta(X)$ a linear function of X may lead to a marginal model where $\eta(X)$ is a quadratic function.

Figure 11.2 characterizes the marginalized random effects model. The inner dashed box shows that the marginal regression model describes systematic variation in the response as a function of covariates. The marginal regression structure is just one facet of the multivariate distribution of $\boldsymbol{Y}_i$ which is assumed to be of GLMM form.

By introducing the marginally specified model, we allow a choice as to whether the marginal mean structure or the conditional mean structure is the focus of modelling when using a latent variable formulation. There exists a general correspondence between $\eta(X)$ and $\Delta(X)$ so that the distinction becomes purely one of where simple regression structure is usefully assumed, and what summaries will be presented through the estimated regression coefficients. The choice between marginal or conditional regression models can now be determined by the scientific objectives of the analysis rather than by the availability of only conditional random effects regression models.

Estimation for marginalized latent variable models is just as computationally demanding as estimation for GLMMs described in Section 11.2. The likelihood function has the same form as the GLMM likelihood detailed in Section 11.2.1. However, $f(Y_{ij} \mid \boldsymbol{X}_i, \boldsymbol{U}_i)$ depends on $\Delta_{ij}(\boldsymbol{X}_i)$ which is a non-linear function of both $\boldsymbol{\beta}^{\mathrm{M}}$ and the variance components $\boldsymbol{\alpha}$. The parameter $\Delta_{ij}(\boldsymbol{X}_i)$ can be recovered using numerical integration to solve the one-dimensional convolution equation (11.3.9). Algorithm details are described in Heagerty (1999) and Heagerty and Zeger (2000). Similar to the GLMM, ML estimation for the marginalized random effects model is currently limited to low-dimensional random effects distributions due to the intractability of the likelihood function.

11.3.4 *Marginalized transition models*

In Chapter 10 we describe how transition models focus on the distribution of Y_{ij} conditional on past outcomes $Y_{ij-1}, Y_{ij-2}, \ldots,$ and covariates $\boldsymbol{X}_i$. These models are particularly attractive for categorical data that exhibit serial dependence since the coefficients of $Y_{ij-1}, Y_{ij-2}, \ldots,$ indicate how strongly the past outcomes predict the current response. However, there are situations where we would not want to condition on past outcomes to make inference regarding a covariate $\boldsymbol{X}_i$. For example, most clinical trials are interested in the impact of treatment on the response at a fixed final follow-up time, or on the entire response profile over time. In this case we would not want to condition on outcomes $Y_{ij-1}, Y_{ij-2}, \ldots,$ measured after baseline when making inference regarding the effect of treatment on Y_{ij} since earlier outcomes should be properly considered as intermediate variables and not controlled for.

The attractive characterization of serial dependence that a transition model provides can be combined with a marginal regression structure by adopting a marginalized transition model (Azzalini, 1994; Heagerty, 2002). In this section we first review the first-order Markov chain models of Azzalini (1994) and describe an alternative, but equivalent, model specification in terms of the combination of a marginal regression model used to characterize the dependence of the response on covariates, and a transition model (Chapter 10), used to capture the serial dependence in the response process and identify a likelihood function. We then generalize the first-order marginalized transition model to allow pth-order dependence.

Azzalini (1994) introduced a binary Markov chain model to accommodate the serial dependence that is common in longitudinal data. A first-order Markov model assumes that the current response variable is dependent on the history only through the immediate previous response, $\mathrm{E}(Y_{ij} \mid Y_{ik},\, k < j) = \mathrm{E}(Y_{ij} \mid Y_{ij-1})$. The transition probabilities $p_{ij,0} = \mathrm{E}(Y_{ij} \mid Y_{ij-1} = 0)$ and $p_{ij,1} = \mathrm{E}(Y_{ij} \mid Y_{ij-1} = 1)$ define the Markov process but do not directly parameterize the marginal mean. Azzalini (1994) parameterizes the transition probabilities through two assumptions. First, a marginal mean regression model is adopted which constrains the transition probabilities to satisfy

$$\mu_{ij}^{\mathrm{M}} = p_{ij,1} \cdot \mu_{ij-1}^{\mathrm{M}} + p_{ij,0} \cdot \left(1 - \mu_{ij-1}^{\mathrm{M}}\right). \tag{11.3.10}$$

Second, the transition probabilities are structured through assumptions on the pairwise odds ratio

$$\Psi_{ij} = \frac{p_{ij,1}/(1 - p_{ij,1})}{p_{ij,0}/(1 - p_{ij,0})}, \tag{11.3.11}$$

which quantifies the strength of serial correlation. The simplest dependence model assumes a time-homogeneous association, $\Psi_{ij} = \Psi_0$, however, models that allow Ψ_{ij} to depend on covariates or to depend on time are also possible.

The transition probabilities, and therefore the likelihood, can be recovered as a function of the marginal means, μ_{ij}^{M}, and the odds ratios Ψ_{ij}. Azzalini (1994) provides details on the calculations required for ML estimation and establishes the orthogonality of the marginal mean and the odds ratio parameter in the restricted case of a time-constant (scalar) dependence model.

Heagerty and Zeger (2000) view the approach of Azzalini (1994) as combining a marginal mean model that captures systematic variation in the response as a function of covariates, with a conditional mean model that describes serial dependence and identifies the joint distribution of $\boldsymbol{Y}_i$. The first-order marginalized transition model, or MTM(1), is specified by first assuming a regression structure for the marginal mean, $\mathrm{E}(Y_{ij} \mid \boldsymbol{X}_i)$, using a generalized linear model, $h(\mu_{ij}^{\mathrm{M}}) = \boldsymbol{x}_{ij}'\boldsymbol{\beta}^{\mathrm{M}}$. Next, serial dependence is specified by assuming a Markov structure, or equivalently by assuming a regression model for how strongly Y_{ij-1} predicts Y_{ij}. Heagerty and Zeger (2000) describe the dependence model using a model for the conditional expectation $\mu_{ij}^{C} = \mathrm{E}(Y_{ij} \mid \boldsymbol{X}_i, Y_{ik}, k < j)$ with logit link

$$\text{logit}\{\mathrm{E}(Y_{ij} \mid \boldsymbol{X}_i, \mathcal{H}_{ij})\} = \Delta_{ij}(\boldsymbol{X}_i) + \gamma_{ij,1} \cdot y_{ij-1}, \tag{11.3.12}$$

where $\mathcal{H}_{ij} = \{Y_{ik} \colon k < j\}$ and $\gamma_{ij,1} = \log \Psi_{ij}$. The log odds ratio $\gamma_{ij,1}$ is simply a logistic regression coefficient in the model that conditions on both $\boldsymbol{X}_i$ and Y_{ij-1}. The parameter $\Delta_{ij}(\boldsymbol{X}_i)$ equals $\text{logit}(p_{ij,0})$ and is determined implicitly by $\boldsymbol{\beta}^{\mathrm{M}}$ and $\gamma_{ij,1}$ through the marginal regression equation and equation (11.3.12). Furthermore, a general regression model can be specified for $\gamma_{ij,1}$,

$$\gamma_{ij,1} = \boldsymbol{Z}'_{ij,1}\boldsymbol{\alpha}_1, \tag{11.3.13}$$

where the parameter $\boldsymbol{\alpha}_1$ determines how the dependence of Y_{ij} on Y_{ij-1} varies as a function of covariates, $\boldsymbol{Z}_{ij,1}$. For example, $\gamma_{ij,1} = \alpha_j$, allows serial dependence to change over time, and $\gamma_{ij,1} = \alpha_0 + \alpha_1 Z_i$ allows subjects for whom $Z_i = 1$ to have a different serial correlation as compared to subjects for whom $Z_i = 0$. In general, $\boldsymbol{Z}_{ij}$ is a subset of $\boldsymbol{X}_i$ since we assume that equation (11.3.12) denotes the conditional expectation of Y_{ij} given both $\boldsymbol{X}_i$ and $\boldsymbol{Z}_{ij}$.

In summary, the marginalized transition model separates the specification of the dependence of Y_{ij} on $\boldsymbol{X}_i$ (regression) and the dependence of Y_{ij} on the history $Y_{ij-1}, Y_{ij-2}, \ldots, Y_{i1}$ (auto-correlation) to obtain a fully specified parametric model for longitudinal binary data. A first-order model assumes that Y_{ij} is conditionally independent of $Y_{ij-2}, \ldots, Y_{i1}$ given Y_{ij-1}. The transition model intercept, $\Delta_{ij}(\boldsymbol{X}_i)$, is determined such that both the marginal mean structure and the Markov dependence structure are simultaneously satisfied.

Equations (11.3.12) and (11.3.13) indicate how the first-order dependence model can naturally be extended to provide a marginalized transition model of general order, p. We assume that Y_{ij} depends on the history only through the previous p responses, $Y_{ij-1}, \ldots, Y_{ij-p}$. A pth-order dependence model, or MTM(p) can be specified through the pair of regressions:

$$h\{\mathrm{E}(Y_{ij} \mid \boldsymbol{X}_i)\} = \boldsymbol{x}'_{ij}\boldsymbol{\beta}^{\mathrm{M}} \tag{11.3.14}$$

$$\text{logit}\{\mathrm{E}(Y_{ij} \mid \boldsymbol{X}_i, \mathcal{H}_{ij})\} = \Delta_{ij}(\boldsymbol{X}_i) + \sum_{k=1}^{p} \gamma_{ij,k} \cdot y_{ij-k} \tag{11.3.15}$$

and we can further assume that the dependence parameters follow regression structure

$$\gamma_{ij,k} = \boldsymbol{Z}'_{ij,k}\boldsymbol{\alpha}_k, \quad k = 1, \ldots, p. \tag{11.3.16}$$

For example, a second-order (additive) marginalized transition model assumes: $\text{logit}\{\mu_{ij}^{\text{C}}\} = \Delta_{ij}(\boldsymbol{X}_i) + \gamma_{ij,1} \cdot y_{ij-1} + \gamma_{ij,2} \cdot y_{ij-2}$, and $\gamma_{ij,1} = \boldsymbol{Z}'_{ij,1}\boldsymbol{\alpha}_1$, $\gamma_{ij,2} = \boldsymbol{Z}'_{ij,2}\boldsymbol{\alpha}_2$. Although μ_{ij}^{C} can also depend on the interaction $Y_{ij-1} \cdot Y_{ij-2}$, we assume an additive model for simplicity of presentation.

In the MTM(2) the mean parameter $\boldsymbol{\beta}^{\text{M}}$ describes changes in the average response as a function of covariates, without controlling for previous response variables. Figure 11.3 is a diagram that represents a second-order marginalized transition model. The inner dashed box indicates that the regression parameter $\boldsymbol{\beta}^{\text{M}}$ models the marginal relationship between the response and covariates. Markov transition assumptions are represented by the directed edges connecting Y_{ij-k} to Y_{ij}. The dependence parameters γ_1 and γ_2 describe serial dependence by quantifying how strongly the immediate past predicts the present.

The parameter space for the marginalized transition model is subject only to the constraint that the generalized linear model for μ_{ij}^{M} must yield $\mu_{ij}^{\text{M}} \in [0, 1]$. Using a logistic link for the transition model, μ_{ij}^{C}, implies that the parameters $\boldsymbol{\alpha}_k$ are unconstrained. For a given mean model ($\boldsymbol{\beta}^{\text{M}}$) and dependence model ($\boldsymbol{\alpha}_k$) the intercept parameter $\Delta_{ij}(\boldsymbol{X}_i)$ is fully

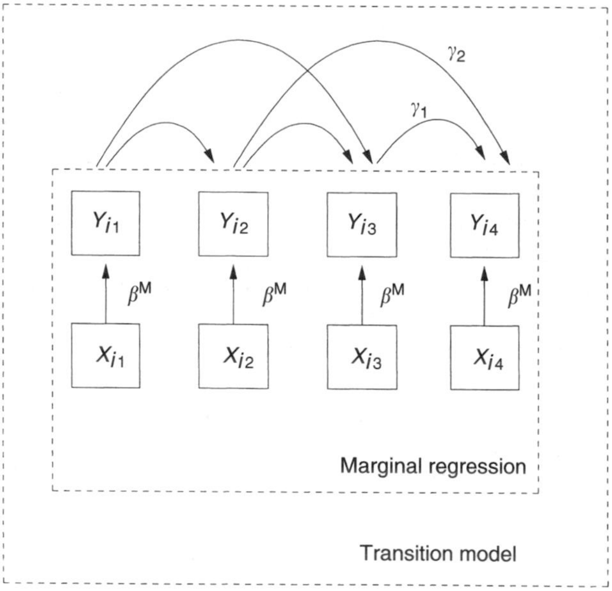

Fig. 11.3. Diagram representing a second-order marginalized transition model. The inner dashed box indicates that the model specifies a marginal generalized linear model, $h\{\text{E}(Y_{ij} \mid \boldsymbol{X}_i)\} = \boldsymbol{x}'_{ij}\boldsymbol{\beta}^{\text{M}}$, induced from an underlying transition model, $\text{E}(Y_{ij} \mid \boldsymbol{X}_i, Y_{ik}\, k < j)$.

constrained and must yield the proper marginal expectation μ_{ij}^{M} when μ_{ij}^{C} is averaged over the distribution of the history. For any finite values of $\boldsymbol{\alpha}_k$, as $\Delta_{ij}(\boldsymbol{X}_i)$ ranges from $-\infty$ to $+\infty$ the induced marginal mean monotonically increases from 0 to 1. Therefore, given any finite valued dependence model and any probability distribution for the history, a unique $\Delta_{ij}(\boldsymbol{X}_i)$ can be identified that satisfies both the transition model and the marginal mean assumptions.

One disadvantage to directly using a transition model with p lagged response variables is that the information in $(Y_{i1}, \ldots, Y_{ip})$ is conditioned upon, and therefore does not contribute to the assessment of covariate effects. With an MTM(p) approach the information in the initial responses regarding μ_{ik}^{M}, and thus $\boldsymbol{\beta}^{\mathrm{M}}$, is included through lower order marginalized transition models involving $\mathrm{E}(Y_{ik} \mid \boldsymbol{X}_{ik}, Y_{ik-1}, \ldots, Y_{i1})$ for $k < p$. For example, when using an MTM(2) the likelihood for the initial responses, (Y_{i1}, Y_{i2}), is obtained by factorization into $\Pr(Y_{i1} \mid \boldsymbol{X}_{i1})$ (determined entirely by μ_{i1}^{M}), and $\Pr(Y_{i2} \mid \boldsymbol{X}_{i2}, Y_{i1})$ which involves μ_{i2}^{M} and the conditional model: $\operatorname{logit} \mathrm{E}(Y_{i2} \mid \boldsymbol{X}_{i2}, Y_{i1}) = \Delta_{i2}(\boldsymbol{X}_i) + \tilde{\gamma}_{i2,1} \cdot Y_{i1}$. Note that $\tilde{\gamma}_{i2,1}$ is distinct from the first-order coefficient $\gamma_{ij,1}$, $j > 2$, in the MTM(2) dependence model, $\operatorname{logit}(\mu_{ij}^{\mathrm{C}}) = \Delta_{ij}(\boldsymbol{X}_i) + \gamma_{ij,1} \cdot Y_{ij-1} + \gamma_{ij,2} \cdot Y_{ij-2}$, since this model involves Y_{ij-2} in addition to Y_{ij-1}. Therefore, in applications we estimate separate lower order dependence parameters.

To carry out estimation within this general class of models, note that the MTM(p) likelihood factors into the distribution of the first p response variables times the subsequent Bernoulli likelihood contributions with parameters μ_{ij}^{C} for $j = (p+1), \ldots, n_i$:

$$
\begin{aligned}
&\Pr(Y_{i1}, Y_{i2}, \ldots, Y_{in_i} \mid \boldsymbol{X}_i) \\
&\quad = \Pr(Y_{i1}, Y_{i2}, \ldots, Y_{ip} \mid \boldsymbol{X}_i) \cdot \Pr(Y_{ip+1}, Y_{ip+2}, \ldots, Y_{in_i} \mid \mathcal{H}_{ip+1}, \boldsymbol{X}_i) \\
&\quad = \Pr(Y_{i1}, Y_{i2}, \ldots, Y_{ip}) \cdot \prod_{j=p+1}^{n_i} \Pr(Y_{ij} \mid \mathcal{H}_{ij}, \boldsymbol{X}_i) \\
&\quad = \Pr(Y_{i1}, Y_{i2}, \ldots, Y_{ip}) \cdot \prod_{j=p+1}^{n_i} \{\mu_{ij}^{\mathrm{C}}\}^{Y_{ij}} \{1 - \mu_{ij}^{\mathrm{C}}\}^{1-Y_{ij}}.
\end{aligned}
$$

The basic maximization algorithm starts with a model for $\Pr(Y_{i1}, \ldots, Y_{ip})$ using lower order marginalized transition model assumptions. The key to subsequent likelihood evaluation is that transition probabilities, μ_{ij}^{C}, can be sequentially recovered as a function of the parameters $\boldsymbol{\beta}^{\mathrm{M}}$ and $\boldsymbol{\alpha}_1, \ldots, \boldsymbol{\alpha}_p$. The dependence parameters enter into μ_{ij}^{C} directly but the intercept $\Delta_{ij}(\boldsymbol{X}_i)$ is an implicit function of $\boldsymbol{\beta}$ and $\boldsymbol{\alpha}_1, \ldots, \boldsymbol{\alpha}_p$. We obtain

$\Delta_{ij}(\boldsymbol{X}_i)$ by solving the marginal constraint equation:

$$\mu_{ij}^{\mathrm{M}} = \sum_{y_{ij-1},\ldots,y_{ij-p}} \Pr(Y_{ij} = 1 \mid Y_{ij-1} = y_{j-1}, \ldots, Y_{j-p} = y_{j-p})$$
$$\times \Pr(Y_{ij-1} = y_{j-1}, \ldots, Y_{ij-p} = y_{ij-p}).$$

In order to obtain a solution we require the initial state probability $\Pr(Y_{i1} = y_{i1}, \ldots, Y_{ip} = y_{ip})$ from which all subsequent p-dimensional probabilities can be obtained by multiplying $\Pr(Y_{ik} = y_{ik}, \ldots, Y_{ik+(p-1)} = y_{ik+(p-1)})$ times μ_{ik+p} and then summing over y_{ik}. Details for MTM(2) estimation are provided in Heagerty (2002).

The computational complexity of MTM(p) likelihood evaluation for subject i is $O(n_i 2^p)$. Calculations required to compute and update the p-dimensional history are $O(2^p)$ and each observation requires such calculations. Therefore, with a fixed dependence order the computational burden only increases linearly with the length of the observation series, n_i. The order of alternative likelihood methods is generally much greater with the iterative proportional fitting algorithm of Fitzmaurice and Laird (1993) requiring exponentially increasing computational time, $O(2^{n_i})$.

Azzalini (1994) suggested that the MTM(1) has general robustness properties but only established a consistency result for a restricted scenario. By viewing the MTM(1) as adopting a logistic regression for μ_{ij}^{C} allows us to show that the MTM(1) is a special case of the mixed-parameter model of Fitzmaurice and Laird (1993) with $\boldsymbol{\gamma} = \mathrm{vec}(\gamma_{ij,1})$ the canonical log-linear interaction parameter. Appendix 1 of Heagerty (2002) provides details that show $\boldsymbol{\beta}^{\mathrm{M}}$ and $\boldsymbol{\alpha}_1$ are orthogonal. The implication of orthogonality is that the ML estimate, $\hat{\boldsymbol{\beta}}^{\mathrm{M}}$, remains consistent for $\boldsymbol{\beta}^{\mathrm{M}}$ even if the dependence model is incorrectly specified. Use of the MTM(1) ML estimate $\hat{\boldsymbol{\beta}}^{\mathrm{M}}$ and a sandwich variance estimator (Huber, 1967; White, 1982; Royall, 1986) provides a likelihood motivated version of GEE appropriate in serial data situations since the point estimate $\hat{\boldsymbol{\beta}}^{\mathrm{M}}$ will be consistent and valid standard errors can be obtained without requiring correct Markov order or correct modelling of $\gamma_{ij,1}$. For general pth-order models, $\boldsymbol{\beta}^{\mathrm{M}}$ and $(\boldsymbol{\alpha}_1, \ldots, \boldsymbol{\alpha}_p)$ may not be orthogonal, and consistent estimation of mean regression parameters requires appropriate dependence modelling.

One practical advantage of marginalized transition modelling is that several simple procedures can be used to assess the dependence model assumptions. First, to establish the appropriate order we can use direct transition models and regress Y_{ij} on $\boldsymbol{X}_{ij}$ and prior responses. Second, approximate score tests for an additional lagged response (increased order from p to $p + 1$) take simple forms. For example, using a MTM(p) we can test the assumption $\alpha_{p+1} = \gamma_{ij,p+1} = 0$ with the statistic

$$U_{p+1} = \sum_{i=1}^{m} \sum_{j=p+2}^{n_i} Y_{ij-(p+1)}(Y_{ij} - \hat{\mu}_{ij}^{\mathrm{C}}),$$

where $\hat{\mu}_{ij}^{\mathrm{C}}$ is the fitted conditional mean obtained from the MTM(p) model. This statistic only approximates the likelihood score statistic because it ignores $\partial\Delta_{ij}/\partial\alpha_{p+1}$. The approximate score statistic is intuitive since it simply evaluates the correlation between the $(p+1)$ lagged response and the conditional residual obtained by fitting a marginalized transition model with the first p lagged responses.

11.3.5 *Summary*

In this section we have introduced marginalized models for categorical longitudinal data. These models separate specification of the average response, μ_{ij}^{M}, from the dependence among the repeated measurements. Dependence is characterized by a second regression model for $\mu_{ij}^{\mathrm{C}} = \mathrm{E}(Y_{ij} \mid \boldsymbol{X}_i, \boldsymbol{A}_{ij})$ where additional variables in $\boldsymbol{A}_{ij}$ are introduced to structure correlation. Marginalized models expand analysis options to allow flexible likelihood-based estimation of marginal regression parameters.

11.4 Examples

11.4.1 *Crossover data*

We now revisit the two period crossover data (Example 1.5) using GLMMs, and marginalized models.

GLMMs. In Section 9.3.3 we analysed the 2×2 crossover data using a GLMM with a random intercept. In Table 11.1 we present estimates obtained using PQL, fixed quadrature, adaptive quadrature, and posterior summaries obtained using MCMC. For Bayesian analysis we use independent normal priors with standard deviation $= 10^2$ for the regression coefficients, and a gamma prior for the precision, $1/G \sim \Gamma(1, 1)$. Not surprisingly, we find that PQL greatly underestimates the random effects standard deviation, $G^{1/2}$, relative to the numerical ML estimators. We find only minor differences between estimates obtained using fixed and adaptive quadrature. The posterior mean for $G^{1/2}$ is larger than the MLE by $(5.82 - 4.84)/4.84 = 20\%$. This is typical when posterior distributions are skewed – the median of $G^{1/2}$ is 5.09 with a 95% posterior credible region (2.48, 13.48).

Marginalized models. In Section 8.2.3 we analysed the crossover data with GEE, using the pairwise odds ratio to model within-subject correlation. In Table 11.2 we display estimates obtained using marginal quasi-likelihood

Table 11.1. Likelihood-based estimates for a GLMM analysis of crossover data. Quadrature methods are based on 20 point Gauss–Hermite quadrature.

	PQL		Fixed, quadrature		Adaptive quadrature		Bayes MCMC	
	Est.	SE	Est.	SE	Est.	SE	Mean	SD
Conditional mean $\boldsymbol{\beta}^{\mathrm{C}}$								
Intercept	0.768	(0.396)	2.153	(1.031)	2.170	(1.098)	2.644	(1.684)
Treatment	0.692	(0.420)	1.841	(0.928)	1.836	(0.900)	2.249	(1.322)
Period	−0.356	(0.419)	−1.020	(0.836)	−1.016	(0.795)	−1.330	(1.160)
Variance components								
$G^{1/2}$	1.448	(0.602)	4.969	(2.263)	4.843	(1.747)	5.824	(2.925)
log-likelihood			−68.17		−68.15			

Table 11.2. Likelihood-based estimates for marginalized model analysis of crossover data.

	MQL		Marginalized GLMM		Marginalized transition	
	Est.	SE	Est.	SE	Est.	SE
Marginal mean $\boldsymbol{\beta}^{\mathrm{M}}$						
Intercept	0.668	(0.356)	0.651	(0.275)	0.674	(0.278)
Treatment	0.569	(0.379)	0.577	(0.227)	0.569	(0.231)
Period	−0.295	(0.378)	− 0.326	(0.222)	− 0.295	(0.229)
Variance components						
$G^{1/2}$	1.239	(0.549)	5.439	(3.718)		
α_1					3.562	(0.907)
log-likelihood			−68.11		−68.32	

(MQL), and two different marginalized models. Recall from Section 9.2.2 that penalized quasi-likelihood (PQL) is a method for obtaining approximate ML inference for GLMMs. In discussing the development of PQL, Breslow and Clayton (1993) also develop estimating equations that can be used for a marginal mean assumed to be induced via a GLMM. Breslow and Clayton (1993) refer to these estimating equations as MQL, and note the relationship to methods discussed in Zeger *et al.* (1988). The marginalized latent variable model for the crossover data assumes the marginal regression structure and

$$\text{logit } \mathrm{E}(Y_{ij} \mid \boldsymbol{X}_i, A_i) = \Delta_{ij}(\boldsymbol{X}_i) + G^{1/2} A_i$$

for a standard normal random effect A_i. In this specification we see that the variance component, $G^{1/2}$, characterizes the magnitude of subject-to-subject variation in the log odds of response that is unmeasured, or not explained by the covariates $\boldsymbol{X}_i$. The marginalized GLMM regression estimates, $\hat{\boldsymbol{\beta}}^{\mathrm{M}}$ in Table 11.2 are nearly identical to the estimates obtained using GEE (Table 8.2), and the variance component estimate, $\hat{G}^{1/2}$ is similar to that obtained with a classical conditionally specified GLMM.

We can also use either a marginalized log-linear model, or marginalized transition model for analysis. In the case where $n_i = 2$ these two approaches are identical. For analysis we use

$$\text{logit } \mathrm{E}(Y_{i2} \mid \boldsymbol{X}_i, Y_{i1}) = \Delta_{i2}(\boldsymbol{X}_i) + \alpha_1 \cdot Y_{i1},$$

where α_1 is the log odds ratio measuring the association between Y_{i1} and Y_{i2} that is not explained by covariates. Again, we obtain ML estimates for marginal regression parameters that are similar to GEE estimates. The estimate $\hat{\alpha}_1 = 3.562$ indicates striking dependence, or concordance, between Y_{i1} and Y_{i2}.

In smaller sample sizes it is often desirable to consider inference based on the likelihood function directly rather than the Wald statistic. In this data set we have a total of $m = 67$ subjects. Figure 11.4 shows a profile likelihood curve for the treatment parameter in the marginal regression model. The MLE, $\hat{\beta}_1^{\mathrm{M}} = 0.569$, is indicated by a vertical dotted line. A dashed line shows the quadratic approximation to the log-likelihood that is the basis for Wald inference. The solid line is $\log L_p(\beta_1^{\mathrm{M}}) = \log L\{\boldsymbol{y}; \hat{\boldsymbol{\delta}}(\beta_1^{\mathrm{M}})\}$, the log-likelihood maximized over $(\beta_0^{\mathrm{M}}, \beta_2^{\mathrm{M}}, \alpha_1)$ for fixed values of β_1^{M}. This profile curve can be used for interval estimation based on likelihood ratio test inversion since the difference between the maximum, $\log L\{\boldsymbol{y}; \hat{\boldsymbol{\delta}}(\hat{\beta}_1^{\mathrm{M}})\}$, and $\log L_p(\beta_1^{\mathrm{M}} = b)$ represents the likelihood ratio test of $H_0\colon \beta_1^{\mathrm{M}} = b$. The horizontal dotted line is at $(\log L\{\boldsymbol{y}; \hat{\boldsymbol{\delta}}(\hat{\beta}_1^{\mathrm{M}})\} - 3.84/2)$, and characterizes a confidence interval based on the critical value of a $\chi^2(df = 1)$. We find excellent agreement between the Wald and likelihood ratio-based inference for β_1^{M} near zero but find differences for β_1^{M} greater than 1.0 that lead to a slightly wider confidence interval.

Summary. We have demonstrated that it is feasible to obtain likelihood-based inference using either a conditionally specified-regression coefficient with a GLMM, or using marginalized models. The marginalized models adopt the dependence formulation of random effects models, or of log-linear models, but directly structure the induced marginal means via a regression model.

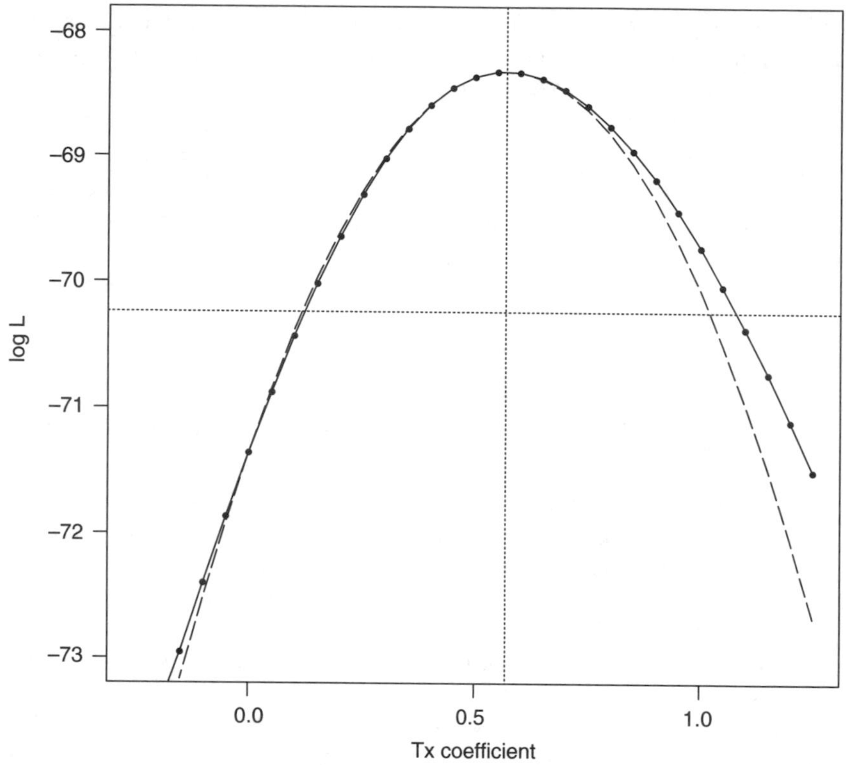

Fig. 11.4. Profile likelihood for the marginal treatment parameter using a marginalized log-linear model likelihood (——), and the quadratic approximation based on the MLE and the model-based information (- - - - - -).

11.4.2 *Madras schizophrenia data*

The Madras Longitudinal Schizophrenia Study investigated the course of positive and negative psychiatric symptoms over the first year after initial hospitalization for disease (Thara, 1994). Scientific interest is in factors that correlate with the course of illness. Our analysis addresses whether the longitudinal symptom prevalence differs across patient subgroups defined by age-at-onset and gender. To statistically address the primary question we use GLMMs and marginalized models to estimate the interaction between time and age-at-onset, and the interaction between time and gender in a logistic regression model. We compare parameter estimates obtained using ML under different dependence assumptions, and estimates obtained using GEE.

The Madras Longitudinal Study collected data on six common schizophrenia symptoms. Symptoms were classified into positive symptoms (hallucinations, delusions, thought disorders) and negative symptoms (flat affect, apathy, withdrawal). Each symptom was recorded every month $j = 0, \ldots, 11$ during the first year following hospitalization for schizophrenia. The prevalence of each positive symptom declines from approximately 70% at initial hospitalization to <20% by the end of the first year, while the prevalence of each negative symptom declines from approximately 40% initially to 10% after one year. Heagerty and Zeger (1998) analysed these data using graphical methods to display the within-subject correlation as a function of the time lag between measurements. The exploratory analysis of the dependence structure suggests strong serial correlation for the positive symptoms and strong long-term correlation for the negative symptoms. Specifically, to characterize the dependence between binary outcomes we use the pairwise log odds ratio $\gamma_{i(j,k)}$ defined by (8.2.2) in Section 8.2.2. In Fig. 11.5 we plot estimates of the pairwise log odds ratio $\log\{\gamma_{i,(j,k)}\}$ versus the time separation $|t_{ij} - t_{ik}|$ for each of the six symptoms. In this figure we display both empirical estimates obtained using crude 2×2 tables, and a smooth function of $|t_{ij} - t_{ik}|$ based on regression spline methods described in Heagerty and Zeger (1998). For the symptom 'thoughts' we find the pairwise log odds ratio between observations 1 month apart is approximately 3.0, but this association decays to approximately 1.0 for observations 5 months apart, and further decays to 0 for observations 10 months apart. Serial dependence models such as the MTM(p) appear appropriate for this symptom and the other two positive symptoms.

For regression analysis we focus on the outcome 'thought disorders'. Not surprisingly, for this specific symptom a large fraction of the $N = 86$ subjects are symptomatic at the time of hospitalization ($56/86 = 65\%$ at month $= 0$). The crude prevalence of thought disorders decreases during the first year with only $6/69 = 9\%$ presenting symptoms at month $= 11$. To evaluate if the course of recovery differs for subjects with early age-at-onset or for women we fit logistic regression models with main effects for month ($j = 0, \ldots, 11$), age ($1 =$ age-at-onset less than 20 years old, $0 =$ age-at-onset ≥ 20 years old), gender ($0 =$ male, $1 =$ female), and the interaction between time and the two subject-level covariates. Evaluation of the interaction terms determines whether the rate of recovery appears to differ by subgroup.

The majority of subjects have complete data but 17/86 subjects have only partial follow-up that ranges from 1 to 11 months. Regression analysis of subject discontinuation (drop-out) suggests that subjects who currently have symptoms, $Y_{ij} = 1$, are at increased risk to drop-out at time $j + 1$ (odds ratio 1.716, p-value $= 0.345$). Women are also at increased risk to discontinue (odds ratio $= 2.375$, p-value $= 0.11$). The potential association between drop-out and the observed outcome data warrant consideration of an analysis that is valid if the drop-out mechanism is MAR. Without special modification GEE is valid only if missing data are missing completely at

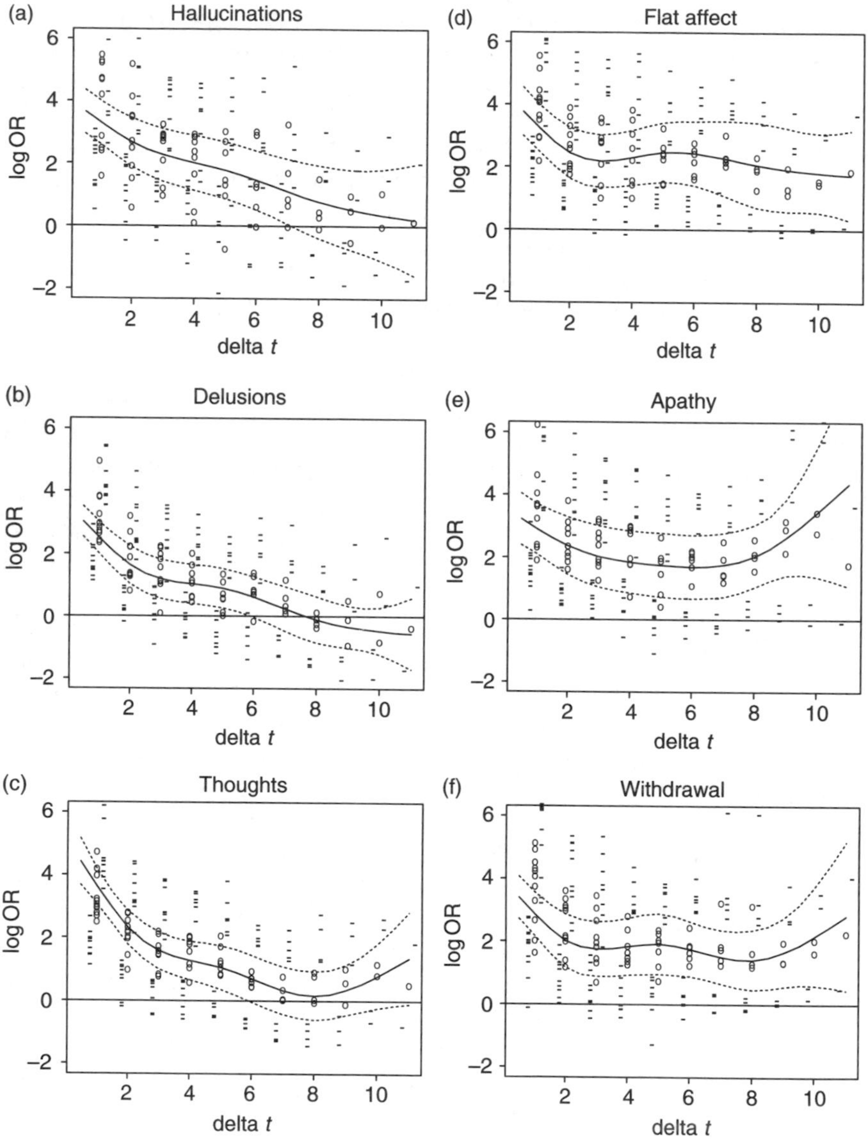

Fig. 11.5. Serial dependence for the Madras schizophrenia data. Pairwise log odds ratios are plotted against the time lag for each of six symptoms. Solid lines are based on a natural spline model using knots at $t = 3, 5, 7$ months. The dashed lines are pointwise 95% confidence bands. Also shown are the crude pairwise log odds ratios and corresponding asymptotic 95% confidence limits. The 'o' represents the crude zero-cell corrected log odds ratio computed from a 2×2 table of Y_{ij} versus Y_{ik}. The '$-$' represent the confidence limits for these point estimates.

random (MCAR). See Chapter 13 for further discussion of missing data issues.

GLMMs. We first consider analysis of the schizophrenia symptom data using GLMMs. Our primary interest is in a group-by-time model that includes month, age, gender, and both month : age and month : gender product terms:

$$\begin{aligned}\mu_{ij}^{\mathrm{C}} &= \mathrm{E}(Y_{ij} \mid \mathrm{month}_{ij}, \mathrm{age}_i, \mathrm{gender}_i, U_{ij}),\\ \mathrm{logit}(\mu_{ij}^{\mathrm{C}}) &= \beta_0^{\mathrm{C}} + \beta_1^{\mathrm{C}} \cdot \mathrm{month}_{ij} + \beta_2^{\mathrm{C}} \cdot \mathrm{age}_i + \beta_3^{\mathrm{C}} \cdot \mathrm{gender}_i\\ &\quad + \beta_4^{\mathrm{C}} \cdot \mathrm{month}_{ij} \cdot \mathrm{age}_i + \beta_5^{\mathrm{C}} \cdot \mathrm{month}_{ij} \cdot \mathrm{gender}_i + U_{ij}.\end{aligned}$$

Table 11.3 presents estimates using a random intercept model, $U_{ij} \equiv U_{i0}$. Similar to the crossover data we find that PQL underestimates the variance component, with $\hat{G}^{1/2} = 1.827$, versus $\hat{G}^{1/2} = 2.222$ using adaptive quadrature. Our Bayesian analysis adopts independent priors for the regression parameters, β_j^{C} (normal with a standard deviation of 10^2), and specifies a gamma prior for the precision ($G \sim \Gamma(2, 2)$). The estimates obtained using MCMC are quite similar to the ML estimates. Since the conditionally specified GLMM uses a single regression equation that contains both covariates and random effects, the regression estimates $\hat{\beta}^{\mathrm{C}}$ need to be interpreted recognizing that U_{ij} is controlled for. However, in the random intercept model each subject is assumed to have the same change in their log odds

Table 11.3. Likelihood-based estimates for a GLMM analysis of Madras schizophrenia data using random intercepts, $\mathrm{Var}(U_{i0}) = G$.

	PQL		Adaptive quadrature*		Bayes MCMC	
	Est.	SE	Est.	SE	Mean	SD
Conditional mean $\boldsymbol{\beta}^{\mathrm{C}}$						
Intercept	1.005	(0.388)	1.087	(0.457)	1.085	(0.477)
Month	−0.387	(0.048)	−0.437	(0.055)	−0.439	(0.057)
Age	1.180	(0.570)	1.438	(0.678)	1.511	(0.683)
Gender	−0.748	(0.533)	−0.931	(0.632)	−0.965	(0.649)
Month·Age	−0.204	(0.087)	−0.251	(0.100)	−0.262	(0.100)
Month·Gender	−0.079	(0.081)	−0.086	(0.090)	−0.089	(0.092)
Variance components						
$G^{1/2}$	1.827	(0.643)	2.222	(0.285)	2.259	(0.288)

*The maximized log-likelihood using adaptive quadrature is −369.88.

of symptoms over time:

$$\text{logit}(\mu_{ij+1}^{\text{C}}) - \text{logit}(\mu_{ij}^{\text{C}}) = \beta_1^{\text{C}} + \beta_4^{\text{C}} \cdot \text{age}_i + \beta_5^{\text{C}} \cdot \text{gender}_i$$

since the random intercept, U_{i0} is cancelled when computing the within-subject difference. The coefficient of month·age measures the difference in the common rate of recovery among early age-at-onset subjects relative to common rate of recovery among the late age-at-onset subjects and appears statistically significant using the random intercept model ($Z = -0.251/0.100 = -2.51$, $p = 0.012$, based on MLE).

We relax the random intercept assumption to allow either random intercepts and slopes (random lines), or to allow autocorrelated random effects. Results are presented in Table 11.4. In the random lines model we assume

$$\text{logit}\{\text{E}(Y_{ij} \mid \boldsymbol{X}_i, \boldsymbol{U}_i)\} = \boldsymbol{x}_{ij}'\boldsymbol{\beta}^{\text{C}} + U_{i0} + U_{i1} \cdot t_{ij},$$

where $t_{ij} = (j-1)$ represents the month of observation. This model assumes that each patient is following their own linear recovery course, and has a

Table 11.4. Likelihood-based estimates for a GLMM analysis of Madras schizophrenia data using random intercepts and slopes, $\text{var}(U_{i0}) = G_{11}$, $\text{var}(U_{i1}) = G_{22}$, $\text{corr}(U_{i0}, U_{i1}) = R$, and with random autocorrelated random effects $\text{cov}(U_{ij}, U_{ik}) = G \cdot \rho^{|j-k|}$.

	Adaptive quadrature*		Bayes MCMC			
	Est.	SE	Mean	SD	Mean	SD
Conditional mean $\boldsymbol{\beta}^{\text{C}}$						
Intercept	1.620	(0.684)	1.805	(0.780)	2.162	(1.304)
Month	−0.620	(0.129)	−0.709	(0.152)	−1.002	(0.266)
Age	1.616	(0.978)	1.801	(1.107)	2.641	(1.748)
Gender	−0.953	(0.922)	−1.108	(1.064)	−0.976	(1.731)
Month·Age	−0.212	(0.180)	−0.223	(0.224)	−0.429	(0.303)
Month·Gender	−0.188	(0.175)	−0.227	(0.211)	−0.369	(0.297)
Variance components						
$G_{11}^{1/2}$	3.490	(0.555)	3.895	(0.640)		
R	−0.691		−0.604	(0.140)		
$G_{22}^{1/2}$	0.534	(0.101)	0.662	(0.114)		
$G^{1/2}$					6.322	(1.284)
ρ					0.856	(0.031)

*The maximized log-likelihood using adaptive quadrature is −345.94.

subject-specific rate of recovery:

$$\text{logit}(\mu^{\text{C}}_{ij+1}) - \text{logit}(\mu^{\text{C}}_{ij}) = \beta^{\text{C}}_1 + \beta^{\text{C}}_4 \cdot \text{age}_i + \beta^{\text{C}}_5 \cdot \text{gender}_i + U_{i1}.$$

The coefficients of month·age and month·gender now represent differences in the average rate of recovery rather than differences in a common rate of recovery. The maximized log likelihood increases from −369.88 for the random intercept model to −345.94 for the random lines model – a large increase in model fit. Allowing heterogeneity among subjects in regression slopes increases the standard error of the time main effect and the interaction term coefficient estimates. While a random intercept model indicates a significant month·age interaction, the estimate using a more appropriate random lines model is no longer significant ($Z = -0.212/180 = -1.18$, $p = 0.238$, based on MLE). Once again, the estimates obtained using MCMC are comparable to the MLEs.

Finally, we consider the autocorrelated random effects model

$$\text{logit}\{\text{E}(Y_{ij} \mid \boldsymbol{X}_i, \boldsymbol{U}_i)\} = \boldsymbol{x}'_{ij}\boldsymbol{\beta}^{\text{C}} + U_{ij},$$

where $\text{cov}(U_{ij}, U_{ik}) = G \cdot \rho^{|t_{ij}-t_{ik}|}$. The random intercept model is actually a special case of the autocorrelated random effects model where $\rho = 1$, or all U_{ij} are perfectly correlated. The autocorrelated random effects model is prohibitive to fit using ML since the dimension of the random effects in this example is $n_i = 12$. Bayesian estimation using MCMC is feasible. Table 11.4 presents posterior means and standard deviations using vague independent priors for β^{C}_j, a uniform prior for ρ, and a gamma prior (a $\Gamma(2, 2)$ prior) for $G^{1/2}$ that is truncated to lie on $(0.01, 20)$. The correlation parameter ρ has a posterior mean of 0.856 with a posterior standard deviation of 0.031. The posterior 95% credible region (0.792, 0.913) is relatively far from the value that defines the random intercepts model, $\rho = 1$. The standard deviation of the random serial process is estimated as 6.322 (posterior mean). This estimate is substantially larger than the estimated standard deviation in the random intercepts model, or the estimated standard deviation for $U_{i0}+U_{i1} \cdot t_{ij}$ in the random lines model which ranges from 3.490 when $t_{ij} = 0$, to 5.702 when $t_{ij} = 11$ (based on MLEs). In general, the posterior point estimates are larger using the autocorrelated random effects model relative to the random intercept or random line models. For example, comparing posterior means for the coefficient of month · age we find the random lines estimate is $|-0.223+0.429|/|-0.429| = 48\%$ smaller than the autocorrelated process model estimate.

Regression parameter interpretation in this model is somewhat complicated for cluster-level covariates since the regression coefficients are defined in a conditional model that controls for U_{ij}, a random effect which varies over both subjects and time (see Heagerty and Zeger (2000) for a detailed discussion). However, for time contrasts this regression model specifies

$$\text{logit}(\mu_{ij+1}^{\text{C}}) - \text{logit}(\mu_{ij}^{\text{C}}) = \beta_1^{\text{C}} + \beta_4^{\text{C}} \cdot \text{age}_i + \beta_5^{\text{C}} \cdot \text{gender}_i + (U_{ij+1} - U_{ij}).$$

Averaging over time, j, or subject i yields $\beta_1^{\text{C}} + \beta_4^{\text{C}} \cdot \text{age}_i + \beta_5^{\text{C}} \cdot \text{gender}_i$, again providing the interpretation of these parameters as the average rate of recovery among specific covariate subgroups. In summary, GLMMs can be used to compare groups over time and allow a variety of dependence models to be considered through different random effect assumptions. However, as we see in this example, changes in the dependence structure need to be considered when interpreting the estimated regression coefficients obtained using different heterogeneity models.

Marginalized models. We now use marginalized models for analysis of the symptom data. We specify:

$$\begin{aligned}\mu_{ij}^{\text{M}} &= \text{E}(Y_{ij} \mid \text{month}_{ij}, \text{age}_i, \text{gender}_i),\\ \text{logit}(\mu_{ij}^{\text{M}}) &= \beta_0^{\text{M}} + \beta_1^{\text{M}} \cdot \text{month}_{ij} + \beta_2^{\text{M}} \cdot \text{age}_i + \beta_3^{\text{M}} \cdot \text{gender}_i\\ &\quad + \beta_4^{\text{M}} \cdot \text{month}_{ij} \cdot \text{age}_i + \beta_5^{\text{M}} \cdot \text{month}_{ij} \cdot \text{gender}_i.\end{aligned}$$

In the marginal model we essentially use the subscript i to identify a specific covariate subgroup rather than an individual, and characterize the difference in the prevalence of symptoms over time for subgroups:

$$\text{logit}(\mu_{ij+1}^{\text{M}}) - \text{logit}(\mu_{ij}^{\text{M}}) = \beta_1^{\text{M}} + \beta_4^{\text{M}} \cdot \text{age}_i + \beta_5^{\text{M}} \cdot \text{gender}_i.$$

In contrast to the GLMMs the interpretation of the parameters in the marginal mean do not depend on the specific correlation model that is chosen for analysis.

Table 11.5 presents GEE estimates for the marginal mean model,

$$\text{logit}(\mu_{ij}^{\text{M}}) = \boldsymbol{x}_{ij}'\boldsymbol{\beta}^{\text{M}}.$$

There is a non-significant suggestion that the rate of recovery (time slope) is faster among women, but recovery does not appear to depend on age-at-onset. Using GEE with a working AR(1) model yields a coefficient for the age by month interaction of $\hat{\beta}_4^{\text{M}} = -0.101$ with a Z statistic based on empirical standard errors of $-0.101/0.089 = 1.19$, p-value $= 0.235$. The gender by month interaction is weakly suggestive with $\hat{\beta}_5^{\text{M}} = -0.150$, $Z = -0.150/0.089 = -1.69$, p-value $= 0.091$. However, if a working independence model is used we obtain $\hat{\beta}_5^{\text{M}} = -0.113$ with $Z = -0.113/0.096 = 1.18$, p-value $= 0.238$. Unfortunately, the choice of working dependence model can impact point estimates and significance levels, and without objective criterion we cannot formally choose among various asymptotically valid estimators.

Table 11.5. GEE estimates for a logistic regression analysis of schizophrenia symptoms. Model based and empirical standard errors are presented.

	GEE – independence			GEE – AR(1)*		
Variable	Coef.	Mod. SE	Emp. SE	Coef.	Mod. SE	Emp. SE
Marginal mean $\boldsymbol{\beta}^{\mathrm{M}}$						
Intercept	0.643	(0.202)	(0.305)	0.553	(0.296)	(0.291)
Month	−0.254	(0.038)	(0.059)	−0.235	(0.053)	(0.055)
Age	0.811	(0.305)	(0.493)	0.638	(0.440)	(0.461)
Gender	−0.388	(0.286)	(0.449)	−0.161	(0.412)	(0.420)
Month·Age	−0.137	(0.064)	(0.094)	−0.101	(0.089)	(0.085)
Month·Gender	−0.113	(0.063)	(0.096)	−0.150	(0.090)	(0.089)

*The estimated lag-1 correlation is $\hat{\rho} = 0.590$.

By using a likelihood-based method rather than a semi-parametric method we are able to compare alternative dependence models using likelihood ratios. Table 11.6 presents ML estimates adopting both first-order and second-order marginalized transition models. The simplest marginalized transition model is the first-order time homogeneous dependence model, $\gamma_{ij,1} = \alpha_{1,0}$. Table 11.6 presents the mean regression and dependence parameter estimates for this model. Point estimates and standard errors for $\boldsymbol{\beta}^{\mathrm{M}}$ are quite close to those obtained using GEE. The estimated first-order coefficient $\hat{\alpha}_{1,0} = 3.166$ indicates that the odds of symptoms at month $= t$ are exp(3.166) times greater among subjects who previously had symptoms, $Y_{j-1} = 1$, compared to subjects who previously did not have symptoms, $Y_{j-1} = 0$. Recall that since the MTM(1) has $\boldsymbol{\beta}^{\mathrm{M}}$ orthogonal to $\boldsymbol{\alpha}$, the resulting ML estimates, $\hat{\boldsymbol{\beta}}$, are consistent even if the dependence model is incorrectly specified.

To evaluate the specification of the dependence order we can compute score tests using only the MTM(1) fit, or use likelihood ratio tests comparing second-order to first-order models. The score test of $\gamma_{ij,2} = \alpha_{2,0} = 0$ obtained from model 1 is 1.428 with p-value = 0.232. Model 2 is a second-order marginalized transition model with scalar first- and second-order coefficients. The first-order coefficient model includes the variable 'initial', an indicator variable for month = 1, allowing $\boldsymbol{\alpha}_1$ to be used for both the second-order model, $Y_{ij} \mid Y_{ij-1}, Y_{ij-2}$, and the initial state, $Y_{i1} \mid Y_{i0}$, which is a purely first-order distribution. The second-order coefficient, $\hat{\alpha}_{2,0} = 0.650$, is significant based on the Wald statistic, $Z = 0.650/0.295 = 2.20$, p-value = 0.028. Comparison of deviances yields, $\Delta D = 2\times(337.19 - 334.44) = 5.50$, p-value = 0.064 on 2 degrees of freedom.

Table 11.6. Generalized estimating equations and ML estimates using marginalized transition models for schizophrenia symptoms.

	MTM(1)		MTM(2)			
Variable	Coef.	SE	Coef.	SE	Coef.	SE
Marginal mean $\boldsymbol{\beta}^{\mathrm{M}}$						
Intercept	0.534	(0.300)	0.576	(0.301)	0.568	(0.295)
Month	−0.236	(0.054)	−0.238	(0.052)	−0.234	(0.054)
Age	0.650	(0.442)	0.588	(0.439)	0.619	(0.434)
Gender	−0.142	(0.413)	−0.150	(0.412)	−0.161	(0.407)
Month · Age	−0.112	(0.086)	−0.101	(0.086)	−0.100	(0.091)
Month · Gender	−0.144	(0.083)	−0.140	(0.084)	−0.149	(0.089)
First-order coefficient $\boldsymbol{\alpha}_1$						
Intercept	3.166	(0.228)	2.911	(0.291)	2.099	(0.559)
Initial			−0.260	(0.633)	0.403	(0.740)
Month					0.156	(0.096)
Second-order coefficient $\boldsymbol{\alpha}_2$						
Intercept			0.650	(0.295)	0.597	(0.293)
log-likelihood	−337.19			−334.44		−332.93

We can allow the dependence to change over time using the second-order model, $\gamma_{ij,1} = \alpha_{1,0} + \alpha_{1,1} \cdot \text{initial} + \alpha_{1,3}\text{month}$, and $\gamma_{ij,2} = \alpha_{2,0}$, which allows the coefficient of Y_{ij-1} to depend on time (we could also allow the second-order coefficient to depend on time). Model 3 yields a maximized log-likelihood of -332.93 and $\hat{\alpha}_{1,3} = 0.156$, $Z = 0.156/0.096 = 1.625$, and reduction in deviance of $\Delta D = 2 \times (334.44 - 332.93) = 3.02$ on one degree of freedom (p-value $= 0.082$) relative to Model 2. Model 3 also achieves the smallest AIC value among the first-order and second-order models considered. A score test for third-order effects leads to 0.072, indicating the adequacy of a second-order model. The observed time trend in serial dependence is expected in situations where patients stabilize (either with or without symptoms).

Finally, having settled on a dependence model we can assess whether the difference in recovery rates comparing early age-at-onset to late age-at-onset subjects (β_4) and comparing women to men (β_5) are significant. Using Model 3 we obtain $\hat{\beta}_4 = -0.100$, with $Z = -0.100/091 = -1.10$, $p = 0.271$, and $\hat{\beta}_5 = -0.149$, with $Z = -0.149/089 = -1.67$, $p = 0.094$. Although both early age-at-onset subjects and women appear to have faster recovery rates, subgroup differences in recovery are not significant at the nominal 0.05 level.

Marginalized transition models fitted using ML permit a thorough model-based analysis of schizophrenia symptoms. We use the maximized log-likelihood to establish an appropriate dependence model, and then evaluate the evidence regarding differences in the disease course across subgroups defined by age-at-onset and gender. We find that a second-order time inhomogeneous dependence model is appropriate. Corresponding regression estimates of the marginal mean structure indicate that the rate of recovery does not vary significantly among the covariate subgroups.

Summary. We have used both GLMMs and marginalized models to compare covariate subgroups over time. In the GLMM we interpret the coefficient of month as an average within-subject change in the log odds of symptoms for subjects in the reference group (age = 0, gender = 0), while in the marginalized models we interpret the coefficient of month as the change in the log odds of symptoms over time for the reference group. Primary scientific interest is in the interaction terms which have parallel interpretations in terms of differences in average rates of recovery for conditional regression coefficients, $\boldsymbol{\beta}^{C}$, or as differences in the changes in the prevalence log odds across patient subgroups. Using likelihood-based methods we can compare the maximized log-likelihood for the various models. The GLMMs yield −369.88 and −345.94 for the random intercept and random slope models, respectively. The marginalized transition models yield −337.19 for the MTM(1) and −332.93 for the time inhomogeneous MTM(2). The maximized log-likelihoods suggest that the serial models provide a better fit for this symptom. Based on Fig. 11.5 we anticipate that serial models will fit the positive symptoms (hallucinations, delusion, thoughts) while models for negative symptoms (flat affect, apathy, withdrawal) will require a random intercept to characterize long-term within-subject dependence.

11.5 Summary and further reading

In this chapter we overview ML methods for the analysis of longitudinal categorical data. We focus on the common case of a binary response. We extend the discussion in Chapter 9 of conditionally specified GLMMs to include details regarding ML and Bayesian estimation methods. In Section 11.3 we discuss marginalized models which unify the marginal models discussed in Chapter 8 with the random effects models discussed in Chapter 9 and with the transition models discussed in Chapter 10.

Marginalized models allow a regression structure to be directly assumed for the marginal mean induced from either a log-linear, random effects, or transition model. Alternatively, random effects or transition models can be fit using their conditional mean specification as discussed in Chapters 9 and 10 and then estimates of induced marginal means obtained by marginalizing the fitted (conditional) model (see Lindsey (2000) for details using a transition model). In situations where the marginal structure is of primary interest the drawback of an indirect approach which fits a conditionally specified model and then computes marginal summaries, is that when regression structure is assumed for a conditional mean, μ_{ij}^{C}, then the induced marginal means, μ_{ij}^{M} may not have the same simple regression structure. Therefore, an indirect approach may not facilitate simple covariate adjusted estimates or tests for marginal effects.

Marginal models can be fitted using GEE and the efficiency of GEE relative to likelihood-based alternatives is discussed in Fitzmaurice *et al.* (1993), Fitzmaurice (1995), and Heagerty (2002). A properly specified likelihood leads to efficient parameter estimates, but when misspecified can lead to biased estimates. The bias of misspecified ML estimates for clustered data is discussed in Neuhaus *et al.* (1992), TenHave *et al.* (1999), and Heagerty and Kurland (2001).

In this chapter we have focused on binary response data. Approaches for longitudinal ordinal data are overviewed in Molenberghs and Lesaffre (1999). Heagerty and Zeger (1996) discuss methods based on log-linear models, while Agresti and Lang (1993) and Hedeker and Gibbons (1994) present random effects models.

We have focused on GLMMs and marginalized models. Alternative estimation approaches for hierarchical random effects models are discussed in Lee and Nelder (1996, 2001). Alternative ML approaches that directly model marginal means are found in Molenberghs and Lesaffre (1994, 1999), and Glonek and McCullagh (1995).

12
Time-dependent covariates

12.1 Introduction

One of the main scientific advantages of conducting a longitudinal study is the ability to observe the temporal order of key exposure and outcome events. Specifically, we can determine whether changes in a covariate precede changes in the outcome of interest. Such data provide crucial evidence for a causal role of the exposure (see Chapter 2 in Rothman and Greenland, 1998).

There are important analytical issues that arise with time-varying covariates in observational studies. First, it is necessary to correctly characterize the lag relationship between exposure and the disease outcome. For example, in a recent study of the health effects of air pollution the analysis investigated association between mortality on day t and the value of exposure measured on days t, $t-1$, and $t-2$ (Samet *et al.*, 2000). Subject matter considerations are crucial since the lag time from exposure to health effect reflects the underlying biological latency. Also, the relevance of cumulative exposure or acute (recent) exposure depends on whether the etiologic mechanisms of exposure are transient or irreversible. Second, there is the issue of covariate *endogeneity* where the response at time t predicts the covariate value at times $s > t$. In this case we must decide upon meaningful targets of inference and must choose appropriate estimation methods.

In this chapter we adopt the following notation and definitions. We assume a common set of discrete follow-up times, $t = 1, 2, \ldots, T$, with a well-defined final study measurement time T. Let Y_{it} be the response on subject i at time t. Let X_{it} be a time varying covariate and $\boldsymbol{Z}_i$ a collection of baseline, or time-invariant covariates. For simplicity we assume that only a single time varying covariate is considered for analysis. We also assume that Y_{it} and X_{it} are simultaneously measured, and that for cross-sectional analyses we would correlate Y_{it} directly with X_{it}. However, for etiologic or causal analyses we assume that only previous covariate measurements $X_{it-1}, X_{it-2}, \ldots$ are potential causes of Y_{it}. Thus, in terms of causal ordering we assume that X_{it} represents the exposure directly after Y_{it} rather than before.

Factors that influence the covariate X_{it} need to be determined in order to select appropriate analysis approaches that relate a longitudinal response to a time-dependent covariate. In survival analysis Kalbfleisch and Prentice (1980, p. 124) define an *internal* covariate as 'the output of a stochastic process that is generated by the individual under study' in contrast to an *external* covariate that is not influenced by the individual under study. Similarly, in the econometrics literature the term *endogenous* is typically used to refer to variables that are stochastically determined by measured factors within the system under observation while *exogenous* variables are determined by factors outside the system under study (Amemiya, 1985).

In the econometrics literature precise definitions of covariate exogeneity involve both statements of conditional independence, and statements of parameter separation. Define $\mathcal{H}_i^X(t) = \{X_{i1}, X_{i2}, \ldots, X_{it}\}$ as the history of the covariate through time t, and similarly define $\mathcal{H}_i^Y(t) = \{Y_{i1}, Y_{i2}, \ldots, Y_{it}\}$. A covariate process is exogenous with respect to the outcome process if the covariate at time t is conditionally independent of all preceding response measurements. We define endogenous simply as the opposite of exogenous. Formally the definitions are

$$\text{exogenous:} \quad f(X_{it} \mid \mathcal{H}_i^Y(t), \mathcal{H}_i^X(t-1), \boldsymbol{Z}_i) = f(X_{it} \mid \mathcal{H}_i^X(t-1), \boldsymbol{Z}_i),$$
$$\text{endogenous:} \quad f(X_{it} \mid \mathcal{H}_i^Y(t), \mathcal{H}_i^X(t-1), \boldsymbol{Z}_i) \neq f(X_{it} \mid \mathcal{H}_i^X(t-1), \boldsymbol{Z}_i),$$

where $f(x)$ represents a density function for continuous covariates and probability otherwise. This definition is not the same as that given by Engle *et al.* (1983) since we have not further discussed specific implications of this assumption, nor commented on the relationship of the process X_{it} to parameters of interest (our statement is referred to as 'Granger non-causality' by Engle *et al.* (1983)). Our definition is essentially equivalent to that given for statistical exogeneity by Hernán *et al.* (2001).

One implication of the assumption of exogeneity is the factorization of the likelihood for (X_{it}, Y_{it}):

$$\begin{aligned} f(\boldsymbol{X}_i, \boldsymbol{Y}_i \mid \boldsymbol{Z}_i; \boldsymbol{\theta}) &= \left[\prod_{t=1}^{T} f(Y_{it} \mid \mathcal{H}_i^Y(t-1), \mathcal{H}_i^X(t-1), \boldsymbol{Z}_i; \boldsymbol{\theta})\right] \\ &\quad \times \left[\prod_{t=1}^{T} f(X_{it} \mid \mathcal{H}_i^X(t-1), \boldsymbol{Z}_i; \boldsymbol{\theta})\right] \\ &= \mathcal{L}_Y(\boldsymbol{\theta}) \times \mathcal{L}_X(\boldsymbol{\theta}). \end{aligned}$$

If we further assume that $\boldsymbol{\theta} = (\boldsymbol{\theta}_1, \boldsymbol{\theta}_2)$, where $\boldsymbol{\theta}_1$ and $\boldsymbol{\theta}_2$ are variation independent parameters (i.e. $(\boldsymbol{\theta}_1 \in \boldsymbol{\Theta}_1) \times (\boldsymbol{\theta}_2 \in \boldsymbol{\Theta}_2)$, and that $\boldsymbol{\theta}_1$ is the parameter of interest, then Engle *et al.* (1983) define the process X_{it} as *strongly exogenous* for the parameter $\boldsymbol{\theta}_1$. One motivation for introducing the concept of strong exogeneity is that when the assumption is satisfied, likelihood-based inference regarding $\boldsymbol{\theta}_1$ can condition on X_{it} without loss of information, and therefore analysis can proceed without having to specify an explicit model for X_{it}.

A second important implication of exogeneity is that the expectation of Y_{it} conditional on the entire covariate process $(X_{i1}, X_{i2}, \ldots, X_{iT})$ will depend only on the covariates prior to time t. Formally, when a process is exogenous

$$\mathrm{E}(Y_{it} \mid X_{i1}, X_{i2}, \ldots, X_{it}, \ldots, X_{iT}, \boldsymbol{Z}_i) = \mathrm{E}(Y_{it} \mid X_{i1}, X_{i2}, \ldots, X_{it-1}, \boldsymbol{Z}_i).$$

Exogeneity is actually a stronger statement since it implies that Y_{it} is conditionally independent of all future covariates given both past outcomes and covariates, that is, $Y_{it} \perp \{X_{it}, \ldots, X_{iT}\} \mid \mathcal{H}_i^Y(t-1), \mathcal{H}_i^X(t-1)$.

In Example 1.1 we model CD4+ counts as a function of time since seroconversion. Any analysis that uses scheduled observation times, t_{ij}, as a time-dependent covariate can safely assume exogeneity – time is external to the system under study and not stochastic. An example of a random time-dependent covariate is the treatment assignment at time t_j in the crossover trial, Example 1.5. However, in a randomized study the determination of the treatment arm or treatment order is independent of outcomes by design and therefore exogenous. Finally, in the Indonesian children's health study we use the time-dependent xerophthalmia status, X_{it}, as a predictor of respiratory infection, Y_{it}. We can empirically check for endogeneity in this example by regressing X_{it} on both $Y_{it-1}, Y_{it-2}, \ldots$, and $X_{it-1}, X_{it-2}, \ldots$. After controlling for prior xerophthalmia status we find no significant association between current xerophthalmia status and past illness.

In Section 12.3 we discuss some general issues regarding the analysis of time-dependent covariates. When covariates are exogenous, analysis can focus on specifying the dependence of Y_{it} on $X_{it-1}, X_{it-2}, \ldots$. We discuss methods that can be used to characterize such lagged dependencies in Section 12.4. When a covariate is endogenous we are confronted with choosing both meaningful targets of inference and valid methods of estimation – these are discussed in Section 12.5.

12.2 An example: the MSCM study

Alexander and Markowitz (1986) studied the relationship between maternal employment and paediatric health care utilization. The investigation was motivated by the major social and demographic changes that have occurred in the US since 1950. For example, in 1950 only 12% of married women with preschool children worked outside the home while in 1980 approximately 45% of mothers with children under the age of six were part of the labour force. A significant body of research has examined the effect of mothers' work on cognitive and social aspects of child development while only limited prior research investigated the impact on paediatric care utilization. The Mothers' Stress and Children's Morbidity Study (MSCM) enrolled $N = 167$ preschool children between the ages of 18 months and 5 years that attended an inner-city paediatric clinic. To be eligible for the study children needed to be living with their mother and free of chronic conditions. At entry, mothers provided demographic and background information regarding their family and their work outside the home. During 4 weeks of follow-up daily measures of maternal stress and child illness were recorded. A final data source included a medical record review to document health care utilization. We use these data to illustrate statistical issues that pertain to regression analysis with time-dependent covariates. The specific scientific questions that we consider include:

1. Is there an association between maternal employment and stress?
2. Is there an association between maternal employment and child illness?
3. Do the data provide evidence that maternal stress causes child illness?

A total of 55 mothers were employed outside the home ($55/167 = 33\%$). We will refer to mothers that work outside the home as 'employed', and will refer to mothers that do not work outside the home as 'non-employed'. The analysis data contains additional baseline covariates including self-reported maternal and child health, child race, maternal educational attainment, marital status, and household size. Time-dependent measures for household i included daily ratings of child illness, Y_{it}, and maternal stress, X_{it}, during a 28-day follow-up period $t = 1, 2, \ldots, 28$. In the first week of follow-up the prevalence of maternal stress was 17% but declined to 12%, 12%, and 10% in weeks 2 through 4. The prevalence of child illness similarly declined slightly from 16% in the first week to 14%, 11%, and 11% in the subsequent weeks. Figure 12.1 shows the crude weekly stress and illness prevalence for families with employed mothers and for non-employed mothers. For illness we find large day-to-day variation but observe a trend of slightly decreased prevalence among children whose mothers are employed. The time course for stress is more complicated with employed mothers initially having a higher rate of stress but after week 14 the employed mothers report less stress than non-employed mothers.

To meaningfully address the association between maternal employment and either stress or illness we need to control for several potential confounders. For example, Table 12.1 shows that the majority of working mothers were high school graduates while only 41% of non-employed mothers were high school graduates. Also, compared to the non-employed mothers the employed mothers were more likely to be married (58% versus 43%) and to be white (62% versus 37%). Since stress may be in the causal pathway that leads from employment to illness we do not adjust for

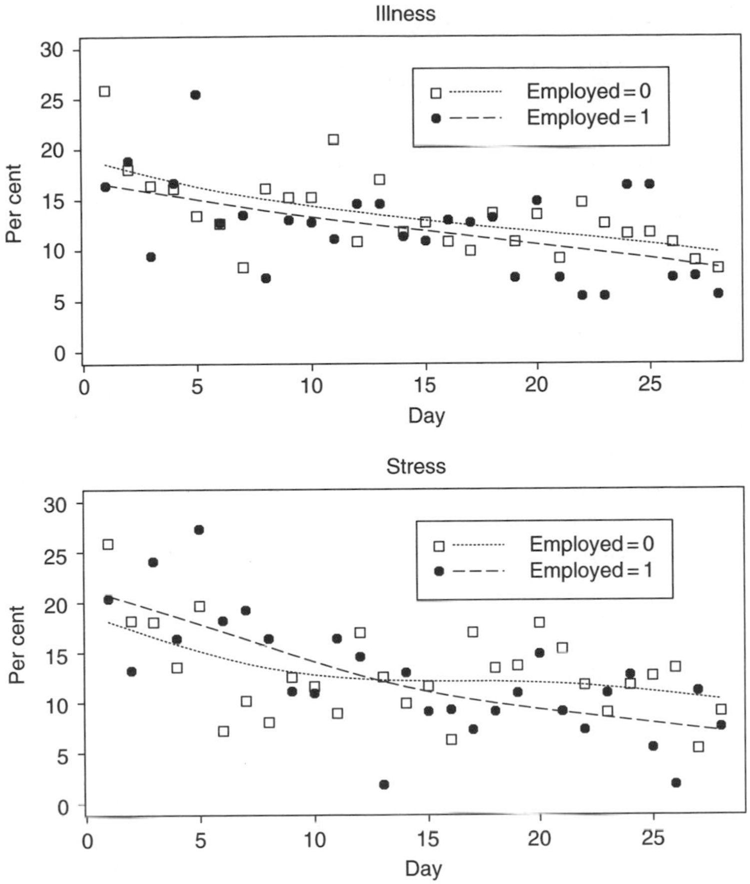

Fig. 12.1. The prevalence of maternal stress and child illness in the MSCM study during the 28 days of follow-up for those families where the mother worked outside the home (employed = 1) and those families where the mother did not (employed = 0).

any of the daily stress indicators when evaluating the dependence of illness on employment. Similarly, we do not adjust for illness in the analysis of employment and stress. Therefore, the only time-dependent variable in our initial analyses is the study day (time) – a non-stochastic time-dependent covariate.

Table 12.2 presents unadjusted and adjusted log odds ratios for the primary exposure variable, maternal employment, and both of the longitudinal outcomes. Using generalized estimating equation (GEE) with working independence the crude association that adjusts for a common temporal trend indicates that working mothers are slightly less likely to

Table 12.1. Covariate summaries for mothers who were employed outside the home and those who were not.

	Employed = 1 $n = 55$ (%)	Employed = 0 $n = 112$ (%)
Married		
0 = no	42	57
1 = yes	58	43
Maternal health		
1, 2 = fair/poor	9	17
3 = good	33	34
4 = very good	47	32
5 = excellent	11	17
Child health		
1, 2 = fair/poor	7	5
3 = good	7	16
4 = very good	55	46
5 = excellent	31	33
Race		
0 = white	62	37
1 = non-white	38	63
Education		
0 ≤ high school	16	59
1 = HS graduate	84	41
Household size		
0 = less than 3	38	31
1 = 3 or more	62	69

have ill children (estimated odds ratio = $\exp(-0.12) = 0.89$) but are nearly equivalent in their rates of reporting stress. Adjustment for covariates has a minor impact on the coefficient of employment in the analysis of illness and indicates a non-significant difference between employed and non-employed mothers. In the adjusted analysis of stress we find a different time pattern for employed and non-employed mothers with a significant group-by-time interaction. Therefore, using GEE we conclude that there is a significant decline in the rate of child illness over the 28 days of follow-up but that there is no significant difference between employed and non-employed mothers. For stress we find a difference in the rate of decline comparing employed and non-employed mothers with a negative but non-significant time (week) coefficient of -0.14 for non-employed mothers, and a time (week) coefficient of -0.14–$0.20 = -0.34$ for the employed mothers. The regression methods

Table 12.2. Logistic regression analysis of the association between employment and both longitudinal illness and stress using GEE with an independence working correlation matrix. Time is modelled using the variable week = (day-14)/7.

	Coef.	SE	*Z*	Coef.	SE	*Z*	Coef.	SE	*Z*
Illness									
Intercept	−1.86	(0.11)	−16.44	−0.50	(0.39)	−1.26	−0.50	(0.39)	−1.26
Employed	−0.12	(0.17)	− 0.69	−0.14	(0.17)	−0.83	−0.15	(0.18)	−0.83
Week	−0.19	(0.05)	− 3.59	−0.19	(0.05)	−3.59	−0.19	(0.06)	−3.06
Married				0.55	(0.15)	3.69	0.55	(0.15)	3.69
Maternal health				−0.06	(0.10)	−0.57	−0.06	(0.10)	−0.57
Child health				−0.32	(0.09)	−3.68	−0.32	(0.09)	−3.68
Race				0.48	(0.16)	2.91	0.48	(0.16)	2.90
Education				−0.01	(0.20)	−0.04	−0.01	(0.20)	−0.04
House size				−0.75	(0.16)	−4.84	−0.75	(0.16)	−4.84
Week × employed							−0.02	(0.12)	−0.17
Stress									
Intercept	−1.91	(0.10)	−18.50	−0.13	(0.45)	−0.29	−0.12	(0.45)	−0.27
Employed	−0.04	(0.20)	− 0.20	−0.25	(0.19)	−1.28	−0.28	(0.19)	−1.42
Week	−0.20	(0.05)	− 4.37	−0.21	(0.05)	−4.41	−0.14	(0.06)	−2.49
Married				0.34	(0.16)	2.12	0.34	(0.16)	2.12
Maternal health				−0.29	(0.10)	−2.91	−0.29	(0.10)	−2.91
Child health				−0.26	(0.10)	−2.57	−0.26	(0.10)	−2.58
Race				0.21	(0.18)	1.17	0.21	(0.18)	1.18
Education				0.52	(0.18)	2.85	0.52	(0.18)	2.86
House size				−0.46	(0.16)	−2.78	−0.46	(0.16)	−2.79
Week × employed							−0.20	(0.10)	−2.13

that we have introduced in Chapter 7 are well suited for analyses that focus on the characterization and comparison of groups over time.

The final scientific question seeks to determine the casual effect of stress on child illness. Figure 12.2 shows raw stress and illness series for 12 randomly selected families. We find a large amount of variation in the reporting of stress. For example, one subject (#219) reports no stress during follow-up while another subject (#156) reports 3 days of stress in the first week, 1 day in the second week, 5 days in the third week, and 3 days in week four. Analysis of these data raises several questions:

1. What is the cross-sectional association between stress on day t and illness on day t?
2. Does illness at day t depend on prior stress measured on day $(t-k)$ for $k = 1, 2, \ldots$?
3. What are the factors that influence maternal stress on day t? Does child illness on day $(t-k)$ for $k = 0, 1, 2, \ldots$ predict maternal stress?

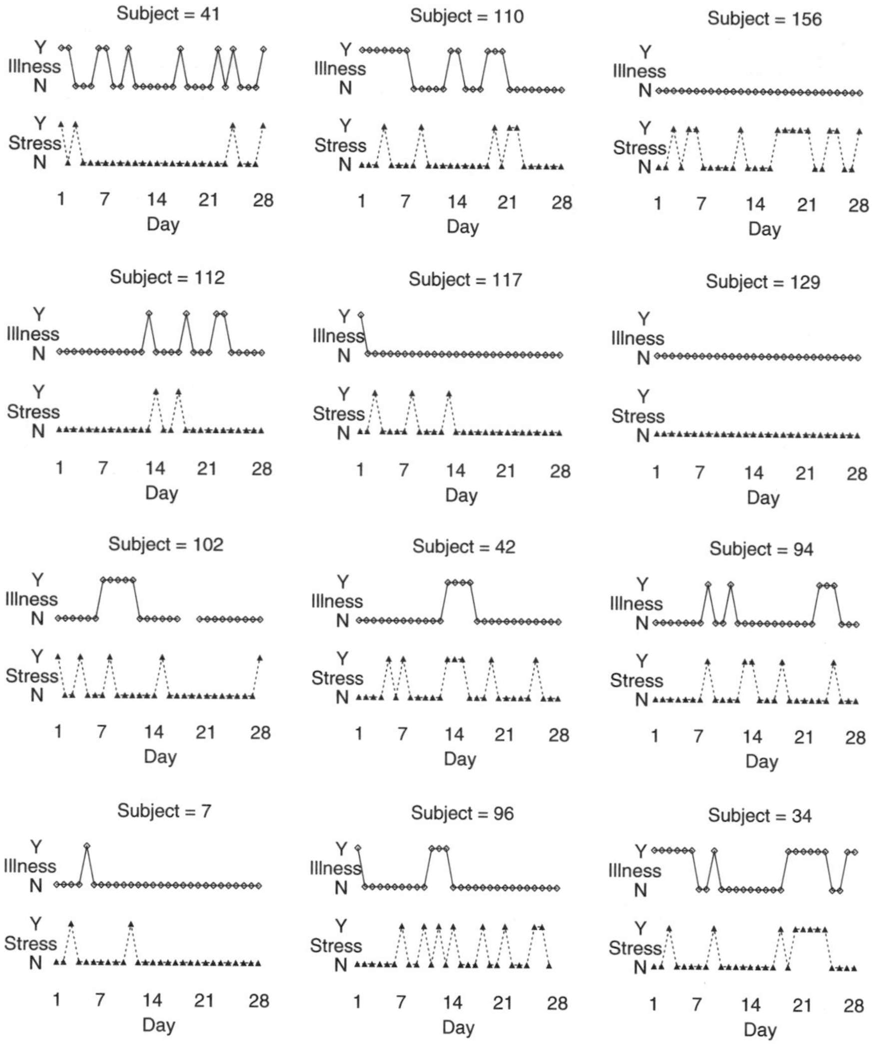

Fig. 12.2. A random sample of data from the MSCM study. The presence or absence of maternal stress and child illness is displayed for each day of follow-up.

The first question considers the marginal association between a longitudinal response variable and a time-dependent covariate. In Section 12.3 we discuss regression methods that can be used in this context. The second question deals with the analysis of a stochastic time-dependent covariate and the specification of covariate lags. This issue has received attention in time-series literature, but we only discuss methods for finite lag models since longitudinal series are typically short and methods for infinite series are not necessary. Finally, question three addresses whether the covariate

X_{it} is *endogenous* meaning that it is both a predictor of the outcome of interest, and is predicted by the outcome measured at earlier occasions. Certain authors refer to scenarios where the covariate influences the response, and the response influences the covariate as *feedback* (Zeger and Liang, 1991). In this situation the response at time $t-1$, Y_{it-1}, may be both an intermediate variable for the outcome at time t, Y_{it}, and a confounder for the exposure at time t, X_{it}. This situation leads to a consideration of proper targets of inference and appropriate methods of estimation and is discussed in Section 12.5.

12.3 Stochastic covariates: full and partly conditional means

With longitudinal data and a time-varying exposure or treatment there are several possible conditional expectations that may be of scientific interest and thus identify useful regression models. We distinguish between *partly conditional* and *fully conditional* regression models since the taxonomy identifies models whose parameters have different interpretations, and relates to assumptions required for valid use of covariance weighted estimation, such as with linear mixed models, or with non-diagonal GEE working models. For example, if we are interested in the relationship between a response on day t and an exposure on the same day, then we can use $\mathrm{E}(Y_{it} \mid X_{it})$ to characterize whether the average response varies as a function of concurrent exposure measurement. We may also hypothesize a lag between exposure and ultimate impact on the response so focus our analysis on $\mathrm{E}(Y_{it} \mid X_{it-1})$, or more generally on $\mathrm{E}(Y_{it} \mid X_{it-k})$ for some value of k. Alternatively, the entire exposure history may predict outcome and therefore we model $\mathrm{E}(Y_{it} \mid X_{i1}, X_{i2}, \ldots, X_{it-1})$, perhaps allowing a simple dependence of Y_{it} on the cumulative exposure, $X_{it}^* = \sum_{s<t} X_{is}$. Finally, we may target analysis toward the average response given the entire covariate process, $\mathrm{E}(Y_{it} \mid X_{is},\ s = 1, 2, \ldots, T)$. Neuhaus and Kalbfleisch (1998) discuss one such model for clustered data where both X_{it} and $\bar{X}_i = (1/n_i)\sum_s X_{is}$ are used as predictors for Y_{it}.

Following Pepe and Couper (1997), we classify $\mathrm{E}(Y_{it} \mid X_{is}\ s = 1, 2, \ldots, T)$ as the *full covariate conditional mean* and refer to $\mathrm{E}[Y_{it} \mid \text{subset}\ (X_{i1}, \ldots, X_{in_i})]$ for proper (non-exhaustive) covariate subsets as a *partly conditional mean.* The cross-sectional mean $\mathrm{E}(Y_{it} \mid X_{it})$ is one partly conditional mean, as are the conditional expectations that include only a single lagged covariate, or that include the entire covariate history prior to time t. The first consideration for regression analysis of longitudinal data with time-varying covariates is determination of the target of inference – that is, whether the full covariate conditional mean is of interest, or whether a certain partly conditional mean captures relationships of primary interest. The second issue is identification of valid and efficient estimation methods.

When the covariate process is endogenous the full covariate conditional mean, $\mathrm{E}(Y_{it} \mid X_{is} \;\; s = 1,2,\ldots,T)$, may depend on any or all covariates X_{is}. However, when a covariate is exogenous we know that $\mathrm{E}(Y_{it} \mid X_{is} \;\; s = 1,2,\ldots,T) = \mathrm{E}(Y_{it} \mid X_{it-1}, X_{it-2}, \ldots, X_{i1})$. If we further assume that only the k most recent exposures predict the response then we obtain further simplification: $\mathrm{E}(Y_{it} \mid X_{it-1}, X_{it-2}, \ldots, X_{it-k}, \ldots, X_{i1}) = \mathrm{E}(Y_{it} \mid X_{it-1}, X_{it-2}, \ldots, X_{it-k})$. Therefore, under specific model assumptions such as exogeneity and a finite covariate lag, the partly conditional mean $\mathrm{E}(Y_{it} \mid X_{it-1}, X_{it-2}, \ldots, X_{it-k})$ may equal the full covariate conditional mean.

In some situations we may simply be interested in the cross-sectional association between Y_{it} and X_{it}. In Section 12.3.1 we discuss estimation issues for cross-sectional models. However, many longitudinal studies are interested in assessing the impact of prior exposure on current health status, and thus focus on characterizing $\mathrm{E}(Y_{it} \mid X_{it-1}, \ldots, X_{i1})$. In Section 12.4 we discuss regression methods using single or multiple lagged covariate values. Although in general we may not believe that future exposure causally influences current health status, when the covariate process is *endogenous*, the fact that $[X_{it} \mid \mathcal{H}_i^Y(t), \mathcal{H}_i^X(t-1)]$ depends on $\mathcal{H}_i^Y(t)$ implies that $\mathrm{E}(Y_{it} \mid X_{is} \;\; s = 1,2,\ldots,T) \neq \mathrm{E}(Y_{it} \mid X_{is} \;\; s < t)$. This identifies one important scenario where the full covariate conditional mean is not equal to the scientifically desired partly conditional mean. Section 12.5 discusses methods of analysis when a covariate is endogenous.

12.3.1 *Estimation issues with cross-sectional models*

In Chapter 4 we showed that the multivariate Gaussian likelihood equations take the form

$$\sum_{i=1}^{m} \boldsymbol{X}_i' \boldsymbol{W}_i (\boldsymbol{Y}_i - \boldsymbol{X}_i \boldsymbol{\beta}) = \boldsymbol{0},$$

where $\boldsymbol{W}_i = [\mathrm{Var}(\boldsymbol{Y}_i \mid \boldsymbol{X}_i)]^{-1}$. We noted that the resulting weighted least squares solution to these equations enjoys a consistency robustness since the estimator using a general weight matrix $\boldsymbol{W}_i$ remains unbiased even when $\boldsymbol{W}_i \neq [\mathrm{Var}(\boldsymbol{Y}_i \mid \boldsymbol{X}_i)]^{-1}$. Similarly, in Chapter 8 we introduced estimating equation methods where the regression estimator is defined as the solution to the estimating equation

$$\boldsymbol{S}_{\boldsymbol{\beta}}(\boldsymbol{\beta}, \boldsymbol{W}) \equiv \sum_{i=1}^{m} \left(\frac{\partial \boldsymbol{\mu}_i}{\partial \boldsymbol{\beta}} \right)' \boldsymbol{W}_i (\boldsymbol{Y}_i - \boldsymbol{\mu}_i) = \boldsymbol{0}.$$

Consistency of the weighted least squares estimator, and the GEE regression estimator relies on the assumption that $\boldsymbol{S}_{\boldsymbol{\beta}}(\boldsymbol{\beta}, \boldsymbol{W})$ is 'unbiased', that is, has expectation equal to zero.

Pepe and Anderson (1994) have clarified that to ensure that $\mathrm{E}[\boldsymbol{S}_{\boldsymbol{\beta}}(\boldsymbol{\beta}, \boldsymbol{W})] = 0$ it is sufficient to assume

$$\mu_{it} \equiv \mathrm{E}(Y_{it} \mid X_{it}) = \mathrm{E}(Y_{it} \mid X_{i1}, X_{i2}, \ldots, X_{iT}). \tag{12.3.1}$$

Furthermore, if this condition is not satisfied but substantive interest is in the cross-sectional association between X_{it} and Y_{it} then working independence GEE should be used otherwise biased regression estimates may obtain. We refer to (12.3.1) as the *full covariate conditional mean* (FCCM) assumption. Although Pepe and Anderson (1994) focused on the use of GEE, the issue that they raise is important for all longitudinal data analysis methods including likelihood-based methods such as linear and generalized linear mixed models.

To understand the importance of the FCCM condition we consider the sums represented by matrix multiplications in the estimating function $\boldsymbol{S}_{\boldsymbol{\beta}}(\boldsymbol{\beta}, \boldsymbol{W})$:

$$\boldsymbol{S}_{\boldsymbol{\beta}}(\boldsymbol{\beta}, \boldsymbol{W}) = \sum_{i=1}^{m} \left(\frac{\partial \boldsymbol{\mu}_i}{\partial \boldsymbol{\beta}}\right)' \boldsymbol{W}_i(\boldsymbol{Y}_i - \boldsymbol{\mu}_i), \tag{12.3.2}$$

$$= \sum_{i=1}^{m} \left[\sum_{j=1}^{n_i}\sum_{k=1}^{n_i} x_{ij} w_{ijk}^{*}(Y_{ik} - \mu_{ik})\right], \tag{12.3.3}$$

where $w_{ijk}^{*} = \frac{\partial \eta_{ij}}{\partial \mu_{ij}} \cdot w_{ijk}$, and w_{ijk} is the (j,k) element of the weight matrix $\boldsymbol{W}_i$. In order to ensure that $\mathrm{E}[\boldsymbol{S}_{\boldsymbol{\beta}}(\boldsymbol{\beta}, \boldsymbol{W})] = 0$ we can consider the expectation of each summand in (12.2.3):

$$\begin{aligned}\mathrm{E}[x_{ij} w_{ijk}^{*}(Y_{ik} - \mu_{ik})] &= \mathrm{E}\left\{\mathrm{E}[x_{ij} w_{ijk}^{*}(Y_{ik} - \mu_{ik}) \mid X_{i1}, X_{i2}, \ldots, X_{in_i}]\right\} \\ &= \mathrm{E}\left\{x_{ij} w_{ijk}^{*}(E[Y_{ik} \mid X_{i1}, X_{i2}, \ldots, X_{in_i}] - \mu_{ik})\right\}.\end{aligned}$$

If the FCCM condition is satisfied then $\mu_{ik} = \mathrm{E}(Y_{ik} \mid X_{i1}, X_{i2}, \ldots, X_{in_i})$ and the estimating function is unbiased. However, if $\mu_{ik} = \mathrm{E}(Y_{ik} \mid X_{ik}) \neq \mathrm{E}(Y_{ik} \mid X_{i1}, X_{i2}, \ldots, X_{in_i})$ then the estimating function will likely be biased and result in inconsistent estimates for the cross-sectional mean structure. Finally, if a diagonal weight matrix is used then $\boldsymbol{S}_{\boldsymbol{\beta}}(\boldsymbol{\beta}, \boldsymbol{W})$ simplifies to

$$\boldsymbol{S}_{\boldsymbol{\beta}}(\boldsymbol{\beta}, \boldsymbol{W}) = \sum_{i=1}^{m} \left[\sum_{j=1}^{n_i} x_{ij} w_{ijj}^{*}(Y_{ij} - \mu_{ij})\right] \tag{12.3.4}$$

and $\boldsymbol{S}_{\boldsymbol{\beta}}(\boldsymbol{\beta}, \boldsymbol{W})$ will have zero expectation provided that $\mu_{ij} = \mathrm{E}(Y_{ij} \mid X_{ij})$. In this case the FCCM condition is not required for consistent cross-sectional estimation.

12.3.2 *A simulation illustration*

To illustrate the FCCM assumption and the failure of methods that use non-diagonal covariance weighting we simulated data under the following mechanism:

$$Y_{it} = \gamma_0 + \gamma_1 X_{it} + \gamma_2 X_{it-1} + b_i + e_{it}, \tag{12.3.5}$$

$$X_{it} = \rho X_{it-1} + \epsilon_{it}, \tag{12.3.6}$$

$$b_i, e_{it}, \epsilon_{it} \sim \text{mutually independent mean zero.} \tag{12.3.7}$$

This model represents the plausible scenario where a time-dependent covariate has an autoregressive structure and a response variable depends on both current and lagged values of the covariate. The model yields the full conditional and cross-sectional mean models

$$\mathrm{E}(Y_{it} \,|\, X_{i1}, \ldots, X_{in}) = \gamma_0 + \gamma_1 X_{it} + \gamma_2 X_{it-1},$$
$$\mathrm{E}(Y_{it} \,|\, X_{it}) = \beta_0 + \beta_1 X_{it},$$

where $\beta_0 = \gamma_0$ and $\beta_1 = \gamma_1 + \rho \cdot \gamma_2$. The induced cross-sectional model remains linear in X_{it}.

In many applications the cross-sectional association between X_{it} and Y_{it} is of substantive interest. For example, in assessing the predictive potential of biomarkers for the detection of cancer, the accuracy of a marker is typically characterized by the cross-sectional sensitivity and specificity. Although alternative predictive models may be developed using longitudinal marker series, these models would not apply to the common clinical setting where only a single measurement is available.

Pepe and Anderson (1994) conclude that using longitudinal data to estimate a cross-sectional model requires that either the FCCM assumption be verified or that working independence GEE be used. To demonstrate the bias that manifests through covariance weighting we generated data under models (12.3.5)–(12.3.7) with $b_i \sim N(0,1)$, $e_{it} \sim N(0,1)$, and $\epsilon_{i0} \sim N(0,1)$, $\epsilon_{it} \sim N(0, 1-\rho^2)$. Under these assumptions it can be shown that

$$\mathrm{E}[x_{it-1} w^*_{it-1,t}(Y_{it} - \beta_0 - \beta_1 X_{it})] = w^*_{it-1,t} \cdot \gamma_2 \cdot (1 - \rho^2)$$

indicating the potential for bias if the covariates are time varying ($\rho \neq 1$), Y_{it} is predicted by X_{it-1} ($\gamma_2 \neq 0$), and a non-diagonal weight matrix is used ($w^*_{it-1,t} \neq 0$).

For a range of correlations ($\rho = 0.9$–0.1) we simulated 1000 data sets each of which contained data on $m = 200$ subjects with up to 10 observations per subject. The number of observations for each subject, n_i, was generated as a uniform random variable between 2 and 10, representing data missing completely at random for a final scheduled follow-up of

Table 12.3. Average estimates of β_1 in the linear model $\mathrm{E}(Y_{it} \mid X_{it}) = \beta_0 + \beta_1 X_{it}$ based on models (12.3.5)–(12.3.7) with $\gamma_0 = 0$, $\gamma_1 = 1$, and $\gamma_2 = 1$ for different values of the covariate auto-correlation.

	$\rho = 0.9$ $\beta_1 = 1.9$	$\rho = 0.7$ $\beta_1 = 1.7$	$\rho = 0.5$ $\beta_1 = 1.5$	$\rho = 0.3$ $\beta_1 = 1.3$	$\rho = 0.1$ $\beta_1 = 1.1$
Independence	1.90	1.70	1.50	1.30	1.10
Exchangeable	1.73	1.51	1.33	1.19	1.01
AR(1)	1.73	1.36	1.11	0.89	0.74

$T = 10$. We estimated the cross-sectional regression coefficient β_1 using GEE with working independence, compound symmetric (exchangeable), and AR(1) correlation structures. Table 12.3 shows the simulation results indicating that GEE using either exchangeable or AR(1) correlation structures lead to biased estimates of β_1. For example, when $\rho = 0.7$ the exchangeable GEE estimator is negatively biased with a mean of 1.51, and a relative bias of $(1.51 - 1.7)/1.7 = -11\%$, while the AR(1) GEE estimator is similarly negatively biased with a mean estimate of 1.36, and a relative bias of $(1.36 - 1.7)/1.7 = -20\%$. These simulations illustrate that if regression analysis involves a time-dependent covariate then either the FCCM condition should be verified, or a working independence GEE estimator should be used.

12.3.3 *MSCM data and cross-sectional analysis*

The results of GEE analysis of child illness, Y_{it}, and maternal stress, X_{it}, are presented in Table 12.4. The children of mothers who report stress on day $= t$ are estimated to have an illness odds of $\exp(0.66) = 1.93$ the odds of illness among children of mothers that do not report stress. Unless we can verify the FCCM assumption, the GEE exchangeable and GEE AR(1) estimates cannot be assumed valid. Table 12.4 shows that we obtain smaller estimated regression coefficients using non-diagonal covariance weighting schemes. In particular, using an AR(1) correlation yields a coefficient estimate $(0.37 - 0.66)/0.66 = 43\%$ smaller than the working independence estimate. In the next section we evaluate the FCCM assumption and find that illness, Y_{it}, is associated with lagged maternal stress, X_{it-k} for $k = 1, 2, \ldots, 7$. In addition, stress appears strongly autocorrelated. Therefore we suspect that GEE estimators based on non-diagonal weight matrices are biased. There are important limitations to the cross-sectional summaries that we use independence estimating equations (IEE) to obtain. The cross-sectional association does not imply causation and it is equally plausible that stress causes illness or that illness causes stress. In order

Table 12.4. GEE analysis of child illness, Y_{it}, and stress, X_{it}, using different working correlation models. Time is modelled using week = (day-14)/7. Analysis also adjusts for employment, marital status, maternal and child health, race, education, and household size (not shown).

	Working correlation					
	Independence		Exchangeable		AR(1)	
	Est.	SE	Est.	SE	Est.	SE
Stress (X_{it})	0.66	(0.14)	0.52	(0.13)	0.37	(0.12)
Week	−0.18	(0.05)	−0.18	(0.05)	−0.20	(0.05)
			$\hat{\rho} = 0.07$		$\hat{\rho} = 0.40$	

to infer cause we need to address the temporal ordering of exposure and outcome.

12.3.4 *Summary*

Analysis of stochastic time-dependent covariates requires consideration of the dependence of the response at time t, Y_{it}, on both current, past, and future covariate values. We have shown that GEE with working independence can provide valid estimates for the cross-sectional association between Y_{it} and X_{it} but that covariance weighted estimation can lead to bias. One solution is to consider specification of the regression model as fully conditional on all of the covariates. In our simulation example in Section 12.3.2 this would require inclusion of the necessary current and lagged covariates. However, in other situations there is feedback where the current response influences future covariate values, and satisfying the FCCM condition would require conditioning on the future covariates. This may not be desirable and therefore alternative methods would need to be considered. Pepe and Anderson (1994) discuss the FCCM assumptions required to use GEE with general covariance weighting and offer GEE with working independence as a 'safe' analysis choice. Related work is presented in Emond *et al.* (1997) and Pan *et al.* (2000). The FCCM condition is also discussed for general clustered data analysis where separate 'within-cluster' covariates, or $(X_{ij} - \bar{X}_i)$, and 'between-cluster' covariates, or $\bar{X}_i$, may have different coefficients. In this case the full conditional mean μ_{ij} is a function of X_{ij} and the covariate values for all other observations, X_{ik}, $k \neq j$, through $\bar{X}_i$. See Palta *et al.* (1997) or Neuhaus and Kalbfleisch (1998) for further discussion.

12.4 Lagged covariates

In many applications an entire covariate history $X_{i1}, X_{i2}, \ldots, X_{it}$ is available and considered as potentially predictive of the response Y_{it}. In chronic disease epidemiology it is common to use cumulative exposure, $X_{it}^* = \sum_{s<t} X_{is}$, such as pack-years smoked, as the appropriate summary of the exposure history. In other settings, only a small subset of recent covariate values, $X_{it-1}, X_{it-2}, \ldots, X_{it-k}$, are used since an acute effect is hypothesized (Samet *et al.*, 2000). In either case, use of more than a single lagged covariate value can lead to highly correlated predictors, to questions regarding choice of the number of lagged covariates, and to specification of the structure for the coefficients of the lagged covariates. In this section we first review methods that can be used for a single lagged covariate, X_{it-k} but possibly with different choices of the lag $k = 1, 2, \ldots,$ and then we discuss use of multiple lagged covariates. To emphasize that in most applications one would only use exposure that occurred prior to the measurement time t to predict Y_{it}, we choose to discuss models such as $\mathrm{E}(Y_{it} \mid X_{it-k})$ rather than assume X_{it} represents the relevant summary of $\mathcal{H}_i^X(t-1)$ that would be used as a predictor at time t.

12.4.1 *A single lagged covariate*

In certain applications there is *a priori* justification to consider the covariate at a single lag time k time units prior to the assessment of disease status. For example, many pharmacologic agents are quickly cleared from the body so may only yield short duration effects. In this case analysis can use any of the methods discussed in Chapters 7–10 provided the FCCM condition is satisfied or appropriate alternative methods are selected, such as GEE with working independence. It is perhaps more common that the appropriate lag is unknown and several different choices are considered. If regression methods are used for a single time $t^\star$ then we can formulate a general model using a lagged covariate as

$$h(\mu_{it^\star}) = \beta_0 + \beta_1(k) \cdot X_{it^\star-k} + \boldsymbol{\beta}_2' \cdot \boldsymbol{Z}_i,$$

where $\boldsymbol{Z}_i$ represents a collection of additional time-invariant covariates, and $\mu_{it^\star} = \mathrm{E}(Y_{it^\star} \mid X_{it^\star-k}, \boldsymbol{Z}_i)$. In this model the coefficient $\beta_1(k)$ explicitly depends on the choice of the lag, k.

When interest is in the coefficient function $\beta_1(k)$ and comparisons between the coefficient at different lags k and $k^\star$, then *partly conditional* methods described by Pepe *et al.* (1999) can be used. Such methods allow inference on $\beta_1(k)$ by forming the observations $(Y_{it^\star}, X_{it^\star-k}, \boldsymbol{Z}_i)$ using multiple values of k and then using GEE with working independence. More generally, consider the partly conditional generalized linear model:

$$h\{\mathrm{E}(Y_{it} \mid X_{is}, \boldsymbol{Z}_i)\} = \beta_0(t,s) + \beta_1(t,s) \cdot X_{is} + \boldsymbol{\beta}_2'(t,s) \cdot \boldsymbol{Z}_i.$$

Here the coefficient of the covariate X_{is} may depend on both the response time t and/or the covariate time s. In certain applications we may assume that $\beta(t,s)$ is only a function of the lag, $(t-s)$, and may restrict analysis to pairs such that $t > s$. Pepe *et al.* (1999) refer to this as a partly conditional model since only a single covariate time is included as a predictor, rather than the covariate history $\{X_{is}\ s < t\}$, or the entire covariate process $\{X_{is}\ s = 1, 2, \ldots, T\}$ when modelling Y_{it}.

Given functional forms for the covariate functions $\beta_j(t,s)$ the partly conditional model can be estimated using GEE with working independence by constructing an expanded data set containing $(Y_{it}, X_{is}, \boldsymbol{Z}_i)$ for all pairs (t,s) and may contain n_i^2 records per subject derived from n_i observations. Using GEE allows the sandwich variance estimator to validly compute standard errors and make inference on the coefficient functions.

The partly conditional models that use a single value of the covariate process are strongly related to measures of cross-correlation (Diggle, 1990) and can be viewed as providing a generalized cross-association measure. To recognize this, recall that the cross-correlation $\rho(s,t) = \text{corr}(Y_{it}, X_{is})$ is related to $\beta_1(s,t)$, where $\text{E}(Y_{it} \mid X_{is}) = \beta_0(s,t) + \beta_1(s,t) \cdot X_{is}$ since $\beta_1(s,t) = \rho(s,t) \cdot \sigma_t^Y / \sigma_s^X$, $\sigma_t^Y = \sqrt{\text{Var}(Y_{it})}$, and $\sigma_s^X = \sqrt{\text{Var}(Y_{is})}$. Similarly, when Y_{it} and X_{it} are binary, the logistic partly conditional model specifies $\beta_1(s,t)$ which is the pairwise log odds ratio (Heagerty and Zeger, 1998). Therefore, the partly conditional models provide a method for characterizing the association between two stochastic processes that uses the flexibility of a regression formulation to capture the temporal structure of association between continuous, discrete, or mixed variables.

12.4.2 *Multiple lagged covariates*

When interest is in using the entire covariate history $\{X_{is}\ s < t\}$ as a predictor then methods that use multiple lagged covariates may be needed. The time series literature has considered models for both infinite and finite covariate lags. Since longitudinal data are typically short series we review a finite lag proposal that uses a lower dimensional model for the coefficients of lagged covariates. In *distributed lag models* (Almon, 1965; Dhrymes, 1971) lagged coefficients are assumed to follow a lower order smooth parametric function. For example, with a finite lag L a polynomial model with $p < L$ can be used to obtain smooth regression coefficients:

$$h\{\text{E}(Y_{it} \mid X_{is}\ s < t\,)\} = \beta_0 + \beta_1 \cdot X_{it-1} + \beta_2 \cdot X_{it-2} + \cdots + \beta_L \cdot X_{it-L},$$
$$\beta_j = \gamma_0 + \gamma_1 \cdot j + \gamma_2 \cdot j^2 + \cdots + \gamma_p \cdot j^p.$$

Polynomial models, and spline models (linear, cubic, natural) all permit use of standard software since the distributed lag model can be represented as a linear model with appropriate basis elements,

$\boldsymbol{Z}_j = [Z_0(j), Z_1(j), Z_2(j), \ldots, Z_p(j)]$. For example, in the polynomial model $Z_l(j) = j^l$. The regression model for μ_{it} is then a linear model with sums of the products $Z_l(j) \cdot X_{it-j}$ as covariates:

$$\beta_j = \boldsymbol{Z}_j'\gamma,$$

$$\begin{aligned} h(\mu_{it}) &= \beta_0 + \sum_{j=1}^{L} \beta_j \cdot X_{it-j} = \beta_0 + \sum_{j=1}^{L} [\boldsymbol{Z}_j'\gamma] \cdot X_{it-j}, \\ &= \beta_0 + \sum_{l=0}^{p} \gamma_l \left[\sum_{j=1}^{L} Z_l(j) \cdot X_{it-j} \right], \\ &= \beta_0 + \sum_{l=0}^{p} \gamma_l X_{it,l}^*, \end{aligned}$$

where $X_{it,l}^* = \sum_{j=1}^{L} Z_l(j) \cdot X_{it-j}$. In matrix form we obtain $\boldsymbol{\beta} = \boldsymbol{Z}'\boldsymbol{\gamma}$, and $h(\boldsymbol{\mu}_i) = \boldsymbol{X}_i\boldsymbol{\beta} = \boldsymbol{X}_i\boldsymbol{Z}'\boldsymbol{\gamma} = (\boldsymbol{X}_i^*)'\boldsymbol{\gamma}$.

Although distributed lag models permit parsimonious modelling of multiple lagged measurements, the specification of both the number of lagged covariates and the degrees of freedom for the coefficient model need to be considered. Selection of the number of lagged covariates, L, or the order of the coefficient model, p, may be determined using likelihood ratio tests for nested models, or using score or Wald tests (Godfrey and Poskitt, 1975) or through consideration of a loss function (Amemiya and Morimune, 1974).

12.4.3 *MSCM data and lagged covariates*

We first consider estimation of the association between illness, Y_{it}, and stress, X_{it-k}, using a single lagged stress covariate. We specify a logistic regression that adjusted for baseline covariates, $\boldsymbol{Z}_i$:

$$\text{logit E}(Y_{it} \mid X_{it-k}, \boldsymbol{Z}_i) = \beta_0(k) + \beta_1(k) \cdot X_{it-k} + \boldsymbol{\beta}_2'(k) \cdot \boldsymbol{Z}_i$$

and used GEE with working independence for inference. In Fig. 12.3 we display the point estimates and 95% confidence intervals for $\beta_1(k)$, $k = 1, 2, \ldots, 7$, based on separate fitted models for each value of k. Next we specify a parametric function for $\beta_0(k)$ and $\beta_1(k)$ and assume a constant β_2. Using natural splines with knots at $t_j = 4, 8, 12, 16$ we estimate a lag coefficient function, $\hat{\beta}_1(k)$, and pointwise standard errors using all possible pairs (Y_{it}, X_{is}) such that $t > s$. Figure 12.3 shows the estimated coefficient function and reveals a decaying association that is not significantly different from 0 after $k = 9$.

To investigate whether maternal stress measured on the previous 7 days is predictive of current child illness we use logistic regression controlling for

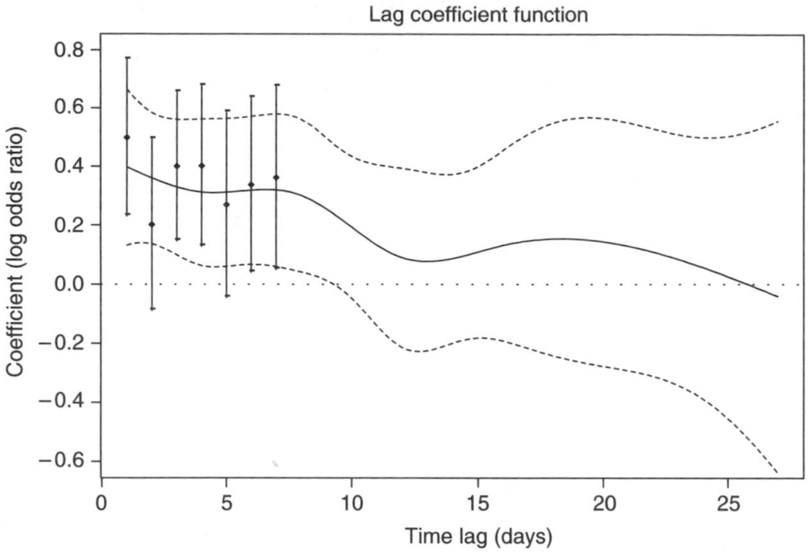

Fig. 12.3. Coefficients of lagged stress in logistic regression models for illness that use a single lagged covariate, X_{it-k} for $k = 1, 2, \ldots$. Shown is a smooth lag function with pointwise 95% confidence intervals, and the individual estimates for $k = 1, 2, \ldots, 7$.

baseline covariates. To account for the potential correlation in the longitudinal response we rely on empirical standard errors from GEE with working independence for inference. Table 12.5 shows the fitted coefficients for the lagged covariates X_{it-j} for $j = 1, 2, \ldots, 7$. Using separate unconstrained coefficients we obtain a significant positive coefficient for X_{it-1} but obtain a non-significant negative coefficient for X_{it-2}. Coefficient estimates for X_{it-3} through X_{it-7} vary between 0.18 and 0.25. Alternatively, we adopt a distributed lag model using a natural cubic spline model for the coefficients β_j and using knots at $j = 3$ and $j = 5$ requires only four estimated parameters rather than seven. Figure 12.4 shows the fitted coefficients and 95% confidence intervals using this model, and fitted coefficients from a monotone model that assumes $\beta_j = \gamma_0 + \gamma_1 \cdot (1/j)$. The constraints imposed by the spline models lead to less variation in the estimated coefficients of X_{it-j}. The model assumptions also lead to decreased standard errors for the fitted stress coefficients, $\hat{\beta}_j = \boldsymbol{Z}'_j\hat{\gamma}$. The monotone model yields $\hat{\beta}_j = 0.19 + 0.03 \cdot (1/j)$ and exhibits minimal variation in the estimates. One disadvantage of the spline models is that the parameterization does not lead to directly interpretable parameters. The fitted values from an alternative step function model, $\beta_j = \gamma_0 + \gamma_1 \cdot (j \geq 2) + \gamma_2 \cdot (j \geq 5)$ is shown in Table 12.5. This model indicates that lagged stress is positively correlated with illness and yields lag coefficient values of 0.32, 0.13, and 0.23. Testing $\gamma_1 = 0$

Table 12.5. Coefficients of lagged stress, X_{it-k}, as predictors of child illness, Y_{it}. Estimates are from a logistic regression using GEE with working independence and adjusting for week, employment status, marital status, maternal, and child health at baseline, race, education, and household size.

	Coefficient model					
	Saturated parameters = 7		Natural spline parameters = 4		Step function parameters = 3	
	Est.	SE	Est.	SE	Est.	SE
X_{it-1}	0.34	(0.16)	0.24	(0.16)	0.32	(0.16)
X_{it-2}	−0.05	(0.15)	0.14	(0.12)	0.13	(0.10)
X_{it-3}	0.18	(0.13)	0.11	(0.12)	0.13	(0.10)
X_{it-4}	0.25	(0.13)	0.17	(0.09)	0.13	(0.10)
X_{it-5}	0.22	(0.14)	0.25	(0.12)	0.23	(0.11)
X_{it-6}	0.19	(0.14)	0.26	(0.11)	0.23	(0.11)
X_{it-7}	0.25	(0.14)	0.21	(0.13)	0.23	(0.11)

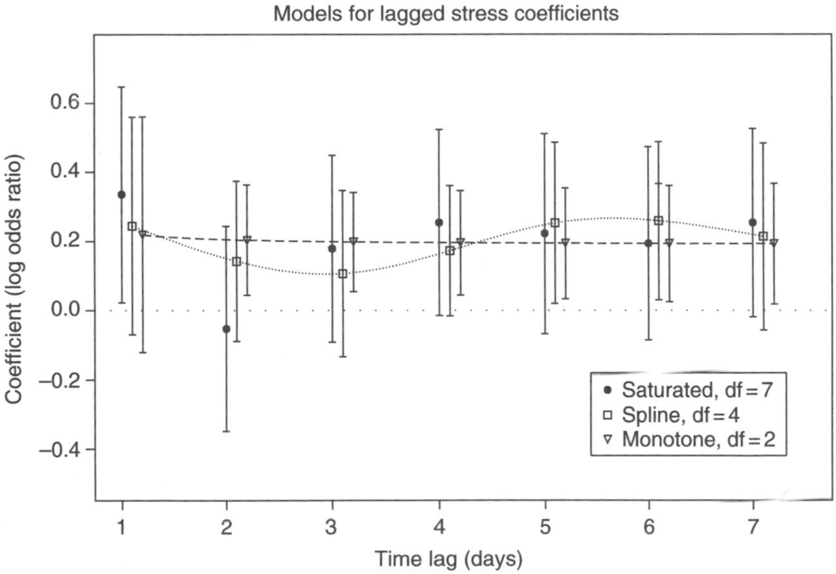

Fig. 12.4. Logistic regression analysis of lagged stress, X_{it-k}, as predictors of child illness using distributed lag models.

evaluates H_0: $\beta_1 = (\beta_2 = \beta_3 = \beta_4)$ versus H_1: $\beta_1 \neq (\beta_2 = \beta_3 = \beta_4)$ and yields a non-significant result with a Z value of -1.18. Similarly, γ_2 tests whether the common value $\beta_2 = \beta_3 = \beta_4$ equals the common value of the later coefficients $\beta_5 = \beta_6 = \beta_7$. We fail to reject equality of these coefficients (Z for $\hat{\gamma}_2$ is 0.66). Each of these models suggests an association between maternal stress in the previous week and current child illness although the statistical significance of the fitted coefficients varies depending on the specific model choice.

Since we choose to use GEE with an independence working correlation model for estimation we cannot use the maximized log-likelihood or information criterion such as AIC or BIC to compare the adequacy of different distributed lag models. As an alternative we can assess the predictive accuracy of each model by deleting individual subjects, re-fitting the model, and comparing observed and fitted outcome vectors. We use the c-index, or area under the ROC curve, as a global summary of model accuracy (Harrell *et al.*, 1984). The c-index is 64.1% for the saturated model with 7 degrees of freedom, and is 63.8% for the spline model ($p = 4$), and 64.2% for the monotone model ($p = 2$). Thus, these models provide nearly identical predictive accuracy with the monotone model only slightly favoured.

Figure 12.5 shows fitted models using $k = 1, 2, \ldots, L$ lagged stress variables for different choices of L. We can read this plot from right to left to determine the first model that has a significant coefficient for the last

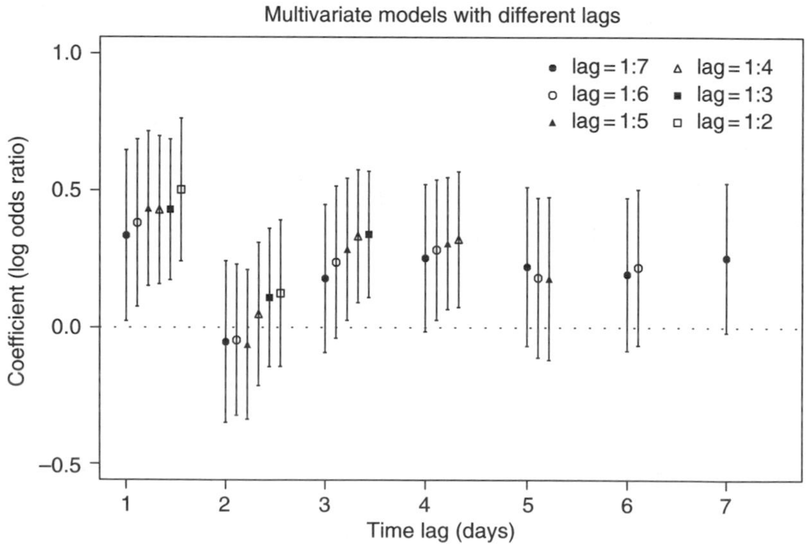

Fig. 12.5. Coefficients of lagged stress in logistic regression models for illness using L lagged covariates, X_{it-k} for $k = 1, 2, \ldots, L$ for different choices of L.

lag. In the model with $L = 7$ we see that the confidence interval for β_7 crosses 0 indicating non-significance. Similarly, for $L = 5$ and $L = 6$ we find that the confidence interval for β_L intersects 0. These evaluations represent Wald-based hypothesis tests for nested models, and we first reject with $L = 4$ where $\hat{\beta}_4$ is significant. Finally, Fig. 12.5 shows the changes in the coefficient estimates as we change the order L of the covariate lag. In general, the value of the coefficient for each remaining term increases as we decrease L and remove more distant lagged covariates.

12.4.4 *Summary*

In this section we first discussed estimation of the coefficient, $\beta_1(k)$, of a single covariate measured k time units prior to the response Y_{it}. Either separate parameters for every value k can be estimated using standard methods, or a smooth covariate function can be estimated by adopting a partly conditional regression model. Partly conditional models can be used to characterize the longest lag at which X_{it-k} and Y_{it} remain associated. Similarly, using multiple lagged covariates we discussed both saturated methods that allow a separate coefficient for each covariate lag, and distributed lag models that adopt regression structure for the lag coefficients. Models with multiple lagged covariates can be useful to describe the association between the full covariate process and the response process, or can be used to parsimoniously predict the response as a function of the complete covariate history.

12.5 Time-dependent confounders

Traditional epidemiologic regression analysis considers a classification of variables that are related to both an exposure of interest and the outcome as either confounders or intermediate variables. A confounder is loosely defined as a variable that is associated with both the exposure of interest and the response, and which if ignored in the analysis will lead to biased exposure effect estimates. An intermediate variable is one that is in the causal pathway from exposure to outcome and an analysis of exposure should not control for such a variable since the effect of exposure mediated through the intermediate variable is lost. In longitudinal studies a variable can be both a confounder and an intermediate variable, leading to analytical challenges. For example, using data from an observational study of HIV infected patients we may hope to determine the magnitude of benefit (or harm) attributable to treatment with AZT on either patient survival or longitudinal measures such as CD4 count. However, we may find that the CD4 count at time t predicts both later CD4 counts and subsequent treatment choices. In this case CD4 at time $s < t$ is the response variable for treatment received prior to s, but is also a predictor of, and therefore a potential confounder for, treatment given at future times, $t > s$.

A naive regression of CD4 at time t on treatment received prior to time t may reveal a lower mean CD4 among treated subjects. Such a finding may simply reflect the fact that patients who are more sick are the ones that are given treatment. In the subsections that follow we first summarize issues using a simple example, then we discuss methods of estimation and apply these methods to the MSCM data. Although the methods that we describe have been developed for general analysis with a time-dependent confounder, in this section we focus on the special case of an endogenous covariate. A more general and theoretical treatment can be found in Robins *et al.* (1999) and the references therein.

12.5.1 *Feedback: response is an intermediate and a confounder*

To clarify the issues that arise with time-dependent covariates consider a single pair of study times, $t = 1, 2$, with exposure and outcome measurements (X_{t-1}, Y_t). Let Y_t be a disease or symptom severity indicator (1 = disease/symptoms present, 0 = disease/symptoms absent) and let $X_t = 1$ if treatment is given and 0 otherwise. Assume that the exposure X_{t-1} precedes Y_t for $t = 1, 2$ and that Y_1 either precedes or is simultaneously measured with X_1. Figure 12.6 presents a directed graph that represents the sequential conditional models:

$$\text{logit } \mathrm{E}(Y_1 \mid X_0 = x_0) = -0.5 - 0.5 \cdot x_0, \tag{12.5.1}$$

$$\text{logit } \mathrm{E}(X_1 \mid Y_1 = y_1, X_0 = x_0) = -0.5 + 1.0 \cdot y_1, \tag{12.5.2}$$

$$\text{logit } \mathrm{E}(Y_2 \mid \mathcal{H}_1^X = h_1^X, Y_1 = y_1) = -1.0 + 1.5 \cdot y_1 - 0.5 \cdot x_1, \tag{12.5.3}$$

where $\mathcal{H}_1^X = \{X_0, X_1\}$ and $h_1^X = \{x_0, x_1\}$. These models specify a beneficial effect of treatment X_0 on the outcome at time 1 with a log odds ratio of -0.5 in the model $[Y_1 \mid X_0]$. However, the second model specifies that the treatment received at time 2 is strongly dependent on the outcome at time one. For either $X_0 = 0$ or $X_0 = 1$ if patients have a poor initial response ($Y_1 = 1$) they are more likely to receive treatment at time 2 than if they responded well ($Y_1 = 0$). Finally, the response at the second time is strongly correlated with the initial response and is influenced by treatment at time 2.

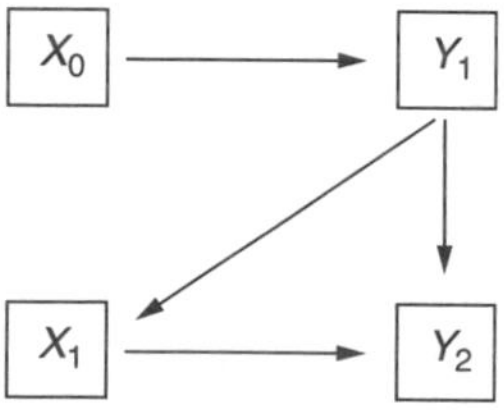

Fig. 12.6. Time-dependent covariate, X_{t-1}, and response Y_t.

Table 12.6. Expected counts when 500 subjects are initially treated, $X_0 = 1$, and 500 subjects are not treated, $X_0 = 0$, when treatment at time 2, X_1, is predicted by the outcome at time 1, Y_1, according to the model given by (12.5.1)–(12.5.3).

X_0	**0**								**1**							
n	500								500							
Y_1	**0**				**1**				**0**				**1**			
n	311				189				365				135			
X_1	**0**		**1**		**0**		**1**		**0**		**1**		**0**		**1**	
n	194		117		71		118		227		138		51		84	
Y_2	**0**	**1**	**0**	**1**	**0**	**1**	**0**	**1**	**0**	**1**	**0**	**1**	**0**	**1**	**0**	**1**
n	142	52	96	21	27	44	59	59	166	61	113	25	19	32	42	42

$$\mathrm{E}(Y_2 \mid x_0 = 1, x_1 = 1) = (25 + 42)/(138 + 84) = 0.30$$
$$\mathrm{E}(Y_2 \mid x_0 = 1, x_1 = 0) = (61 + 32)/(227 + 51) = 0.33$$
$$\mathrm{E}(Y_2 \mid x_0 = 0, x_1 = 1) = (21 + 59)/(117 + 118) = 0.34$$
$$\mathrm{E}(Y_2 \mid x_0 = 0, x_1 = 0) = (52 + 44)/(194 + 71) = 0.36$$

Table 12.6 shows the expected counts for each treatment/outcome path if 500 subjects initially received treatment and 500 subjects did not. This table illustrates the benefit of treatment at time 1 on the first response, Y_1, showing that only 134 subjects (27%) are expected to have symptoms if initially treated as compared to 189 subjects (38%) among those not treated. The apparent benefit of treatment is diminished by the second measurement time with 30% of patients showing symptoms among those receiving treatment at both times ($X_0 = X_1 = 1$) versus 36% among those not receiving treatment at either time ($X_0 = X_1 = 0$).

The conditional distributions in (12.5.1)–(12.5.3) lead to a marginal distribution of Y_2 conditional on the treatment at times 1 and 2 represented by the regression structure:

$$\text{logit } \mathrm{E}(Y_2 \mid \mathcal{H}_1^X = h_1^X) = -0.56 - 0.13 \cdot x_0 - 0.10 \cdot x_1 - 0.04 \cdot x_0 \cdot x_1. \tag{12.5.4}$$

This model indicates a beneficial impact of treatment among those subjects that were observed to have treatment at time 1 and at time 2.

Note that the marginal expectation is computed by taking averages over the distribution of the intermediate outcome. Since the intermediate variable influences both the second outcome and treatment assignment we need to average over Y_1 to obtain both $\Pr(Y_2 \mid X_0, X_1)$ and $\Pr(X_1 \mid X_0)$:

$$\begin{aligned}
\mu_2(x_0, x_1) &= \Pr(Y_2 = 1 \mid X_0 = x_0, X_1 = x_1), \\
\mu_2(1,1) &= \frac{\Pr(Y_2 = 1, X_1 = 1 \mid X_0 = 1)}{\Pr(X_1 = 1 \mid X_0 = 1)}, \\
\Pr(Y_2 = 1, X_1 = 1 \mid X_0 = 1) &= \sum_{y_1=0,1} \Pr(Y_2 = 1 \mid X_1 = 1, Y_1 = y_1, X_0 = 1) \\
&\quad \times \Pr(X_1 = 1 \mid Y_1 = y_1, X_0 = 1) \\
&\quad \times \Pr(Y_1 = y_1 \mid X_0 = 1), \\
\Pr(X_1 = 1 \mid X_0 = 1) &= \sum_{y_1=0,1} \Pr(X_1 = 1 \mid Y_1 = y_1, X_0 = 1) \\
&\quad \times \Pr(Y_1 = y_1 \mid X_0 = 1).
\end{aligned}$$

Suppose that the scientific goal is to determine the effect of treatment at both time 1 and time 2 on the final patient status, Y_2. We may consider reporting the observed marginal means $\mu_2(x_0, x_1)$. However, since Y_1 is correlated with both X_1 and Y_2 we recognize that these observed marginal effects do not account for the confounder Y_1 and therefore do not reflect the causal effect of treatment. The marginal structure does reflect a small beneficial effect of treatment at time 1 in addition to time 2, with the coefficient of X_0 in (12.5.4) equal to -0.13. On the other hand, if analysis controlled for Y_1 then we would obtain the conditional model (12.5.3) that generated the data. In this model which adjusts for Y_1 there is no effect of X_0 on the (conditional) mean of Y_2 since we have conditioned on the intermediate variable Y_1 and blocked the effect of X_0. Therefore, the analysis that adjusts for Y_1 does not reflect the causal effect of both X_0 and X_1 since by conditioning on an intermediate variable it only characterizes direct effects.

This simple illustration forces realization that with longitudinal exposures (treatments) and longitudinal outcomes a variable can be both a confounder and an intermediate variable. No standard regression methods can then be used to obtain causal statements.

12.5.2 *MSCM data and endogeneity*

To determine if there is feedback in the MSCM data we evaluate whether current child illness predicts current and future maternal stress. Note that in our analysis in Section 12.4 we only used lagged values of stress $X_{it-1}, X_{it-2}, \ldots$ and did not use the current value X_{it} to predict Y_{it}. Therefore, if X_{it} is associated with Y_{it} then we have evidence of endogeneity,

Table 12.7. Regression of stress, X_{it}, on illness, Y_{it-k} $k = 0, 1$, and previous stress, X_{it-k} $k = 1, 2, 3, 4+$ using GEE with working independence.

	Est.	SE	Z
Intercept	−1.88	(0.36)	−5.28
Y_{it}	0.50	(0.17)	2.96
Y_{it-1}	0.08	(0.17)	0.46
X_{it-1}	0.92	(0.15)	6.26
X_{it-2}	0.31	(0.14)	2.15
X_{it-3}	0.34	(0.14)	2.42
Mean(X_{it-k}, $k \geq 4$)	1.74	(0.24)	7.27
Employed	−0.26	(0.13)	−2.01
Married	0.16	(0.12)	1.34
Maternal health	−0.19	(0.07)	−2.83
Child health	−0.09	(0.07)	−1.24
Race	0.03	(0.12)	0.21
Education	0.42	(0.13)	3.21
House size	−0.16	(0.12)	−1.28

or feedback, where the response at time t (Y_{it}) influences the covariate at future times (X_{it} is the covariate for time $t + 1$). Table 12.7 presents results from a regression of X_{it} on Y_{it-k} for $k = 0, 1$, prior stress values and covariates. Using GEE with working independence we find a significant association between X_{it} and Y_{it} even after controlling for prior stress variables.

12.5.3 *Targets of inference*

Robins *et al.* (1999) discuss the formal assumptions required to make causal inference from longitudinal data using the concept of counterfactual outcomes (Neyman, 1923; Holland, 1986; Rubin, 1974, 1978). Define $Y_{it}^{(\boldsymbol{x}_t)}$ as the outcome for subject i at time t that would be observed if a given treatment regime $\boldsymbol{x}_t = (x_0, x_1, \ldots, x_{t-1})$ were followed. For example, $Y_{it}^{(0)}$ represents the outcome that would be observed if subject i received no exposure/treatment at all times $s < t$ while $Y_{it}^{(1)}$ represents the outcome that this same subject would have if exposed/treated during all times. For a given subject we can only observe a single outcome at time t for a single specified treatment course, $\boldsymbol{x}_t^*$. All other possible outcomes, $Y_{it}^{(\boldsymbol{x}_t)}$ for $\boldsymbol{x}_t \neq \boldsymbol{x}_t^*$ are not observed and are called counterfactual or potential outcomes.

Defining potential outcomes facilitates definition of estimands that characterize the causal effect of treatment for both individuals and for populations. For example, $Y_{it}^{(1)} - Y_{it}^{(0)}$ represents the causal effect of treatment though time $t-1$ on the ith subject's response at time t. We cannot directly estimate this subject-specific effect since we only observe one potential outcome for each subject. For a well-characterized study population we can also define the average causal effect as $\delta_t = \mathrm{E}[Y_{it}^{(1)} - Y_{it}^{(0)}] = \mathrm{E}[Y_{it}^{(1)}] - \mathrm{E}[Y_{it}^{(0)}]$. Since any study can only observe one outcome per subject, the mechanism that determines which potential outcome is observed, becomes critically important for relating the observed outcomes to the potential outcomes. For example, in a randomized study the average response among treated subjects, $\mathrm{E}(Y_{it} \mid \boldsymbol{x}_t = 1)$, is an unbiased estimate of the mean of $Y_{it}^{(1)}$ in the entire study population since the assignment to treatment is random and unrelated to the outcome or covariates. Thus in a randomized trial with full compliance having m treated and m control subjects the treatment assignment is independent of the potential outcomes $(Y_{it}^{(1)}, Y_{it}^{(0)})$ and therefore the observed treatment effect, $\hat{\delta}_t = \frac{1}{m}\sum_i Y_{it} \cdot \mathbf{1}(\boldsymbol{x}_{it} = 1) - \frac{1}{m}\sum_i Y_{it} \cdot \mathbf{1}(\boldsymbol{x}_{it} = 0)$ is an unbiased estimate of the causal effect δ_t.

In general, we assume that subjects $i = 1, 2, \ldots, m$ are randomly sampled from a population of subjects and that we seek to make inference regarding the effect that a treatment applied to this population would have on the outcome of interest. Let $\boldsymbol{Z}_i$ be a vector of time-invariant baseline covariates. Define $\mu_t^{(\boldsymbol{x}_t)}(\boldsymbol{z}) = \mathrm{E}[Y_t^{(\boldsymbol{x}_t)} \mid \boldsymbol{Z} = \boldsymbol{z}]$ as the average outcome that would be observed at time t within the sub-population defined by $\boldsymbol{Z} = \boldsymbol{z}$ if all subjects followed the treatment path $\boldsymbol{x}_t$. For example, in the MSCM we are interested in the effect of stress so that $\boldsymbol{x}_t = (X_1, X_2, \ldots, X_{t-1})$, a possible pattern of maternal stress exposures, and $\mu_t^{(1)}(\boldsymbol{z})$ represents the prevalence of child illness among children with covariate $\boldsymbol{Z} = \boldsymbol{z}$ if their mother reported stress each day through day $t-1$. Define the causal effect of continuous exposure as $\delta_T(\boldsymbol{z}) = \mu_T^{(1)}(\boldsymbol{z}) - \mu_T^{(0)}(\boldsymbol{z})$, where T represents the end of study (or other specified time).

Robins *et al.* (1999) formalized the definition of 'no unmeasured confounders' that is required in order to estimate causal effects from longitudinal data. Assume that for each time t the exposure X_t is independent of the vector of future potential outcomes given the observed exposure history through time $t-1$, $\mathcal{H}^X(t-1) = (X_0, X_1, \ldots, X_{t-1})$, and the observed outcome history through time t, $\mathcal{H}^Y(t) = (Y_1, Y_2, \ldots, Y_t)$. We state this assumption as

$$\left\{(Y_s^{(0)}, Y_s^{(1)}); s = t+1, t+2, \ldots, T\right\} \perp X_t \mid \mathcal{H}^X(t-1), \mathcal{H}^Y(t). \quad (12.5.5)$$

Note that we are assuming that exposure X_t is ascertained or selected at time t and therefore can causally effect Y_{t+k} but not Y_t. The no unmeasured confounder assumption is also referred to as the sequential randomization assumption. This assumption states that given information through time t, exposure at time X_t does not predict the value of the future potential outcomes. This assumption would be violated, for example, if there existed an unobserved variable u that influenced the likelihood of treatment or exposure and predicted the potential outcomes. A physician who prescribes treatment to the sickest patients is one such mechanism or variable. Although for treated patients we hope that the observed outcome $Y^{(1)}$ is larger than the unobserved outcome $Y^{(0)}$ (assuming a larger value of Y is better), we expect that both $Y^{(1)}$ and $Y^{(0)}$ are lower for patients selected for treatment, $X = 1$, as compared to the potential outcomes $[Y^{(0)}, Y^{(1)}]$ for the more healthy patients that are assigned $X = 0$.

Pearl (2000) cites two main reasons that statisticians have been hesitant to adopt causal models. First, causal inference requires assumptions such as (12.5.5) that are not empirically verifiable. Second, causal statements require new notation. For example, in our simple example given by (12.5.1)–(12.5.3) we structure data such that $\mathrm{E}(Y_2 \mid X_0 = 0, X_1 = 0) = 0.30$ and $\mathrm{E}(Y_2 \mid X_0 = 1, X_1 = 1) = 0.36$. These conditional expectations represent the average of Y_2 among subjects *observed* to receive certain treatment paths. However, causal statements refer to the effect of interventions in the entire population rather than among possibly select, observed subgroups. That is, although we may observe a subgroup that experiences a treatment course, we may not be interested in the mean response in this specific subgroup since it does not generalize to the mean that would be observed if the entire population experienced the same treatment course. Pearl (2000) uses notation such as $\mathrm{E}[Y_2 \mid \mathrm{do}(X_0 = 1, X_1 = 1)]$ to denote the outcome for the entire population, or $\mu_2^{(1)}$ in our notation. Here the notation $\mathrm{do}(X = 1)$ indicates the situation where $X = 1$ was enforced for the entire study population. Pearl's notation emphasizes the fact that we are interested in an average outcome after assignment of the covariate value rather than the average of outcomes in subgroups after simply observing the covariate status.

Table 12.8 presents the outcomes Y_1 and Y_2 determined by the conditional distributions (12.5.1)–(12.5.3) when the covariate values are controlled rather than allowed to be influenced by Y_1. In this case we obtain $\mu_2^{(1)} = \mathrm{E}[Y_2 \mid \mathrm{do}(X_0 = 1, X_1 = 1)] = 0.402$ and $\mu_2^{(0)} = \mathrm{E}[Y_2 \mid \mathrm{do}(X_0 = 0, X_1 = 0)] = 0.267$ giving a causal risk difference of $\delta_2 = 0.267 - 0.402 = -0.135$. We can also calculate the causal odds ratio as $[0.267/(1 - 0.267)]/[0.402/(1 - 0.402)] = 0.542$. The causal effects are actually larger than associational comparisons conveyed by the observed marginal means where we find $\mathrm{E}(Y_2 \mid X_0 = 1, X_1 = 1) - \mathrm{E}(Y_2 \mid X_0 = 0, X_1 = 0) = 0.302 - 0.362 = -0.060$, and the odds ratio is 0.760. The observed mean difference reflects the fact that subjects

Table 12.8. Expected outcomes when treatment is controlled and the causal path leading from Y_1 to X_2 is blocked.

All subjects $X_0 = X_1 = 1$																
X_0	**0**								**1**							
n	0								1000							
Y_1	**0**				**1**				**0**				**1**			
n	0				0				731				269			
X_1	**0**		**1**		**0**		**1**		**0**		**1**		**0**		**1**	
n	0		0		0		0		0		731		0		269	
Y_2	**0**	**1**	**0**	**1**	**0**	**1**	**0**	**1**	**0**	**1**	**0**	**1**	**0**	**1**	**0**	**1**
n	0	0	0	0	0	0	0	0	0	0	598	133	0	0	134	134
$\mu^{(1)} = (133 + 134)/1000 = 0.267$																
All subjects $X_0 = X_1 = 0$																
X_0	**0**								**1**							
n	1000								0							
Y_1	**0**				**1**				**0**				**1**			
n	622				378				0				0			
X_1	**0**		**1**		**0**		**1**		**0**		**1**		**0**		**1**	
n	622		0		378		0		0		0		0		0	
Y_2	**0**	**1**	**0**	**1**	**0**	**1**	**0**	**1**	**0**	**1**	**0**	**1**	**0**	**1**	**0**	**1**
n	455	167	0	0	143	235	0	0	0	0	0	0	0	0	0	0
$\mu^{(0)} = (167 + 235)/1000 = 0.402$																

with a poor response at time 1 were more likely to seek treatment and thus the subgroup with $(X_0 = 1, X_1 = 1)$ represent somewhat sicker subjects (i.e. Y_1 more likely to be 1) as compared to those subjects observed to follow $(X_0 = 1, X_1 = 0)$. Similarly, subjects observed to follow $(X_0 = 0, X_1 = 1)$ are more likely to be subjects with $Y_1 = 1$ as compared to subjects observed to follow $(X_0 = 0, X_1 = 0)$. Note that in order to calculate the causal effects we have substituted the stochastic assignment of treatment at time 1, $[X_1 \mid Y_1, X_0]$, with a deterministic assignment mechanism but have not altered the response models $\Pr(Y_1 \mid X_0)$ or $\Pr(Y_2 \mid Y_1, X_0, X_1)$. This simple example shows that if we can identify the stable building blocks of the data generating process, such as the sequence of conditional distributions in (12.5.1)–(12.5.3), then we may predict the behaviour of the population under alternative, manipulated conditions and thereby provide estimates of causal effects (Pearl, 2000).

12.5.4 *Estimation using g-computation*

There have been several novel approaches proposed for obtaining estimates of causal effects from longitudinal data with time-varying covariates. One approach is termed 'g-computation' and is described in detail for binary response data by Robins *et al.* (1999) or more generally in Robins (1986). In this approach, causal effect estimates are obtained from estimates of the observed response transition model structure under the necessary assumption of no unmeasured confounders, or equivalently sequential randomization (Robins, 1987).

Recall that we are interested in the average response at time T after receiving treatment for all times prior to T, compared to the response at time T after receiving no treatment for all previous occasions. Note that we can decompose the likelihood for a binary response $Y_{i1}, \ldots, Y_{iT}$ and a binary time-dependent covariate $X_{i0}, \ldots, X_{iT-1}$ into the telescoping sequence

$$\mathcal{L} = \prod_{t=1}^{T} \Pr[Y_{it} \mid \mathcal{H}_i^Y(t-1), \mathcal{H}_i^X(t-1), \boldsymbol{Z}_i] \\ \times \Pr[X_{it-1} \mid \mathcal{H}_i^Y(t-1), \mathcal{H}_i^X(t-2), \boldsymbol{Z}_i].$$

This likelihood factors into the likelihood for the response transition model $\mathcal{L}_Y = \prod_{t=1}^{T} \Pr[Y_{it} \mid \mathcal{H}_i^Y(t-1), \mathcal{H}_i^X(t-1), \boldsymbol{Z}_i]$ and the likelihood for the covariate transitions $\mathcal{L}_X = \prod_{t=1}^{T} \Pr[X_{it-1} \mid \mathcal{H}_i^Y(t-1), \mathcal{H}_i^X(t-2), \boldsymbol{Z}_i]$. Unknown parameters in $\mathcal{L}_Y$ and $\mathcal{L}_X$ can be estimated using maximum likelihood as described in Chapter 10.

Under the assumption of no unmeasured confounders given by (12.5.5) the causal effect of treatment can be identified from the observed data since (12.5.5) implies (Robins *et al.*, 1999, p. 690):

$$\Pr[Y_{it}^{(\boldsymbol{x}_t)} \mid Y_{i1}^{(\boldsymbol{x}_t)}, \ldots, Y_{it-1}^{(\boldsymbol{x}_t)}, \boldsymbol{Z}_i] = \Pr[Y_{it} \mid \mathcal{H}_i^Y(t-1), \mathcal{H}_i^X(t-1) = \boldsymbol{x}_t, \boldsymbol{Z}_i].$$

Thus, we can use the distribution of the observed response at time t among subjects with an observed treatment path $\boldsymbol{x}_t$ and observed response history $\mathcal{H}^Y(t-1)$ to estimate the conditional distribution of the counterfactual outcome $Y_t^{(\boldsymbol{x}_t)}$. We obtain the distribution of the outcome at the final time T by using the conditional probabilities to obtain the joint probability for $Y_{i1}^{(\boldsymbol{x}_t)}, \ldots, Y_{it}^{(\boldsymbol{x}_t)}$ and then summing over all possible intermediate paths for the first $t-1$ outcomes, $Y_{i1}^{(x_t)}, \ldots, Y_{it-1}^{(x_t)}$:

$$\mu^{(x_t)}(\boldsymbol{z}) = \Pr[Y_{it}^{(x_t)} = 1 \mid \boldsymbol{Z}_i = \boldsymbol{z}],$$

$$\begin{aligned}\Pr[Y_{it}^{(x_t)} \mid \boldsymbol{Z}_i = \boldsymbol{z}] &= \sum_{\boldsymbol{y}_{t-1}} \Pr[Y_{it}^{(x_t)}, Y_{it-1}^{(x_t)} = y_{t-1}, \ldots, Y_{i1}^{(x_t)} = y_1 \mid \boldsymbol{Z}_i = \boldsymbol{z}], \\ &= \sum_{\boldsymbol{y}_{t-1}} \prod_{s=1}^{t} \Pr[Y_{is}^{(x_t)} \mid Y_{is-1}^{(x_t)} = y_{s-1}, \ldots, Y_{i1}^{(x_t)} = y_1; \boldsymbol{Z}_i = \boldsymbol{z}], \\ &= \sum_{\boldsymbol{y}_{t-1}} \prod_{s=1}^{t} \Pr[Y_{is} \mid \mathcal{H}_i^Y(s-1) = \boldsymbol{y}_{s-1}, \\ &\qquad\qquad \mathcal{H}_i^X(s-1) = \boldsymbol{x}_{s-1}, \boldsymbol{Z}_i = \boldsymbol{z}],\end{aligned}$$

where $\boldsymbol{x}_s$ is the first s elements of the treatment or exposure path of interest, $\boldsymbol{x}_t$. This calculation is a special case of the *g-computational algorithm* formula of Robins (1986). In our simple example this computation is

$$\mu_2^{(1)} = \sum_{y1} \Pr(Y_2 \mid X_1 = 1, Y_1 = y_1, X_0 = 1) \cdot \Pr(Y_1 = y_1 \mid X_0 = 1)$$

since Y_1 is the only intermediate path. Finally, since we can use the observed data to estimate response transition probabilities, $\Pr[Y_{is} \mid \mathcal{H}_i^Y(s-1) = \boldsymbol{y}_{s-1}, \mathcal{H}_i^X(s-1) = \boldsymbol{x}_{s-1}, \boldsymbol{Z}_i = \boldsymbol{z}]$, we can use the observed data to estimate $\mu^{(x_t)}(\boldsymbol{z})$ and $\delta_t(\boldsymbol{z}) = \mu^{(1)}(\boldsymbol{z}) - \mu^{(0)}(\boldsymbol{z})$. In general, the g-computational formula can be evaluated using Monte Carlo to simulate response series $Y_1, \ldots, Y_t$ for given treatment sequences and specified covariates, and then we can marginalize over $Y_1, \ldots, Y_{t-1}$ to obtain $\mu^{(x_t)}(\boldsymbol{z})$. Such calculations make it clear that in estimating the causal effect we are controlling the sequence of exposures, but are allowing the intermediate outcomes Y_s, $s < t$, to unfold and therefore we capture any indirect effects that are mediated by these earlier outcomes.

In summary, if we collect adequate covariates $\boldsymbol{Z}_i$ such that we are willing to assume no unmeasured confounders, then we can use the observed data to model the sequence of conditional distributions, $\Pr[Y_{it} \mid \mathcal{H}_i^Y(t-1), \mathcal{H}_i^X(t-1); \boldsymbol{Z}_i]$, and then use these to calculate probabilities for a final end-point under exposure paths of interest. By so doing we can provide treatment comparisons that are not confounded by exposure feedback. Standard alternatives may not provide a satisfactory solution in this setting. Observed marginal associations are biased since they do not control for the prior outcomes which are exposure confounders. Transition models can control for prior outcomes but only capture the direct effects of exposure and no effects mediated through earlier changes in the outcome.

12.5.5 *MSCM data and g-computation*

Table 12.9 shows estimated coefficients for a transition model with Y_{it} as the response variable and with baseline covariates $\boldsymbol{Z}_i$, lagged illness, Y_{it-k} $k = 1, 2$, and lagged maternal stress, X_{it-k} $k = 1, 2, 3$, as predictors. Although the dominant serial association is first order (the coefficient of Y_{it-1} equals 2.36), we do find significant second-order dependence. Our model includes X_{it-1}, X_{it-2}, and X_{it-3} but only the coefficient of X_{it-3} obtains significance. We performed several checks including assessing further lagged values of both illness and stress but found no substantial departures. Using this model to perform the g-computation involves choosing a final end-point time, identifying a covariate value of interest, $\boldsymbol{Z}_i$, and then generating Markov chains with stress controlled at 1 for all times, and controlled at 0 for all times. Using 28 days as the end-point time, and focusing on $\boldsymbol{Z}_i = \boldsymbol{z}^*$ with employed = 0, married = 0, maternal and child health = 4, race = 0, education = 0, and house size = 0, we obtain $\hat{\mu}^{(1)}(\boldsymbol{z}^*) = 0.189$, and $\hat{\mu}^{(0)}(\boldsymbol{z}^*) = 0.095$. This implies that for this subpopulation, continual maternal stress is associated with a $\hat{\delta}(\boldsymbol{z}) = (0.189 - 0.095) = 0.094$ increase in the prevalence of child illness.

A causal log odds ratio comparing continual stress to no stress over 28 days in the subpopulation $\boldsymbol{Z}_i = \boldsymbol{z}^*$ is estimated from $\hat{\mu}^{(1)}(\boldsymbol{z}^*)$ and $\hat{\mu}^{(0)}(\boldsymbol{z}^*)$ as 0.80. Using a marginal regression model and GEE gives the

Table 12.9. Regression of illness, Y_{it}, on previous illness, Y_{it-k} $k = 1, 2$, and stress, X_{it-k} $k = 1, 2, 3$ using GEE with an independence working correlation matrix.

	Est.	SE	Z
Intercept	−1.83	(0.29)	−6.29
Y_{it-1}	2.36	(0.16)	14.83
Y_{it-2}	0.33	(0.14)	2.31
X_{it-1}	0.24	(0.14)	1.72
X_{it-2}	−0.14	(0.15)	0.93
X_{it-3}	0.40	(0.13)	3.21
Employed	−0.09	(0.13)	−0.70
Married	0.44	(0.12)	3.79
Maternal health	0.01	(0.07)	0.10
Child health	−0.24	(0.06)	−3.90
Race	0.31	(0.13)	2.50
Education	0.01	(0.14)	0.06
House size	−0.53	(0.12)	−4.42

corresponding associational log odds ratio as 1.38 (based on the sum of saturated model coefficients in Table 12.5), and the transition model in Table 12.9 gives a direct effect of only $(0.24 - 0.14 + 0.40) = 0.50$. Here the marginal association appears to overestimate the causal effect which should be anticipated when both $X_{it-k} = 1$ increases the likelihood that $Y_{it} = 1$, and $Y_{it} = 1$ increases the likelihood that $X_{it+k} = 1$. The MSCM analysis results are in contrast to our example given by (12.5.1)–(12.5.3) where X_1 decreased the likelihood that $Y_1 = 1$. Finally, the validity of our causal estimates relies on the assumption of no unmeasured confounders, and on the model form used to estimate $\Pr[Y_{it} \mid \mathcal{H}_i^Y(t-1), \mathcal{H}_i^X(t-1), \boldsymbol{Z}_i]$. One limitation to use of the g-computational algorithm for estimation is that no direct regression model parameter represents the null hypothesis of no causal effect, and thus the approach does not facilitate formal testing.

12.5.6 *Estimation using inverse probability of treatment weights (IPTW)*

One of the advantages of using the g-computational algorithm approach to obtaining estimates of causal effects is the fact that a model for the treatment (or exposure) is not required. Stated alternatively, the likelihood $\mathcal{L}_Y$ contains the parameters necessary to calculate $\delta_t(\boldsymbol{z})$ and the telescoping likelihood corresponding to X_{it} given by $\mathcal{L}_X$ is ancillary. However, the g-computational algorithm is based on an indirect parameterization of $\delta_t(\boldsymbol{z})$ and does not facilitate testing for exposure effects by setting a parameter equal to zero, or permit structuring of exposure effects in the presence of covariates $\boldsymbol{Z}_i$. An alternative approach to estimation based on marginal structural models (MSMs), introduced by Robins (1998) and discussed by Hernán *et al.* (2001), does require a model for the covariate process, but permits direct regression modelling of causal effects. In this section we first describe the basic model and then discuss methods of estimation using inverse probability of treatment weighted GEE.

Marginal structural models specify the average counterfactual outcome directly as a function of exposure and covariates. Define the average outcome if the subpopulation with $\boldsymbol{Z}_i = \boldsymbol{z}$ experienced a treatment regime $\boldsymbol{x}_t$:

$$\mu_t^{(x_t)}(\boldsymbol{z}) = \mathrm{E}[Y_{it}^{(x_t)} \mid \boldsymbol{Z}_i = \boldsymbol{z}].$$

We formulate a regression model for the counterfactual outcomes such as

$$h\{\mu_t^{(x_t)}(\boldsymbol{z})\} = \beta_0 + \beta_1 X_{it}^* + \boldsymbol{\beta}_2' \boldsymbol{Z}_i,$$

where, for example, X_{it}^* represents cumulative exposure, $X_{it}^* = \sum_{s<t} X_{is}$, or any other function of the covariate history. This model parsimoniously

structures the causal effect of exposure and identifies a single parameter, β_1, that can be used to quantify and test the causal effect of exposure.

Estimation for MSMs can be obtained using IPTW estimation. Recall that the key reason we cannot use standard methods such as GEE is due to the fact that the prior response, Y_{it-k}, is a confounder. However, we do not want estimates that control for the prior response since it is also an intermediate variable. In the absence of confounding association implies causation and thus obtaining a population where confounding was non-existent would allow use of standard regression methods. Robins (1998, 1999) and Hernán *et al.* (2001) discuss how to use weights to construct a pseudo-population that has the causal relationship of interest but is free from confounding. Define the *stabilized weights*:

$$\mathrm{SW}_i(t) = \prod_{s<t} \frac{\Pr(X_{is} = x_{is} \mid \mathcal{H}_i^X(s-1) = \boldsymbol{h}_i^X(s-1), \boldsymbol{Z}_i)}{\Pr(X_{is} = x_{is} \mid \mathcal{H}_i^Y(s-1) = \boldsymbol{h}_i^Y(s-1), \mathcal{H}_i^X(s-1) = \boldsymbol{h}_i^X(s-1), \boldsymbol{Z}_i)}.$$

These weights compare the probability of the treatment received through time $t-1$ conditional only on knowledge of the treatment histories to the probability of the treatment received conditional on both treatment and response histories. The weights $\mathrm{SW}_i(t)$ would be identically one if the covariate process was exogenous (by definition) and can therefore be viewed as a measure of endogeneity. In practice, the weights $\mathrm{SW}_i(t)$ will need to be estimated by choosing and fitting models for the numerator, $\Pr(X_{is} \mid \mathcal{H}_i^X(s-1), \boldsymbol{Z}_i)$, and the denominator, $\Pr(X_{is} \mid \mathcal{H}_i^Y(s-1), \mathcal{H}_i^X(s-1), \boldsymbol{Z}_i)$. Correct modelling of the denominator is necessary for consistent parameter estimation, while the numerator can be any function of $(\mathcal{H}_i^X(s), \boldsymbol{Z}_i)$, the choice of which only impacts estimation efficiency not validity. One assumption necessary for use of weighted estimation is that the weights are bounded away from zero, that is: $\Pr(X_{is} \mid \mathcal{H}_i^Y(s-1), \mathcal{H}_i^X(s-1), \boldsymbol{Z}_i) \geq \epsilon > 0$.

GEE with working independence and estimated weights $\widehat{\mathrm{SW}}_i(t)$ can be used to obtain an estimate of the causal regression parameter $\boldsymbol{\beta}$. Weights are necessary to obtain causal estimates, and GEE is used simply to obtain a sandwich variance estimator that accounts for the repeated measures. It is interesting to note that the variance of $\hat{\boldsymbol{\beta}}$ is smaller when weights are estimated, making the sandwich variance estimator conservative. Formal justification for the IPTW estimation is given in Robins (1999) and references therein.

To illustrate that weights can be used to construct a pseudo-population where Y_{it} is still an intermediate but no longer a confounder we return to the simple example given by (12.5.1)–(12.5.3) whose expected counts are shown in Table 12.6. In Table 12.10 we reproduce the expected counts for

Table 12.10. Example of using IPTW to re-weight data and obtain causal effect estimates for a saturated MSM that corresponds to (12.5.1)–(12.5.3).

X_0	Y_1	X_1	Y_2	Expected count	Weight	Re-weighted count
1	1	1	1	41.9	0.712	29.8
1	1	1	0	41.9	0.712	29.8
1	1	0	1	31.6	1.474	46.6
1	1	0	0	19.2	1.474	28.3
1	0	1	1	25.2	1.174	29.6
1	0	1	0	112.8	1.174	132.5
1	0	0	1	61.2	0.894	54.7
1	0	0	0	166.3	0.894	148.7
0	1	1	1	58.8	0.755	44.4
0	1	1	0	58.8	0.755	44.4
0	1	0	1	44.4	1.404	62.3
0	1	0	0	26.9	1.404	37.8
0	0	1	1	21.4	1.245	26.7
0	0	1	0	96.1	1.245	119.6
0	0	0	1	52.1	0.851	44.4
0	0	0	0	141.6	0.851	120.6

$$\mu^{(X_0=1,X_1=1)} = (29.8 + 29.6)/(29.8 + 29.8 + 29.6 + 132.5) = 0.268$$
$$\mu^{(X_0=1,X_1=0)} = (46.6 + 54.7)/(46.6 + 28.3 + 54.7 + 148.7) = 0.364$$
$$\mu^{(X_0=0,X_1=1)} = (44.4 + 26.7)/(44.4 + 44.4 + 26.7 + 119.6) = 0.302$$
$$\mu^{(X_0=0,X_1=0)} = (62.3 + 44.4)/(62.3 + 37.8 + 44.4 + 120.6) = 0.402$$

Y_2 as a function of X_0, Y_1, and X_1. We also compute the stabilized weights $\mathrm{SW}(2) = \Pr(X_1 \mid X_0)/\Pr(X_1 \mid Y_1, X_0)$. Notice that subjects with $(X_0 = 1, Y_1 = 1, X_1 = 1)$ are down-weighted, $\mathrm{SW}(2) = 0.712$, while subjects with $(X_0 = 1, Y_1 = 0, X_1 = 1)$ are up-weighted, $\mathrm{SW}(2) = 1.174$. This suggests that our observed population has an over representation of subjects with $(X_0 = 1, Y_1 = 1, X_1 = 1)$ relative to our desired pseudo-population where Y_1 is not a confounder. Intuitively this reflects the fact that when $Y_1 = 1$, subjects are more likely to obtain $X_1 = 1$, and in order to correct for this selection we up-weight those with $Y_1 = 0$ and down-weight those with $Y_1 = 1$. To verify that the pseudo-population (re-weighted count) has the causal structure of interest we compute the observed means as a function of X_0 and X_1, marginalizing over Y_1. We find agreement (to rounding error) with the g-computation results given in Table 12.8. Note that in the re-weighted population Y_1 no longer is associated with X_1. For example,

$$\begin{aligned}\Pr(X_1 \mid Y_1 = 1, X_0 = 1) &= (29.8 + 29.8)/(29.8 + 29.8 + 46.6 + 28.3) \\ &= 0.443, \\ \Pr(X_1 \mid Y_1 = 0, X_0 = 1) &= (29.6 + 132.5)/(29.6 + 132.5 + 54.7 + 148.7) \\ &= 0.443,\end{aligned}$$

showing that Y_1 does not predict X_1. However, Y_1 does still predict the final outcome and therefore remains an intermediate variable in the pseudo-population. Therefore, in the pseudo-population Y_1 is only an intermediate variable and not a confounder, and we can use standard summaries in the pseudo-population to obtain causal summaries.

12.5.7 *MSCM data and marginal structural models using IPTW*

To obtain MSM estimates for the MSCM data we first estimate $\mathrm{SW}_i(t)$ based on models for the exposure process X_{it}. For the denominator we use the logistic regression model presented in Table 12.7 where Y_{it}, Y_{it-1}, lagged stress, and baseline demographic covariates are used as predictors. For the numerator we use the same regression model except that illness measures are excluded (not shown). Using the estimated weights we then use working independence GEE to obtain estimates of the causal regression parameters and valid (conservative) standard errors. Table 12.11 displays the MSM estimates and standard errors. In this model we use the first three

Table 12.11. MSM estimation of the effect of stress, X_{it-k} $k \geq 1$, on illness, Y_{it}.

	Est.	SE	Z
Intercept	−0.71	(0.40)	−1.77
X_{it-1}	0.15	(0.14)	1.03
X_{it-2}	−0.19	(0.18)	−1.05
X_{it-3}	0.18	(0.15)	1.23
Mean(X_{it-k}, $k \geq 4$)	0.71	(0.43)	1.65
Employed	−0.11	(0.21)	−0.54
Married	0.55	(0.17)	3.16
Maternal health	−0.13	(0.10)	−1.27
Child health	−0.34	(0.09)	−3.80
Race	0.72	(0.21)	3.46
Education	0.34	(0.22)	1.57
House size	−0.80	(0.18)	−4.51

lagged values of maternal stress, X_{it-k} for $k = 1, 2, 3$, and the average of stress indicators prior to $t-4$. We can use this model to estimate the casual effect of continual stress over a 28-day period by summing the coefficients of the stress predictors: $(0.15 - 0.19 + 0.18 + 0.71) = 0.85$. The MSM log odds ratio is comparable to the estimate obtained using the g-computational algorithm (estimate for one covariate subset $= 0.80$ in Section 12.5.5). One advantage of the MSM approach is that we can test the causal null, H_0: $\beta_1 + \beta_2 + \beta_3 + \beta_4 = 0$ using the estimated coefficients and standard errors. We obtain a Z statistic of 1.998 and p-value of 0.046. Therefore, using the MSM we reject the causal null hypothesis of no effect of continuous stress on the likelihood of child illness.

12.5.8 *Summary*

This section has introduced causal targets of inference for analysis of longitudinal data with endogenous covariates. We have demonstrated that standard methods cannot provide causal summaries, and have introduced g-computation and MSM with IPTW as alternative approaches. We have not presented the detailed theory that underlies the causal methodology and refer the interested reader to Robins (1998, 1999), Robins *et al.* (1999), and Hernán *et al.* (2001) for further detail and additional references.

12.6 Summary and further reading

In this chapter we have provided a taxonomy for covariate processes and a taxonomy for conditional means, or regression models. When a covariate process is exogenous analysis focuses on specifying a regression model in terms of cross-sectional associations, $\mathrm{E}(Y_{it} \mid X_{it})$, or in terms of lagged relationships, $\mathrm{E}(Y_{it} \mid X_{it-1}, X_{it-2}, \ldots)$. We have shown that biased estimation can result if GEE with non-diagonal weighting is used unless the model $\mu_{it} = \mathrm{E}(Y_{it} \mid X_{it})$ for cross-sectional models, or $\mu_{it} = \mathrm{E}(Y_{it} \mid X_{it-1}, X_{it-1}, \ldots, X_{it-k})$ for finite lag models, equals the FCCM, $\mathrm{E}(Y_{it} \mid X_{is}\ s = 1, 2, \ldots, T)$. For an exogenous covariate process we need only consider dependence of Y_{it} on $\mathcal{H}_i^X(t-1)$ to satisfy the FCCM condition. Partly conditional and distributed lag regression models can adopt a flexible relationship between past exposure and current outcomes and can be implemented using standard software programs. For endogenous covariates we have shown that a prior response variable can be both a confounder and an intermediate variable. This issue has motivated the development of causal estimation methods by Robins and co-workers. Although we have focused on a single time-dependent endogenous covariate, the same issue of a confounding intermediate variable may arise via a time-dependent covariate that is distinct from the response and the exposure. The methods that we overview have been developed for this more general scenario and are discussed in Robins (1986, 1987, 1998, 1999) and Robins *et al.* (1999) for the case of longitudinal binary response data. Lauritzen (2000) provides an excellent overview of graphical models and causal inference. Finally, we have not discussed another class of methods known as g-estimation and structural nested models. Robins (1999) overviews structural nested models and compares them to both g-computation and MSMs.

13
Missing values in longitudinal data

13.1 Introduction

Missing values arise in the analysis of longitudinal data whenever one or more of the sequences of measurements from units within the study are incomplete, in the sense that *intended* measurements are not taken, are lost, or are otherwise unavailable. The emphasis is important: if we choose in advance to take measurements every hour on one-half of the subjects and every two hours on the other half, the resulting data could also be described as incomplete but there are no missing values in the sense that we use the term; we call such data *unbalanced*. This is not just playing with words. Unbalanced data may raise technical difficulties – we have seen that some methods of analysis can only cope with data for which measurements are made at a common set of times on all units. Missing values raise the same technical difficulties, since of necessity they result in unbalanced data, but also deeper conceptual issues, since we have to ask *why* the values are missing, and more specifically whether their being missing has any bearing on the practical questions posed by the data.

A simple (non-longitudinal) example makes the point explicitly. Suppose that we want to compare the mean concentrations of a hormone in blood samples taken from ten subjects in each of two groups: one a control, the other an experimental treatment intended to suppress production of the hormone. We are presented with ten assayed values of the hormone concentration from the control subjects, eight assayed values from the treated subjects, and are told that the values from the other two treated subjects are 'missing'. If we knew that this was because somebody dropped the test tubes on the way to the assay lab, we would probably be happy to proceed with a two-sample t-test using the 18 non-missing values. If we knew that the missing values were from subjects whose hormone concentrations fell below the sensitivity threshold of the assay, ignoring the missing values would mask the very effect we were looking to detect. Lest this example offend the sophisticated reader, we suggest that more subtle versions of it are not uncommon in real longitudinal studies. For example, it may be that a sequence of atypically low (or high) values on a particular unit foreshadows its removal from the study.

13.2 Classification of missing value mechanisms

Little and Rubin (1987), give a general treatment of statistical analysis with missing values, which includes a useful hierarchy of missing value mechanisms. Let $\boldsymbol{Y}^*$ denote the complete set of measurements which would have been obtained were there no missing values, and partition this set into $\boldsymbol{Y}^* = (\boldsymbol{Y}^{(o)}, \boldsymbol{Y}^{(m)})$ with $\boldsymbol{Y}^{(o)}$ denoting the measurements actually obtained and $\boldsymbol{Y}^{(m)}$ the measurements which would have been available had they not been missing, for whatever cause. Finally, let $\boldsymbol{R}$ denote a set of indicator random variables, denoting which elements of $\boldsymbol{Y}^*$ fall into $\boldsymbol{Y}^{(o)}$ and which into $\boldsymbol{Y}^{(m)}$. Now, a probability model for the missing value mechanism defines the probability distribution of $\boldsymbol{R}$ conditional on $\boldsymbol{Y}^* = (\boldsymbol{Y}^{(o)}, \boldsymbol{Y}^{(m)})$. Little and Rubin classify the missing value mechanism as

- *completely random* if $\boldsymbol{R}$ is independent of both $\boldsymbol{Y}^{(o)}$ and $\boldsymbol{Y}^{(m)}$
- *random* if $\boldsymbol{R}$ is independent of $\boldsymbol{Y}^{(m)}$
- *informative* if $\boldsymbol{R}$ is dependent on $\boldsymbol{Y}^{(m)}$.

It turns out that for likelihood-based inference, the crucial distinction is between random and informative missing values. To see this, let $f(\boldsymbol{y}^{(o)}, \boldsymbol{y}^{(m)}, \boldsymbol{r})$ denote the joint probability density function of $(\boldsymbol{Y}^{(o)}, \boldsymbol{Y}^{(m)}, \boldsymbol{R})$ and use the standard factorization to express this as

$$f(\boldsymbol{y}^{(o)}, \boldsymbol{y}^{(m)}, \boldsymbol{r}) = f(\boldsymbol{y}^{(o)}, \boldsymbol{y}^{(m)}) f(\boldsymbol{r} \mid \boldsymbol{y}^{(o)}, \boldsymbol{y}^{(m)}). \tag{13.2.1}$$

For a likelihood-based analysis, we need the joint pdf of the observable random variables, $(\boldsymbol{Y}^{(o)}, \boldsymbol{R})$, which we obtain by integrating (13.2.1) to give

$$f(\boldsymbol{y}^{(o)}, \boldsymbol{r}) = \int f(\boldsymbol{y}^{(o)}, \boldsymbol{y}^{(m)}) f(\boldsymbol{r} \mid \boldsymbol{y}^{(o)}, \boldsymbol{y}^{(m)}) \mathrm{d}\boldsymbol{y}^{(m)}. \tag{13.2.2}$$

Now, if the missing value mechanism is random, $f(\boldsymbol{r} \mid \boldsymbol{y}^{(o)}, \boldsymbol{y}^{(m)})$ does not depend on $\boldsymbol{y}^{(m)}$ and (13.2.2) becomes

$$\begin{aligned} f(\boldsymbol{y}^{(o)}, \boldsymbol{r}) &= f(\boldsymbol{r} \mid \boldsymbol{y}^{(o)}) \int f(\boldsymbol{y}^{(o)}, \boldsymbol{y}^{(m)}) \mathrm{d}\boldsymbol{y}^{(m)} \\ &= f(\boldsymbol{r} \mid \boldsymbol{y}^{(o)}) f(\boldsymbol{y}^{(o)}). \end{aligned} \tag{13.2.3}$$

Finally, taking logarithms in (13.2.3), the log-likelihood function is

$$L = \log f(\boldsymbol{r} \mid \boldsymbol{y}^{(o)}) + \log f(\boldsymbol{y}^{(o)}), \tag{13.2.4}$$

which is maximized by separate maximization of the two terms on the right-hand side. Since the first term contains no information about the distribution of $\boldsymbol{Y}^{(o)}$, we can ignore it for the purpose of making inferences about $\boldsymbol{Y}^{(o)}$.

Because of the above result, both completely random and random missing value mechanisms are sometimes referred to without distinction as *ignorable*. However, it is important to remember that 'ignorability' in this sense relies on the use of the likelihood function as the basis for inference. For example, the method of generalized estimating equations, as described in Section 8.2.3, is valid only under the stronger assumption that the missing value mechanism is completely random. Also, even within a likelihood-based analysis, the treatment of a random missing value mechanism as ignorable makes several tacit assumptions. The first of these, as emphasized by Little and Rubin, is that $f(\boldsymbol{y}^{(o)})$ and $f(\boldsymbol{r} \mid \boldsymbol{y}^{(o)})$ are separately parameterized, which need not be the case; if there are parameters common to $f(\boldsymbol{y}^{(o)})$ and $f(r \mid \boldsymbol{y}^{(o)})$, ignoring the first term in (13.2.4) leads to a loss of efficiency. Secondly, maximization of the second term on the right-hand side of (13.2.4) implies that the unconditional distribution of $\boldsymbol{Y}^{(o)}$ is the correct inferential focus. Again, this need not be the case; for example, in a clinical trial concerned with a life-threatening condition in which missing values identify patients who have died before the end of the study and $\boldsymbol{Y}^{(o)}$ measures health status, it may be more sensible to make inferences about the distribution of time to survival and the *conditional* distribution of $\boldsymbol{Y}^{(o)}$ given survival rather than about the unconditional distribution of $\boldsymbol{Y}^{(o)}$.

13.3 Intermittent missing values and dropouts

An important distinction is whether missing values occur intermittently or as dropouts. Suppose that we intend to take a sequence of measurements, $Y_1, \ldots, Y_n$, on a particular unit. Missing values occur as *dropouts* if whenever Y_j is missing, so are Y_k for all $k \geq j$; otherwise we say that the missing values are *intermittent*. In general, dealing with intermittent missing values is more difficult than dealing with dropouts because of the wider variety of patterns of missing values which need to be accommodated.

When intermittent missing values arise through a known censoring mechanism, for example, if all values below a known threshold are missing, the EM algorithm (Dempster *et al.*, 1977) provides a possible theoretical framework (Laird, 1988; Hughes, 1999). When intermittent missing values do not arise from censoring, the reason for their being missing is often known, since the subjects in question remain in the study, and in some cases this information will make it reasonable to assume that the missingness is unrelated to the measurement process. In such cases, the resulting data can be analysed by any method which can accommodate unbalanced data. Furthermore, if the method of analysis is likelihood-based, the inferences will be valid under the weaker assumption that the missing value mechanism is random.

In contrast, dropouts are frequently lost to any form of follow-up and we have to admit the possibility that they arise for reasons directly or indirectly connected to the measurement process.

An example of dropout directly related to the measurement process arises in clinical trials, where ethical considerations may require a patient to be withdrawn from a trial on the basis of their observed measurement history. Murray and Findlay (1988) discuss this in the context of long-term trials of drugs to reduce blood pressure where 'if a patient's blood pressure is not adequately controlled then there are ethical problems associated with continuing the patient on their study medication'. Note that a trial protocol which specifies a set of circumstances under which a patient *must* be withdrawn from the trial on the basis of their observed measurement history defines a *random*, and therefore ignorable, dropout mechanism in Little and Rubin's sense.

In contrast, the 'dropouts' in the data on protein content of milk samples arose because the cows in question calved after the beginning of the experiment (Cullis, 1994), and there may well be an indirect link between calving date and milk quality.

When there is any kind of relationship between the measurement process and the dropout process, the interpretation of apparently simple trends in the mean response over time can be problematic, as in the following simulated example.

We simulated two sets of data from a model in which the mean response was constant over time, and the random variation within units followed the uniform correlation model described in Section 4.2.1. In each data-set, up to ten responses, at unit time-intervals, were obtained from each of 100 subjects. Dropouts occurred at random, according to the following model: conditional on the observed responses up to and including time $t-1$, the probability of dropout at time t is given by a logistic regression model,

$$\text{logit}(p_t) = -1 - 2y_{t-1}.$$

In the first simulation, shown in Fig. 13.1, the correlation between any two responses on the same unit was $\rho = 0.9$, and the empirical mean responses, calculated at each time-point from those subjects who had not yet dropped out, show a steadily rising trend. A likelihood-based analysis which ignores the dropout process leads to the conclusion that the mean response is essentially constant over time whereas the empirical means suggest a clearly increasing time-trend. There is no contradiction in this apparent discrepancy: the likelihood-based analysis estimates the mean response which would have been observed had there been no dropouts, whereas the empirical means estimate the conditional mean response in the sub-population who have not dropped out by time t. Another way to explain the discrepancy between the likelihood-based and empirical estimates of the mean response is that the former recognizes the correlation in

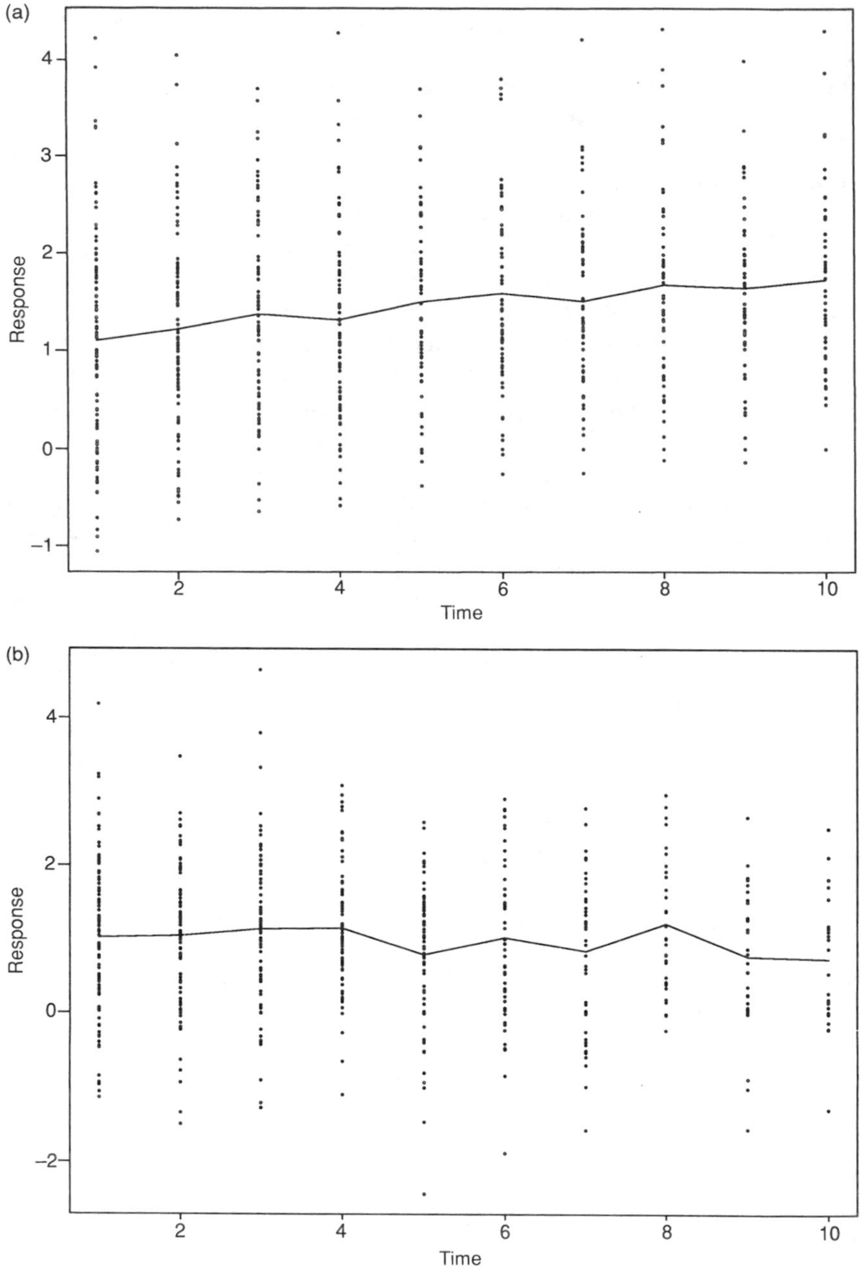

Fig. 13.1. Simulated realizations of a model with a constant mean response, uniform correlation and random dropouts: (a) within-unit correlation $\rho = 0.9$; (b) within-unit correlation $\rho = 0.0$. ......: data; ——: empirical mean response.

the data and, in effect, imputes the missing values for a particular subject taking into account the same subject's observed values. To confirm this, Fig. 13.1(b) shows the result of the second simulation, which uses the same model for measurements and dropouts except that the within-unit correlation is $\rho = 0$. Both the empirical means and a likelihood-based inference now tell the same story – that there is no time-trend in the mean response.

These examples may convince the reader, as they convince us, that it would be useful to have methods for analyzing data with a view to distinguishing amongst completely random, random and informative dropouts. Fortunately, the additional structure of data with dropouts makes this a more tractable problem than in the case of intermittent missing values.

In the rest of this chapter, we concentrate on the analysis of data with dropouts. In Section 13.4 we briefly mention two simple, but in our view inadequate, solutions to the problem. In Section 13.5 we describe methods for testing whether dropouts are completely random. In Section 13.6 we describe an extension to the method of generalized estimating equations which gives consistent inferences under the assumption of random dropouts. In Section 13.7 we review various model-based approaches which can accommodate completely random, random or informative droputs, henceforth abbreviated to CRD, RD and ID respectively.

13.4 Simple solutions and their limitations

13.4.1 *Last observation carried forward*

As the name suggests, this method of dealing with dropouts consists of extrapolating the last observed measurement for the subject in question to the remainder of their intended time-sequence. A refinement of the method would be to estimate a time-trend, either for an individual subject or for a group of subjects allocated to a particular treatment, and to extrapolate not at a constant level, but relative to this estimated trend. Thus, if y_{ij} is the last observed measurement on the ith subject, $\hat{\mu}_i(t)$ is their estimated time-trend and $r_{ij} = y_{ij} - \hat{\mu}_i(t_j)$, the method would impute the missing values as $y_{ik} = \hat{\mu}_i(t_k) + r_{ij}$ for all $k > j$.

Last observation carried forward is routinely used in the pharmaceutical industry, and elsewhere, in the analysis of randomized parallel group trials for which a primary objective is to test the null hypothesis of no difference between treatment groups. In that context, it can be argued that dropout, and the subsequent extrapolation of last observed values, is an inherent feature of the random outcome of the trial for a given subject. Validity of the test for no difference between treatment groups is then imparted by the randomization, without requiring explicit modelling assumptions. A further argument to justify last observation carried forward is that if, for example, subjects are expected to show improvement over the duration of a longitudinal trial (i.e. treatment is beneficial), carrying forward a last observation should result in a conservative assessment of any treatment benefits.

Whilst these arguments are legitimate in particular contexts, we do not recommend last observation carried forward as a general method.

13.4.2 *Complete case analysis*

Another very simple way of dealing with dropouts is to discard all incomplete sequences. This is obviously wasteful of data when the dropout process is unrelated to the measurement process. Perhaps, more seriously, it has the potential to introduce bias if the two processes are related, as the complete cases cannot then be assumed to be a random sample with respect to the distribution of the measurements y_{ij}.

In general, we do not recommend complete case analysis. Perhaps the only exception is when the scientific questions of interest are genuinely confined to the sub-population of completers, but situations of this kind would seem to be rather specialized. There are many instances in which the questions of interest concern the mean, or other properties, of the measurement process conditional on completion, but this is not quite the same thing. In particular, if we accept that dropout is a random event, and if we are prepared to make modelling assumptions about the relationship between the measurement process and the dropout process, then the incomplete data from the subjects *who happened to be dropouts in this particular realization of the trial* provide additional information about the properties of the underlying measurement *process* conditional on completion. This information would be lost in a complete case analysis.

13.5 Testing for completely random dropouts

In this section, we assume that a complete set of measurements on a unit would be taken at times t_j, $j = 1, \ldots, n$, but that dropouts occur. Then, the available data on the ith of m units are $\boldsymbol{y}_i = (y_{i1}, \ldots, y_{in_i})$, with $n_i \leq n$ and y_{ij} taken at time t_j. Units are allocated into a number of different treatment groups. Our objective is to test the hypothesis that the dropouts are completely random, that is, that the probability that a unit drops out at time t_j is independent of the observed sequence of measurements on that unit at times $t_1, \ldots, t_{j-1}$. We view such a test as a preliminary screening device, and therefore wish to avoid any parametric assumptions about the process generating the measurement data. Note that our definition of completely random dropouts makes no reference to the possible influence of explanatory variables on the dropout process. For example, suppose that in a study comparing two groups with different mean response profiles, the dropout rate is higher in the group with the higher mean response. If we ignored the group structure, the dropout process would appear to be informative in the undifferentiated data, even if it were completely random within each group. We therefore recommend that for preliminary screening, the data should first be divided into homogeneous sub-groups.

Let p_{ij} denote the probability that the ith unit drops out at time t_j. Under the assumption of completely random dropouts, the p_{ij} may depend on time, treatment, or other explanatory variables but cannot depend on the observed measurements, $\boldsymbol{y}_i$. The method developed in Diggle (1989) to test this assumption consists of applying separate tests at each time within each treatment group and analysing the resulting sample of p-values for departure from the uniform distribution on $(0, 1)$. Combination of the separate p-values is necessary if the procedure is to have any practical value, because the individual tests are typically based on very few cases and therefore have low power.

The individual tests are constructed as follows. For each of $k = 1, \ldots, (n-1)$, define a function, $h_k(y_1, \ldots, y_k)$. We will discuss the choice of $h_k(\cdot)$ shortly. Now, within each group and for each time-point t_k, $k = 1, \ldots, n-1$, identify the R_k units which have $n_i \geq k$ and compute the set of scores $h_{ik} = h_k(y_{i1}, \ldots, y_{ik})$, for $i = 1, \ldots, R_k$. Within this set of R_k scores, identify those r_k scores which correspond to units with $m_j = k$, that is, units which are about to drop out. If $1 \leq r_k < R_k$, test the hypothesis that the r_k scores so identified are a random sample from the 'population' of R_k scores previously identified. Finally, investigate whether the complete set of p-values observed by applying this procedure to each time within each treatment group behaves like a random sample from the uniform distribution on $(0, 1)$. The implicit assumption that the separate p-values are mutually independent is valid precisely because once a unit drops out it never returns.

Our first decision in implementing this procedure is how to choose the functions $h_k(\cdot)$. Our aim is to choose these so that extreme values of the scores, h_{ik}, constitute evidence against completely random dropouts. A sensible choice is a linear combination,

$$h_k(y_1, \ldots, y_k) = \sum_{j=1}^{k} w_j y_j. \tag{13.5.1}$$

As with any *ad hoc* procedure, the success of this will be influenced by the investigator's ability to pick a set of coefficients which reflect the actual dependence of the dropout probabilities on the observed measurement history. If dropout is suspected to be an immediate consequence of an abnormally low measurement we should choose $w_k = 1$ and all other $w_j = 0$. If it is suspected to be the culmination of a sustained sequence of low measurements we would do better using equal weights, $w_j = 1$ for all j.

The next decision is how to convert the scores, h_{ik}, into a test statistic and p-value. A natural test statistic is $\bar{h}_k$, the mean of the r_k scores corresponding to those units with $n_j = k$ which are about to drop out. If dropouts occur completely at random, the approximate sampling distribution of $\bar{h}_k$ is Gaussian, with mean $\bar{H}_k = R_k^{-1} \sum_{i=1}^{R_k} h_{ik}$, and variance $S_k^2(R_k - r_k)/(r_k R_k)$, where $S_k^2 = (R_k - 1)^{-1} \sum_{i=1}^{R_k} (h_{ik} - \bar{H}_k)^2$. This is a standard result from elementary sampling theory. See, for example, Cochran (1977). However, in the present context some of the r_k and R_k will be small and the Gaussian approximation may then be poor. For an exact test, we can evaluate the complete randomization distribution of each $\bar{h}_k$ under the null hypothesis of random sampling. If $\binom{R_k}{r_k}$ is too large for this to be practical, a feasible alternative procedure is to sample from the randomization distribution. We recompute $\bar{h}_k$ after each of $s - 1$ independent random selections of r_k scores chosen without replacement from the set h_{ik}, $i = 1, \ldots, R_k$, and let x denote the rank of the original $\bar{h}_k$ amongst the recomputed values. Then, $p = x/s$ is the p-value of an exact, Monte Carlo test (Barnard, 1963).

The final stage consists of analysing the resulting set of p-values. Informal graphical analyses, such as a plot of the empirical distribution function of the p-values with different plotting symbols to identify the different treatment groups, can be useful here. Diggle (1989) also suggests a formal test of departure from uniformity using the Kolmogorov–Smirnov statistic; in practice, we will usually have arranged that a preponderance of *small* p-values will lead us to reject the hypothesis of completely random dropouts, and the appropriate form of the Kolmogorov–Smirnov statistic is its one-sided version, $D_+ = \sup\{\hat{F}(p) - p\}$. Another technical problem now arises because each p-value derives from a *discrete* randomization distribution whereas the Kolmogorov–Smirnov statistic tests for departure from a continuous uniform distribution on the interval $0 \leq p \leq 1$. We would not want to overemphasize the formal testing aspect of this procedure, preferring to regard it as a method of exploratory data analysis. Nevertheless, if we do want a formal test we can again use Barnard's Monte Carlo testing idea to give us an exact statement of significance. We simply rank the observed value of D_+ amongst simulated values based on the appropriate set of discrete uniform distributions which hold under the null hypothesis.

Example 13.1. Dropouts in the milk protein data

Recall that these data consist of up to 19 weekly measurements of protein content in milk samples taken from each of 79 cows. Also, the cows were allocated amongst three different treatments, representing different diets, in a completely randomized design. Of the 79 cows, 38 dropped out during the study. There were also 11 intermittent missing values. In Section 5.4 we fitted a model to these data in which, amongst other things, the mean response in each treatment group was assumed to be constant after an initial settling–in period. We noted that an apparent rise in the *observed* mean response near the end of the experiment was not supported by testing against an enlarged model, and speculated that this might be somehow connected to the dropout process. As a first stage in pursuing this question, we now test whether the dropouts are completely random.

The dropouts are confined to four of the last five weeks of the study, and occur in 12 distinct treatment-by-time combinations. To construct the 12 test statistics we use $h_k(y_1, \ldots, y_k) = y_k$, the latest observed measurement, and implement a Monte Carlo test using $s = 999$ random selections from the randomization distribution of $\bar{h}_k$ for each treatment-by-time combination. The resulting p-values range from 0.001 to 0.254. On the basis of these results, we reject firmly the hypothesis of completely random dropouts. For example, if we use the Kolmogorov–Smirnov statistic to test for uniformity of the empirical distribution of the p-values, again via a Monte Carlo implementation with $s = 999$ to take account of the discreteness of the problem, we obtain a p-value of 0.001. Note that 0.001 is the smallest possible p-value for a Monte Carlo test with $s = 999$.

Table 13.1 shows the 12 p-values cross-classified by dropout time and treatment. It is noticeable that the larger p-values predominate in the third treatment group and at the later dropout times, although the second of these features may simply be a result of the reduced power of the tests as the earlier dropouts lead to smaller sample sizes at later times.

We obtained very similar results for the milk protein data when we used $h_k(y_1, \ldots, y_k) = r^{-1} \sum_{j=k-r+1}^{k} y_j$, for each of $r = 2, 3, 4, 5$. The implication is that dropouts predominate amongst cows whose protein measurements in the preceding weeks are below average. Now recall the likelihood-based analysis of these data reported in Section 5.4. There, we accepted a constant mean response model against an alternative which allowed for a rising trend in the mean response, whereas the empirical mean responses suggested a rise towards the end of the experiment. We now have a possible explanation. The likelihood-based analysis is estimating $\mu_1(t)$, the mean response which would apply to a population with no dropouts, whereas the

Table 13.1. Attained significance levels of tests for completely random dropouts in the milk protein data.

Dropout time (wks)	Treatment (diet)		
	Barley	Mixed	Lupins
15	0.001	0.001	0.012
16	0.016	0.001	0.011
17	0.022	0.053	0.254
19	0.032	0.133	0.206

empirical means are estimating $\mu_2(t)$, the mean response of a unit conditional on its not having dropped out by time t. Under completely random dropouts, or under random dropouts with independent measurements at different times, $\mu_1(t) = \mu_2(t)$, whereas under random dropouts with serially correlated measurements, $\mu_1(t) \neq \mu_2(t)$. This underlines the danger of regarding random dropouts as ignorable in the colloquial sense.

Ridout (1991) points out a connection between Diggle's (1989) procedure and logistic regression analysis. At each time-point, we could use the function $h_k(y_1, \ldots, y_k)$ as an explanatory variable in a logistic regression model for the probability of dropout. Thus, if p_k is the probability that a unit will drop out, we assume that

$$\log\{p_k/(1-p_k)\} = \alpha + \beta h_k. \tag{13.5.2}$$

Then, conditional on the observed values, h_{ik}, for all the units who have not dropped out previously, the mean, $\bar{h}$, of those about to drop out is the appropriate statistic to test the hypothesis that $\beta = 0$ (Cox and Snell, 1989, Chapter 2).

Clearly, it is possible to fit the logistic model (13.5.2), or extensions of it, using standard methodology for generalized linear models as suggested by Aitkin *et al.* (1989, Chapter 3). For example, we can introduce an explicit dependence of p_k on time and/or the experimental treatment administered.

Example 13.2. Protein content of milk samples (continued)

We now give the parametric version of the analysis described in Example 13.1. Let p_{gk} denote the probability that a unit in the gth treatment group drops out at the kth time. We assume that

$$\log\{p_{gk}/(1-p_{gk})\} = \alpha_{gk} + \beta_{gk} h_k, \tag{13.5.3}$$

with $h_k(y_1, \ldots, y_k) = y_k$. In this analysis, we consider only those four of the 19 time-points at which dropouts actually occurred, giving a total of 24 parameters. The residual deviances from this 24-parameter model and various simpler models are given in Table 13.2. Note that the analysis is based on 234 binary responses. These consist of 79 responses in week 15, the first occasion on which any units drop out, 59 in week 11 from the units which did not drop out in week 15, and similarly 50 and 46 from weeks 17 and 19; there were no dropouts in week 18.

From lines 1 to 5 in Table 13.2, we conclude first that there is a strong dependence of the dropout probability on the most recently observed measurement; for example, the log-likelihood ratio statistic to test model 5 within model 4 is 197.66 − 119.32 = 78.34 on 1 degree of freedom. We also conclude that the nature of the dependence does not vary between treatments or times; none of lines 1 to 3 gives a significant reduction in the residual deviance by comparison with line 4. The dependence of the

Table 13.2. Analysis of deviance for a logistic regression analysis of dropouts in the milk protein data.

Model for $\log\{p_{gk}/(1-p_{gk})\}$	Residual deviance	df
1. $\alpha_{gk} + \beta_{gk}h_k$	111.97	210
2. $\alpha_{gk} + \beta_g h_k$	116.33	219
3. $\alpha_{gk} + \beta_k h_k$	118.63	218
4. $\alpha_{gk} + \beta h_k$	119.32	221
5. α_{gk}	197.66	222
6. $\alpha_g + \alpha'_k + \beta h_k$	124.16	227
7. $\alpha_g + \beta h_k$	131.28	230
8. $\alpha + \beta h_k$	139.04	232

dropout rate on treatment or time is investigated in lines 6 to 8 of the table where we test different assumptions about the α_{gk} parameters in the model. We now have some evidence that the dropout rate depends on treatment. Comparing lines 7 and 8 the log-likelihood ratio statistic is 7.76 on 2 degrees of freedom, corresponding to a p-value of 0.021. The evidence for a dependence on time is rather weak; from lines 6 and 7 the log likelihood ratio statistic is 7.12 on 3 degrees of freedom, p-value = 0.089.

The parametric analysis in Example 13.2 allows a more detailed description of departures from completely random dropouts than was possible from the non-parametric analysis in Example 13.1. As always, the relative merits of non-parametric and parametric approaches involve a balance between the robustness and flexibility of the non-parametric approach and the greater sensitivity of the parametric approach when the assumed model is approximately correct. Note that in both approaches the implied alternative hypothesis is of random dropouts. This underlines an inherent limitation of any of the methods described in this section – the hypothesis of completely random dropout is seldom of intrinsic scientific interest, and rejection of it does not determine the subsequent strategy for analysis of the data. As we have seen, the distinction between random and informative dropout is at least as important from a practical point of view as is the distinction between completely random and random dropout.

13.6 Generalized estimating equations under a random missingness mechanism

One of the attractions of the method of generalized estimating equations (GEE), as described in Section 8.2.3, is that for problems in which the questions of interest concern the relationship between the population-averaged mean response and a set of explanatory variables, the GEE method provides consistent inference under the minimal assumption that the model for the mean response is correctly specified. In particular, if the analysis assumes a working form for the variance matrix of the response vector which is incorrect, efficiency may be lost but, under reasonably general conditions, consistency is retained. However, the basic form of the GEE method assumes that any dropouts are completely random, otherwise the consistency of the estimating equation is lost.

When data contain dropouts we may still wish to estimate, under minimal assumptions, the mean response which would have prevailed in the absence of dropouts. Robins *et al.* (1995) present an extension of the GEE method to data with random dropouts, which preserves the property of consistent inference about the mean response without requiring correct specification of the covariance structure.

The basic GEE method uses the estimating equation (8.2.4), which we reproduce here as

$$S_{\boldsymbol{\beta}}(\boldsymbol{\beta},\boldsymbol{\alpha}) = \sum_{i=1}^{m} \left(\frac{\partial \boldsymbol{\mu}_i}{\partial \boldsymbol{\beta}}\right)' \text{Var}(\boldsymbol{Y_i})^{-1}(\boldsymbol{Y_i} - \boldsymbol{\mu}_i) = 0. \tag{13.6.1}$$

Recall that in (13.6.1), $\boldsymbol{Y}_i$ denotes the vector of responses on the ith subject, $\boldsymbol{\mu}_i$ the corresponding mean response, and $\boldsymbol{\beta}$ the vector of regression parameters defining the mean response. Expressed informally, the essential idea in Robins *et al.* (1995) is that if p_{ij} denotes the probability that subject i has not dropped out by time t_j, given that subject's observed measurement history $y_{i1}, \ldots, y_{i,j-1}$ and any relevant covariate information, then the observation y_{ij} from this one subject is representative of all subjects with comparable measurement and covariate information who would have been observed had they not dropped out. Hence, to restore the unbiasedness of (13.6.1) *for the complete population* we need to weight the contribution of y_{ij} by the inverse of p_{ij}. This leads to the extended estimating equation,

$$S_{\boldsymbol{\beta}}(\boldsymbol{\beta},\boldsymbol{\alpha}) = \sum_{i=1}^{m} \left(\frac{\partial \boldsymbol{\mu}_i}{\partial \boldsymbol{\beta}}\right)' \text{Var}(\boldsymbol{Y_i})^{-1}P^{-1}(\boldsymbol{Y_i} - \boldsymbol{\mu}_i) = 0, \tag{13.6.2}$$

in which P is a diagonal matrix with non-zero elements p_{ij}. Robins *et al.* (1995) give a careful discussion of the precise conditions under which (13.6.2) does indeed lead to consistent inferences about $\boldsymbol{\beta}$ when the p_{ij} are themsleves estimated from the data using an assumed random dropout model.

This extension to GEE requires, inevitably, that we can consistently estimate the dropout probabilities for each subject given their observed measurement history and any relevant covariates. This makes the method best suited to large-scale studies. Arguably, it is a tall order to fit a parametric dropout model, for which the data necessarily provide relatively sparse information, in circumstances where the analysts are reluctant to commit themselves to a parametric model for the covariance structure. Scharfstein *et al.* (1999) extend this approach to the case of informative dropout and argue in favour of presenting a range of inferences for the quantities of interest based on different values of informative dropout parameters, rather than attempting to estimate aspects of the dropout process on which the data provide little or no information.

The idea of weighting observed measurements in inverse proportion to the corresponding estimated dropout probabilities also appears in Heyting *et al.* (1992).

13.7 Modelling the dropout process

In this section we review a number of approaches to parametric modelling of longitudinal data with potentially informative dropouts, highlighting the practical implications of each approach and the distinctions amongst them in respect of the assumptions which they make about the underlying dropout mechanism. The formal development will be in terms of a continuous response variable. The extension of these ideas to discrete responses will be discussed briefly in Section 13.9.

Following Diggle and Kenward (1994), we adopt the notational convention that for any one subject, the complete set of intended measurements, $Y^* = (Y_1^*, \ldots, Y_n^*)$, the observed measurements $Y = (Y_1, \ldots, Y_n)$ and the dropout time D obey the relationship

$$Y_j = \begin{cases} Y_j^*: & j < D, \\ 0: & j \geq D. \end{cases}$$

We emphasize that in this notation a zero value for Y is simply a code for missingness, not a measured zero. Note also that $2 \leq D \leq n + 1$, with $D = n + 1$, indicating that the subject in question has not dropped out.

13.7.1 *Selection models*

In a *selection model*, the joint distribution of $\boldsymbol{Y}^*$ and D is factorized as the marginal distribution of $\boldsymbol{Y}^*$ and the conditional distribution of D, given Y^*; thus $\mathrm{P}(\boldsymbol{Y}^*, D) = \mathrm{P}(\boldsymbol{Y}^*)\mathrm{P}(D \mid \boldsymbol{Y}^*)$. The terminology is due to Heckman (1976), and conveys the notion that dropouts are *selected* according to their measurement history. Selection models fit naturally into Little and Rubin's hierarchy, as follows: dropouts are completely random if $\mathrm{P}(D \mid \boldsymbol{Y}^*) = \mathrm{P}(D)$, that is, D and $\boldsymbol{Y}^*$ are independent; dropouts are random if $\mathrm{P}(D \mid \boldsymbol{Y}^*) = \mathrm{P}(D \mid Y_1^*, \ldots, Y_{D-1}^*)$; otherwise, dropouts are informative.

Let $\boldsymbol{\theta}$ and $\boldsymbol{\phi}$ denote the parameters of the sub-model for $\boldsymbol{Y}^*$ and of the sub-model for D conditional on $\boldsymbol{Y}^*$, respectively. We now derive the joint distribution of the observable random vector, $\boldsymbol{Y}$, via the sequence of conditional distributions for Y_k given H_k, where $H_k = (Y_1, \ldots, Y_{k-1})$. Let $f_k^*(y \mid H_k; \boldsymbol{\theta}, \boldsymbol{\phi})$ denote the conditional univariate pdf of $\boldsymbol{Y}_k^*$ given H_k and $f_k(y \mid H_k; \boldsymbol{\theta}, \boldsymbol{\phi})$ the conditional pdf of Y_k given H_k. Then,

$$\Pr(Y_k = 0 \mid H_k, Y_{k-1} = 0) = 1, \tag{13.7.1}$$

$$\Pr(Y_k = 0 \mid H_k, Y_{k-1}, \neq 0) = \int p_k(H_k, y; \boldsymbol{\phi}) f_k^*(y \mid H_k; \boldsymbol{\theta}) \mathrm{d}y \tag{13.7.2}$$

and for $y \neq 0$,

$$f_k(y \mid H_k; \boldsymbol{\theta}, \boldsymbol{\phi}) = \{1 - p_k(H_k, y; \boldsymbol{\phi})\} f_k^*(y \mid H_k; \boldsymbol{\theta}, \boldsymbol{\phi}). \tag{13.7.3}$$

Equations (13.7.1–13.7.3) determine the joint distribution of $\boldsymbol{Y}$, and hence the likelihood function for $\boldsymbol{\theta}$ and $\boldsymbol{\phi}$. Suppressing the dependence on the parameters, the joint pdf of a complete sequence, $\boldsymbol{Y}$, is

$$\begin{aligned} f(\boldsymbol{y}) &= f_1^*(y_1) \prod_{k=2}^{m} f_k(y_k \mid H_k) \\ &= f^*(\boldsymbol{y}) \left[\prod_{k=2}^{m} \{1 - p_k(H_k, y_k)\} \right], \end{aligned} \tag{13.7.4}$$

whilst for an incomplete sequence with dropout at the dth time-point,

$$\begin{aligned} f(\boldsymbol{y}) &= \left\{ f_1^*(y_1) \prod_{k=2}^{d-1} f_k(y_k \mid H_k) \right\} \Pr(y_d = 0 \mid H_d, Y_{d-1} \neq 0) \\ &= f_{d-1}^*(\boldsymbol{y}) \left[\prod_{k=2}^{d-1} \{1 - p_k(H_k, y_k)\} \right] \Pr(Y_d = 0 \mid H_d, Y_{d-1} \neq 0), \end{aligned} \tag{13.7.5}$$

where $f_{d-1}^*(\boldsymbol{y})$ denotes the joint pdf of the first $d-1$ elements of $\boldsymbol{Y}^*$ and the product term within square brackets is absent if $d = 2$.

Note that under either CRD or RD, $p_k(H_k, y; \boldsymbol{\phi})$ does not depend on y, the (unobserved) value of the measurement at time t_k. It follows that this term can be brought outside the integral sign on the right-hand side of (13.7.2), which then reduces to

$$\Pr(Y_k = 0 \mid H_{k-1}, Y_{k-1} \neq 0) = p_k(H_k; \boldsymbol{\phi}),$$

since the integrand is now a pdf and integrates to one. This implies that the contribution to the likelihood separates into two components, one for $\boldsymbol{\theta}$ and one for $\boldsymbol{\phi}$. We now consider the form of the resulting likelihood function for a set of data consisting of m units, in which $\boldsymbol{y}_i = \{y_{ij},\ j = 1, \ldots, d_i - 1\}$

represents the sequence of observed measurements on the ith unit, where $d_i = n + 1$ if the unit does not drop out and d_i identifies the dropout time otherwise. Then, the log-likelihood for $(\boldsymbol{\theta}, \boldsymbol{\phi})$ can be partitioned as

$$L(\boldsymbol{\theta}, \boldsymbol{\phi}) = L_1(\boldsymbol{\theta}) + L_2(\boldsymbol{\phi}) + L_3(\boldsymbol{\theta}, \boldsymbol{\phi}),$$

where

$$L_1\boldsymbol{\theta}) = \sum_{i=1}^{m} \log\{f^*_{d_i-1}(\boldsymbol{y}_i)\},$$

$$L_2(\boldsymbol{\phi}) = \sum_{i=1}^{m} \sum_{k=1}^{d_i-1} \log\{1 - p_k(H_k, y_{ik})\}$$

and

$$L_3(\boldsymbol{\theta}, \boldsymbol{\phi}) = \sum_{i:d_i \leq n} \log\{\Pr(D = d_i \mid \boldsymbol{y}_i)\}.$$

Recall that under RD, $L_3(\boldsymbol{\theta}, \boldsymbol{\phi})$ depends only on $\boldsymbol{\phi}$, and can therefore be absorbed into $L_2(\boldsymbol{\phi})$. Hence, under RD,

$$L(\boldsymbol{\theta}, \boldsymbol{\phi}) = L_1(\boldsymbol{\theta}) + L_2(\boldsymbol{\phi}), \tag{13.7.6}$$

and maximization of $L(\boldsymbol{\theta}, \boldsymbol{\phi})$ is equivalent to separate maximization of $L_1(\boldsymbol{\theta})$ and $L_2(\boldsymbol{\phi})$. Hence the dropouts, which only affect $L_2(\boldsymbol{\phi})$, are *ignorable for likelihood-based inference about* $\boldsymbol{\theta}$. Similarly, $L_2(\boldsymbol{\phi})$ in (13.7.6) is the log-likelihood associated with the sub-model for D conditional on the observed elements of $\boldsymbol{Y}^*$, and it follows that the stochastic structure of the measurement process can be ignored *for likelihood-based inference about* $\boldsymbol{\phi}$.

In summary, under random dropout, the log-likelihood associated with a selection model separates into two components, one for the parameters of the measurement sub-model, the other for the parameters of the dropout sub-model, and it is in this sense that the dropout process is ignorable for inferences about the measurement process, and vice versa. Equally, it is clear that this would not hold if there were parameters in common between the two sub-models, or a more general functional relationship between $\boldsymbol{\theta}$ and $\boldsymbol{\phi}$. Moreover, the implicit assumption that the relevant scientific questions are addressed by inference about the $\boldsymbol{Y}^*$ process may not be reasonable in particular applications. For example, if dropouts occur primarily because subjects with a poor response are withdrawn from the study on ethical grounds, it might be relevant to ask what the trial would have shown if these subjects had not been removed, and this is precisely what is addressed by an analysis of the $\boldsymbol{Y}^*$ process. On the other hand, if dropouts occur because some subjects experience an adverse reaction to treatment (as distinct from a poor clinical response), then inferences about $\boldsymbol{Y}^*$ relate to a fictitious population of subjects for whom such adverse reactions do not occur, and it might be of more practical relevance to analyse both the incidence of adverse reactions and the pattern of responses amongst the sub-population of subjects with no adverse reaction. This leads on to the idea of pattern mixture models, which we discuss in Section 13.7.2.

When the dropout process is informative, the log-likelihood for $\boldsymbol{\theta}$ and $\boldsymbol{\phi}$ does not separate and the statistical analysis becomes more complex. From a technical point of view, the need to evaluate the integral (13.7.2) at each dropout time complicates the computation of the likelihood. More fundamentally, the need to model the relationship between an observed event (dropout) and an *unobservable* concomitant (the measurement which would have been observed had the subject not dropped out) typically leads to poor identifiability of the model parameters, making it difficult, or even impossible, to validate the assumed model from the observed data. See, for example, Fitzmaurice *et al.* (1996).

Example 13.3. Protein content of milk samples (continued)

We now fit the Diggle and Kenward model to the milk protein data, our objectives being to establish whether the dropout process is informative, and if so to find out if this affects our earlier conclusions about the mean response profiles.

For the mean response profiles we use a simple extension of the model fitted in Section 5.4, where we implicitly assumed random dropouts. Note that this model allows the possibility of an increase in mean response towards the end of the experiment. If $\mu_g(t)$ denotes the mean response at time t under diet g, we assume that

$$\mu_g(t) = \begin{cases} \beta_{0g} + \beta_1 t, & t \leq 3, \\ \beta_{0g} + 3\beta_1 + \beta_2(t-3) + \beta_3(t-3)^2, & t > 3. \end{cases}$$

In Section 5.4, Example 5.1, we used a model for the covariance structure of the complete measurement process $Y^*(t)$ which included three distinct components of variation: a random intercept component between animals, a serially correlated component within animals, and an uncorrelated measurement error component. However, the estimated component of variation between animals was very small, and in what follows we have chosen to set this component to zero. Finally, for the dropout process we note that all of the dropouts occur in the last five weeks of the experiment. Writing p_k for the probability of dropout at time k, we therefore assume that $p_k = 0$ for $k \leq 14$, whereas for $k \geq 15$,

$$\log\{p_k/(1-p_k)\} = \phi_0 + \phi_1 y_k + \phi_2 y_{k-1}.$$

Table 13.3. Likelihood analysis of dropout mechanisms for the milk protein data.

Dropout mechanism	$2L_{\max}$
ID	2381.63
RD ($\beta_1 = 0$)	2369.32
CRD ($\beta_1 = \beta_2 = 0$)	2299.06

Table 13.3 gives values of twice the maximized log-likelihood for the full model and for the reduced models with $\phi_1 = 0$ (random dropouts) and $\phi_1 = \phi_2 = 0$ (completely random dropouts). Comparison of the RD and CRD lines in Table 13.3 confirms our earlier conclusion that dropouts are not completely random. More interestingly, there is overwhelming evidence in favour of informative dropouts: from the ID and RD lines, the likelihood ratio statistic to test the RD assumption is 12.31 on one degree of freedom, corresponding to a p-value of 0.0005.

In principle, rejection of the RD assumption forces us to reassess our model for the underlying measurement process, $Y^*(t)$. However, it turns out that the maximum likelihood estimates of the parameters are virtually the same as under the RD assumption. This is not surprising, as most of the information about these parameters is contained in the 14 weeks of dropout-free data. With regard to the possibility of an increase in the mean response towards the end of the experiment, the maximum likelihood estimates of β_2 and β_3 are both close to zero, and the likelihood ratio statistic to test $\beta_2 = \beta_3 = 0$ is 1.70 on two degrees of freedom, corresponding to a p-value of 0.43.

In the case of the milk protein data, our reassessment of the dropout process has not led to any substantive changes in our inferences concerning the mean response profiles for the underlying dropout-free process $Y^*(t)$. This is not always so. See Diggle and Kenward (1994) for examples.

Note also that from a scientific point of view, the analysis reported here is suspect, because the 'dropouts' are an artefact of the definition of time as being relative to calving date, coupled with the termination of the study on a fixed calendar date. This leads us on to a discussion of *pattern mixture models* as an alternative way of representing potentially informative dropout mechanisms.

13.7.2 *Pattern mixture models*

Pattern mixture models, introduced by Little (1993), work with the factorization of the joint distribution of $\boldsymbol{Y}^*$ and D into the marginal distribution of D and the conditional distribution of $\boldsymbol{Y}^*$ given D, thus $\mathrm{P}(\boldsymbol{Y}^*, D) = \mathrm{P}(D)\mathrm{P}(\boldsymbol{Y}^* \mid D)$. From a theoretical point of view, it is always possible to express a selection model as a pattern mixture model and vice versa, as they are simply alternative factorizations of the same joint distribution. In practice, the two approaches lead to different kinds of simplifying assumptions, and hence to different analyses.

From a modelling point of view, a possible rationale for pattern mixture models is that each subject's dropout time is somehow predestined, and that the measurement process varies between dropout cohorts. This literal interpretation would seem unlikely to apply very often although, as noted above, one exception is the milk protein data originally analysed by Diggle and Kenward (1994) using a selection model. Because the 'dropout times' correspond precisely to different cohorts, the literal interpretation of a pattern mixture model is exactly right for these data.

The arguments in favour of pattern mixture modelling are usually of a more pragmatic kind. First, classification of subjects in a longitudinal trial according to their dropout time provides an obvious way of dividing the subjects into sub-groups after the event, and it is sensible to ask whether the response characteristics which are of primary interest do or do not vary between these sub-groups; indeed, separate inspection of sub-groups defined in this way is a very natural piece of exploratory analysis which many a statistician would carry out without formal reference to pattern mixture models. See, for example, Grieve (1994).

Second, writing the joint distribution for $\boldsymbol{Y}^*$ and D in its pattern mixture factorization brings out very clearly those aspects of the model which are assumption-driven rather than data-driven. As a simple example, consider a trial in which it is intended to take two measurements on each subject, $\boldsymbol{Y}^* = (Y_1^*, Y_2^*)$, but that some subjects drop out after providing the first measurement. Let $f(\boldsymbol{y} \mid d)$ denote the conditional distribution of $\boldsymbol{Y}^*$ given $D = d$, for $d = 2$ (dropouts) and $d = 3$ (non-dropouts). Quite generally, $f(\boldsymbol{y} \mid d) = f(y_1 \mid d) f(y_2 \mid y_1, d)$ but the data can provide no information about $f(y_2 \mid y_1, 2)$ since, by definition, $D = 2$ means that Y_2^* is not observed.

Extensions of the kind of example given above demonstrate that pattern mixture models cannot be identified without placing restrictions on the conditional distributions $f(\boldsymbol{y} \mid d)$. For example, Little (1993) discusses the use of *complete case missing variable* restrictions, which correspond to assuming that for each $d < n + 1$ and $t \geq d$,

$$f(y_t \mid y_1, \ldots, y_{t-1}, d) = f(y_t \mid y_1, \ldots, y_{t-1}, n + 1).$$

At first sight, pattern mixture models do not fit naturally into Rubin's hierarchy. However, Molenberghs *et al.* (1997) show that random dropout corresponds precisely to the the following set of restrictions, which they call *available case missing value* restrictions:

$$f(y_t \mid y_1, \ldots, y_{t-1}, d) = f(y_t \mid y_1, \ldots, y_{t-1}, D > t).$$

This result implies that the hypothesis of random dropout cannot be tested without making additional assumptions to restrict the class of alternatives under consideration, since the available case missing value restrictions cannot be verified empirically.

The identifiability problems associated with informative dropout models, and the impossibility of validating a random dropout assumption on empirical evidence alone, serve as clear warnings that the analysis of a longitudinal data-set with dropouts needs to be undertaken with extreme caution. However, in the author's opinion this is no reason to adopt the superficially simpler strategy of automatically assuming that dropouts are ignorable.

Example 13.3. Protein content of milk samples (concluded)

The first stage in a pattern mixture analysis of these data is to examine the data separately within each dropout cohort. The result is shown in Fig. 13.2. The respective cohort sizes are 41, 5, 4, 9 and 20, making it difficult to justify a detailed interpretation of the three intermediate cohorts. The two extreme cohorts produce sharply contrasting results. In the first, 19-week cohort the observed mean response profiles are well separated, approximately parallel and show a three-phase response, consisting of a sharp downward trend during the initial three weeks followed by a gentle rising trend which then levels off from around week 14. In the 15-week cohort, there is no clear separation amongst the three treatment groups and the trend is steadily downward over the 15 weeks. We find it hard to explain these results, and have not attempted a formal analysis. It is curious that recognition of the cohort effects in these data seems to make the interpretation more difficult.

13.7.3 *Random effect models*

Random effect models are extremely useful to the longitudinal data analyst. They formalize the intuitive idea that a subject's pattern of responses in a study is likely to depend on many characteristics of that subject, including some which are unobservable. These unobservable characteristics are then included in the model as random variables, that is, as random effects.

It is therefore natural to formulate models in which a subject's propensity to drop out also depends on unobserved variables, that is, on random effects, as in Wu and Carroll (1988) or Wu and Bailey (1989). In the present context, a simple formulation of a model of this kind would be to postulate a bivariate random effect, $\boldsymbol{U} = (U_1, U_2)$ and to model the joint distribution

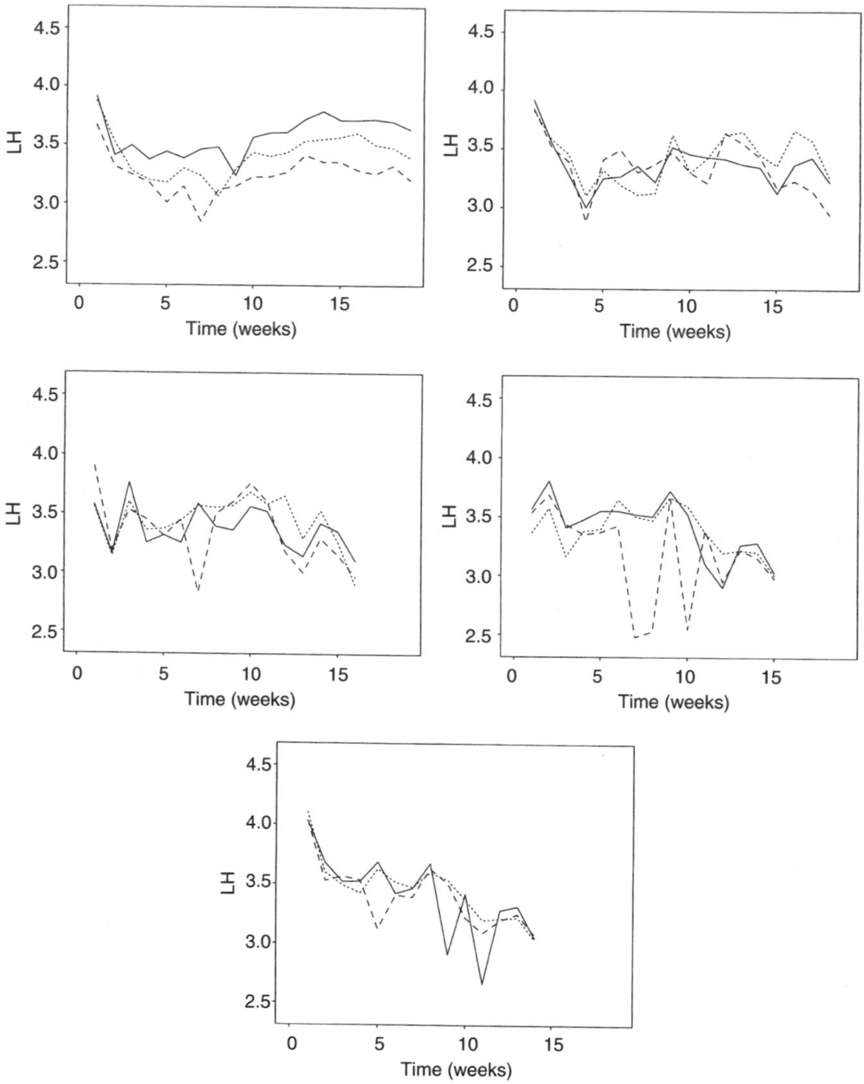

Fig. 13.2. Observed mean response profiles for milk protein data, by dropout cohort.

of $\boldsymbol{Y}^*$, D and $\boldsymbol{U}$ as

$$f(\boldsymbol{y}, d, \boldsymbol{u}) = f_1(\boldsymbol{y} \mid \boldsymbol{u}_1) f_2(d \mid \boldsymbol{u}_2) f_3(\boldsymbol{u}). \tag{13.7.7}$$

In (13.7.7), the dependence between $\boldsymbol{Y}^*$ and D is a by-product of the dependence between $\boldsymbol{U}_1$ and $\boldsymbol{U}_2$, or to put it another way, $\boldsymbol{Y}^*$ and D are conditionally independent given $\boldsymbol{U}$. In terms of Little and Rubin's hierarchy, the dropouts in (13.7.7) are completely random if U_1 and U_2 are independent, whereas if U_1 and U_2 are dependent then in general the dropouts are informative. Strictly, the truth of this last statement depends on the precise formulation of $f_1(\boldsymbol{y} \mid \boldsymbol{u}_1)$ and $f_2(d \mid \boldsymbol{u}_2)$. For example, it would be within the letter, but clearly not the spirit, of (13.7.7) to set either $f_1(\boldsymbol{y} \mid \boldsymbol{u}_1) = f_1(\boldsymbol{y})$ or $f_2(d \mid \boldsymbol{u}_2) = f_2(d)$, in which case the model would reduce trivially to one of completely random dropouts whatever the distribution of $\boldsymbol{U}$.

13.7.4 *Contrasting assumptions: a graphical representation*

In our opinion, debates about the relative merits of selection and pattern mixture models *per se* are unhelpful: models for dropout in longitudinal studies should be considered on their merits in the context of particular applications. In this spirit, Fig. 13.3 shows a schematic view of selection, pattern mixture and random effects models which takes the point of view

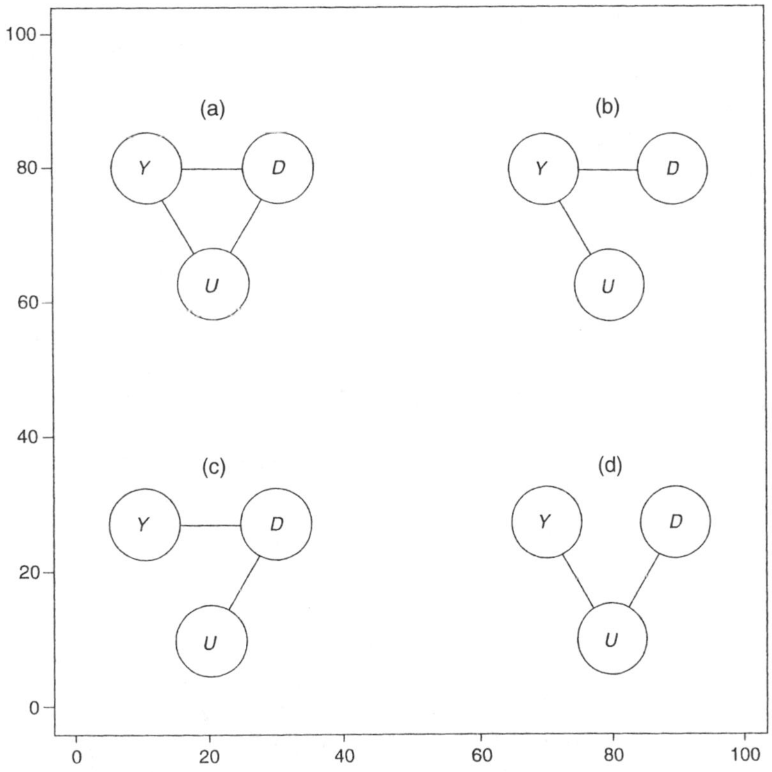

Fig. 13.3. Graphical representation of (a) saturated, (b) selection, (c) pattern mixture and (d) random effects dropout models.

that random effects are almost always with us (whether or not we recognize them in our models), and that one consideration in formulating a model for a longitudinal trial with dropouts would be to think what kinds of causal relationship might plausibly exist amongst *three* sets of random variables: measurements $\boldsymbol{Y}$, dropout times D and random effects $\boldsymbol{U}$. Each diagram in Fig. 13.3 is a conditional independence graph for these three random variables, in which the absence of an edge between two vertices indicates that the two random variables in question are conditionally independent given the third (Whittaker, 1990). The most general kind of model is represented by the complete graph in the top-left panel, whilst the remaining graphs, each of which has a single edge deleted, correspond to selection, pattern mixture and random effects models.

Figure 13.3 is intended as an aid to the kind of thought experiment that the data analyst must conduct in deciding how to deal with dropouts. Fig. 13.3(a) represents a denial that any simplifying assumptions are possible. Under this scenario, we would be more or less compelled to express a model for the data as a collection of joint distributions for $\boldsymbol{Y}$ and $\boldsymbol{U}$ conditional on each of the possible discrete values of D. Fig. 13.3(b) invites interpretation as a causal chain in which random effects or latent subject-specific characteristics, $\boldsymbol{U}$, influence the properties of the measurement process, $\boldsymbol{Y}$, for the subject in question, with propensity to drop out subsequently determined by the realization of the measurement process. In contrast, Fig. 13.3(c) invites the interpretation that the subject-specific characteristics initially determine propensity to drop out, with a consequential variation in the measurement process between different, predestined dropout cohorts. Finally, Fig. 13.3(d) suggests that measurement and dropout processes are a joint response to subject-specific characteristics; we could think of these characteristics as unidentified explanatory variables, discovery of which would convert the model to one in which $\boldsymbol{Y}$ and D were independent, that is, completely random dropout.

Figure 13.3 also prompts consideration of whether selection modelling of the dropout process is appropriate if the measurement sub-model for Y includes measurement error. To be specific, suppose that the measurement sub-model is of the kind described in Section 5.3.2, in which the stochastic variation about the mean response has three components,

$$Y_{ij} = \mu_{ij} + \{\boldsymbol{d}'_{ij}\boldsymbol{U}_i + W_i(t_{ij})\} + Z_{ij}. \qquad (13.7.8)$$

The bracketing of two of the terms on the right-hand side of (13.7.8) is to emphasise that $\{\boldsymbol{d}'_{ij}\boldsymbol{U}_i + W_i(t_{ij})\}$ models the deviation of an individual subject's response trajectory from the population average, whereas Z_{ij} represents additive measurement error, that is, the difference between the observed response y_{ij} and an unobserved true state of nature for the subject in question. In a model of this kind, if dropout is thought to be a response to the subject's true underlying state, it might be more appealing to model the conditional dropout probability as a function of this underlying state rather than as a function of the observed (or missing) y_{ij}, and the conclusion would be that a random effects dropout model is more natural than a selection dropout model.

Even when the above argument applies, a pragmatic reason for cosidering a selection model would be that *if* a random dropout assumption is sustainable the resulting analysis is straightforward, whereas non-trivial random effects dropout models always correspond to informative dropout because the random effects are, by definition, unobserved.

13.8 A longitudinal trial of drug therapies for schizophrenia

In this section we present an analysis, previously reported in Diggle (1998), of data from a randomized trial comparing different drug therapies for schizophrenia, as described in Example 1.7. Table 13.4 lists the data from the first 20 subjects in the placebo arm.

Table 13.4. PANSS scores from a subset of the placebo arm of the longitudinal trial of drug therapies for schizophrenia, from weeks −1, 0, 1, 2, 4, 6 and 8, where −1 is pre-randomization and 0 is baseline. A dash signifies a missing value.

−1	0	1	2	4	6	8
84	112	112	117	—	—	—
68	56	79	89	—	—	—
108	87	104	95	99	—	—
77	69	44	60	58	70	68
79	96	78	84	—	—	—
72	72	64	53	60	98	98
94	106	76	75	84	88	88
104	96	90	—	—	—	—
102	113	105	116	95	113	111
119	111	84	94	83	108	—
94	118	116	153	—	—	—
91	89	90	66	76	101	113
73	72	57	57	53	55	48
71	64	72	65	64	80	—
103	95	110	107	86	95	108
88	97	97	—	—	—	—
122	123	113	104	121	—	—
102	100	90	91	90	98	—
63	77	57	64	52	52	47
115	121	103	84	62	144	—

Recall that, of the 523 patients only 253 are listed as completing the study, although a further 16 provided a complete sequence of PANSS scores. Table 1.6 gives the distribution of the stated reasons for dropout, whilst Table 1.7 gives the numbers of dropouts and completers in each of the six treatment groups. Note that the most common reason for dropout is 'inadequate response,' and that the highest dropout rate occurs in the placebo group, followed by the haloperidol group and the lowest dose risperidone group.

As shown in Fig. 1.6, all six groups show a mean response profile decreasing over time post-baseline, with slower apparent rates of decrease towards the end of the study.

Figure 13.4 shows the observed mean response as a function of time within sub-groups corresponding to the different dropout times, but averaged across all treatments. The mean response profile for the completers is qualitatively similar to all of the profiles shown in Fig. 1.6, albeit with a steeper initial decrease and a levelling out towards the end of the study. Within each of the other dropout cohorts a quite different picture emerges. In particular, in every case the mean score increases immediately prior to dropout. This is consistent with the information that most of the dropouts are due to an inadequate response to treatment. It also underlines the need for a cautious interpretation of the empirical mean response profiles.

Figure 13.4 provides strong empirical evidence of a relationship between the measurement and dropout processes. Nevertheless, we shall initially analyse the measurement data ignoring the dropouts, to provide a basis for comparison with an integrated analysis of measurements and dropouts. From now on, we ignore the pre-baseline measurements because these preceded the establishment of a stable drug regime for each subject.

This phase of the analysis follows the general strategy described in Chapter 5. We first convert the responses to residuals from an ordinary least squares fit to a model which specifies a separate mean value for each combination of time and treatment. We then estimate the variogram of this residual process, under the assumption that the variogram depends only on the time-separation u. The resulting variogram estimate is shown in Fig. 13.5. Its salient features are: a substantial intercept; a relatively smooth increase with u; a maximum value substantially less than the process variance. These features suggest fitting a model of the kind described in Section 5.2.3, whilst the general shape of the variogram appears to be consistent with the Gaussian correlation function (5.2.8). Thus,

$$V(u) = \sigma^2\{\alpha_1 + 1 - \exp(-\alpha_3 u^2)\}$$

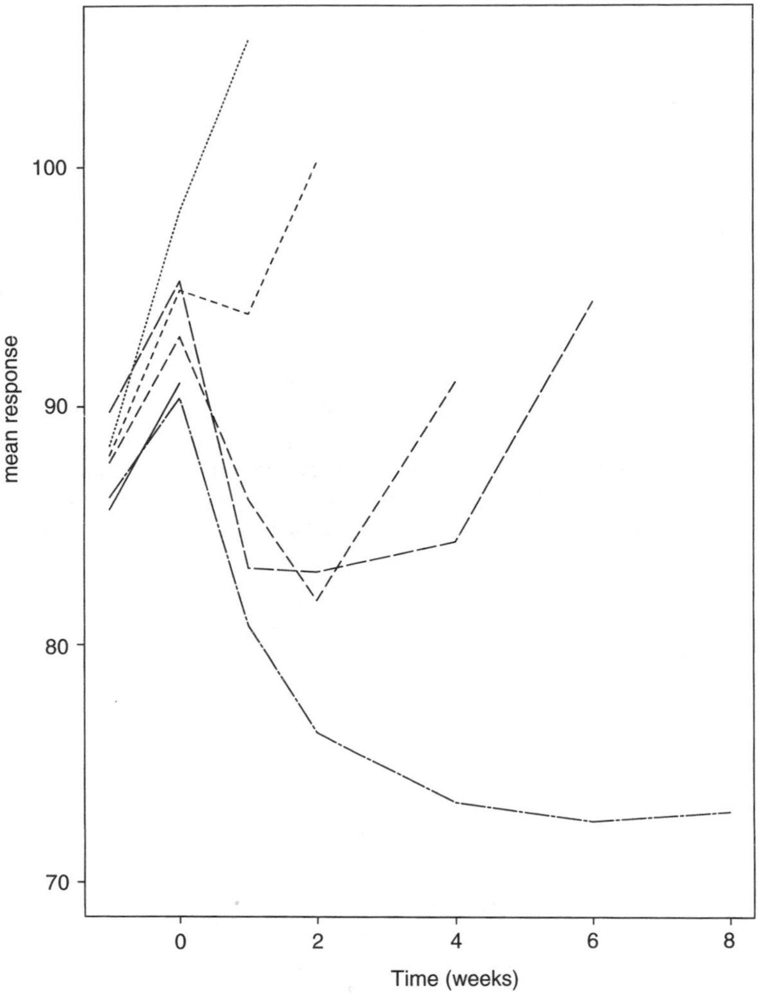

Fig. 13.4. Observed mean responses for the schizophrenia trial data, by dropout cohort an averaged across all treatment groups.

and

$$\text{Var}(Y) = \sigma^2(1 + \alpha_1 + \alpha_2).$$

Recall that the three variance components in this model are σ^2, the variance of the serially correlated component, $\tau^2 = \sigma^2\alpha_1$, the measurement error component, and $\nu^2 = \sigma^2\alpha_2$, the between subject component.

As a model for the mean response profiles $\mu_i(t)$, Fig. 13.6 suggests a collection of convex, non-parallel curves in the six treatment groups. The

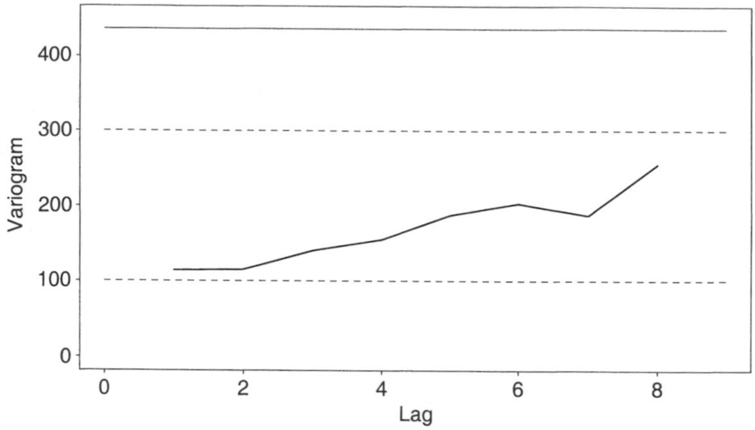

Fig. 13.5. The estimated variogram for the schizophrenia trial data. The horizontal solid line is an estimate of the variance of the measurement process. The dashed horizontal lines are rough initial estimates of the intercept and asymptote of the variogram.

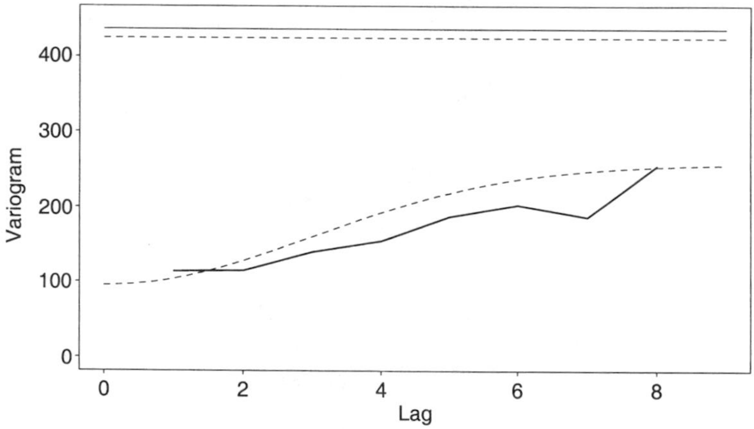

Fig. 13.6. The estimated variogram for the schizophrenia trial data (——), together with a fitted parametric model (------).

simplest model consistent with this behaviour is

$$\mu_i(t) = \mu + \delta_k + \theta_k t + \gamma_k t^2: \quad k = 1, \ldots, 6, \tag{13.8.1}$$

where $k = k(i)$ denotes the treatment group to which the ith subject is allocated. A more sophisticated non-linear model, perhaps incorporating a constraint that the mean response should be monotone and approach a horizontal asymptote as time increases, might be preferable on biological grounds and we shall return to this question in Chapter 14. But for a purely empirical description of the data a low-order polynomial model should be adequate. Note also that, as discussed earlier in this chapter, the empirical man response trajectories are not estimating the $\mu_i(t)$, and should be considered only as rough guides to their general shape.

The focus of scientific interest is the set of mean response curves, $\mu_i(t)$. In particular, we wish to investigate possible simplifications of the assumed mean response model by testing whether corresponding sets of contrasts are significantly different from zero. As described in Section 5.3.3, two ways of implementing tests of this kind are to use the quadratic form T_0 defined at (5.3.14) or the log-likelihood ratio statistic W_k defined at (5.3.15).

For the current example, two different kinds of simplification are of potential interest. First, we can ask whether the quadratic terms are necessary, that is, whether or not the six quadratic parameters γ_k in (13.8.1) are all zero. The quadratic form statistic is $T_0 = 16.97$ on 6 degrees of freedom, correponding to a p-value of 0.009, so we retain the quadratic terms in the model. Second, in Fig. 1.6 the differences amongst the mean response curves for the four risperidone treatments were relatively small. Also, when we fitted the model (13.8.1) we found that the estimated values of the risperidone parameters were not related in any consistent way to the corresponding dose levels. This suggests a possible simplification in which all four risperidone doses are considered as a single group. Within the overall model (13.8.1) the reduction from the original six to three groups is a linear hypothesis on 9 degrees of freedom (3 each for the constant, linear and quadratic effects). The quadratic form statistic is $T_0 = 16.38$, corresponding to a p-value of 0.059. We therefore arrive at a model of the form (13.8.1), but with $k = 1, 2$ and 3 corresponding to haloperidol, placebo and risperidone, respectively.

The parameter estimates for this model are shown in Table 13.5. Note that the treatment code is 1 = haloperidol, 2 = placebo, 3 = risperidone, and that estimation of the mean response parameters incorporates the constraint that $\delta_1 = 0$, that is, δ_2 and δ_3 represent the differences between the intercepts in the placebo and haloperidol groups, and in the the risperidone and haloperidol groups, respectively. The random allocation of patients to treatment groups should result in estimates $\hat{\delta}_2$ and $\hat{\delta}_3$ close to zero, and this is indeed the case, both estimates being less than two standard errors in magnitude. The evidence for curvature in the mean response profiles is not strong; the log-likelhood ratio test of the hypothesis that the quadratic parameters are all zero is $D = 8.72$ on 3 degrees of freedom, corresponding to a p value of 0.033.

How well does the model fit the data? Figure 13.6 shows the correspondence between non-parametric and parametric maximum likelihood estimates of the variogram. The fit is reasonably good, in that the values of $V(u)$ are closely modelled throughout the observed range of time-lags in

Table 13.5. Parameter estimates for the measurement model fitted to the schizophrenia trial data, under random dropout assumption and under informative dropout assumption

	Parameter	Estimate	SE
Mean response	μ	88.586	0.956
$\mu_i(t) = \mu + \delta_k + \theta_k t + \gamma_k t^2 : k = 1, 2, 3$	δ_1	0	0
	δ_2	0.715	1.352
	δ_3	−0.946	0.552
	θ_1	−0.207	0.563
	θ_2	0.927	0.589
	θ_3	−2.267	0.275
	γ_1	−0.113	0.081
	γ_2	−0.129	0.088
	γ_3	0.106	0.039
Covariance structure	σ^2	170.091	
$\gamma(u) = \sigma^2\{\alpha_1 + 1 - \exp(-\alpha_3 u^2)\}$	α_1	0.560	
$\text{Var}(Y) = \sigma^2(1 + \alpha_1 + \alpha_2)$	α_2	0.951	
	α_3	0.056	

the data. Notice, however, that the estimate of α_1 involves an extrapolation to zero time-lag which is heavily influenced by the assumed parametric form of the correlation function.

Figure 13.7 shows the observed and fitted mean responses in the haloperidol, placebo and risperidone groups. On the face of it, the fit is qualitatively wrong, but the diagram is not comparing like with like. As discussed in Section 13.7, the observed means are estimating the mean response at each observation time conditional on not having dropped out prior to the observation time in question, whereas the fitted means are actually estimating what the mean response would have been had there been no dropouts. Because, as Fig. 13.4 suggested and as we shall shortly confirm, dropout is asociated with an atypically high response, the non-dropout subpopulation becomes progressively more selective in favour of low responding subjects, leading to a correspondingly progressive reduction in the observed mean of the non-dropouts relative to the unconditional mean. Note in particular that the fitted mean in the placebo group is approximately constant, whereas a naive interpretation of the observed mean would have suggested a strong placebo effect.

It is perhaps worth emphasizing that the kind of fitted means illustrated in Fig. 13.7 would be produced routinely by software packages

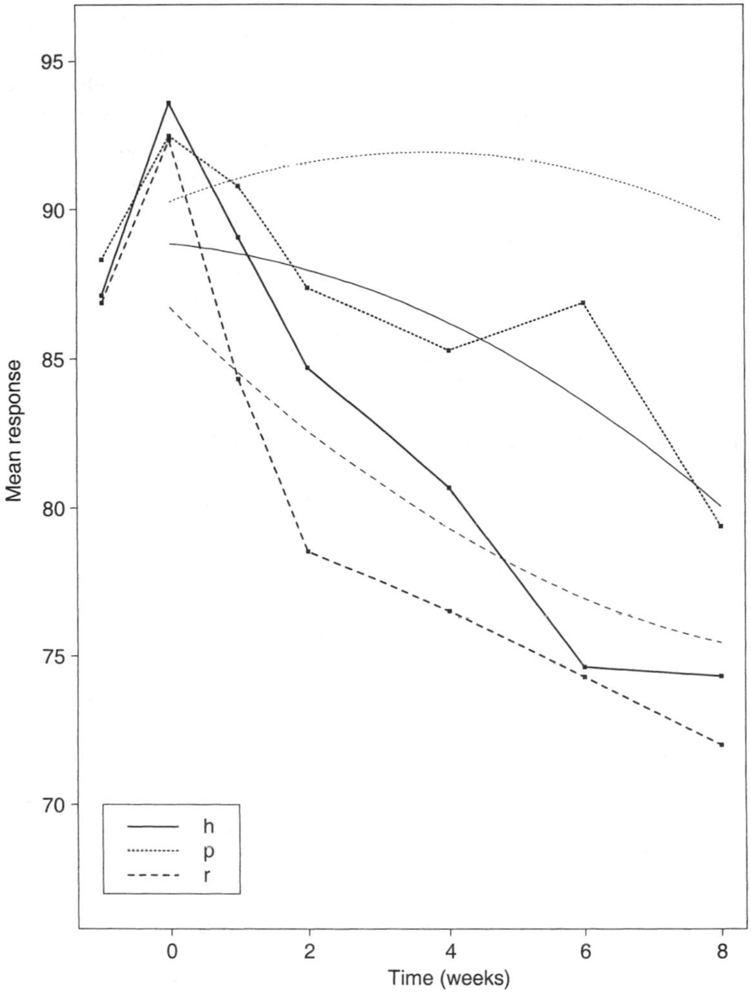

Fig. 13.7. Observed and fitted means in the placebo (**......**), haloperidol (**——**) and risperidone (**------**) treatment groups, compared with fitted means (......, —— and ------, respectively) from an analysis ignoring dropouts.

which include facilities for modelling correlated data. They are the result of a likelihood-based fit to a model which recognizes the likely correlation between repeated measurements on the same subject but treats missing values as ignorable in the Little and Rubin sense. As discussed in Section 13.7, estimates of this kind may or may not be appropriate to the scientific questions posed in a particular application, but in any event the qualitative discrepancy between the observed and fitted means surely deserves further investigation.

We therefore proceed to a joint analysis of measurements and dropouts. The empirical behaviour of Fig. 13.4, in which the mean response within each dropout cohort shows a sharp increase immediately before dropout, coupled with the overwhelming preponderance of 'inadequate response' as the stated reason for dropout, suggests modelling the probability of dropout as a function of the measured response, that is, a selection model. In the first instance, we fit a simple logistic regression model for dropout, with the most recent measurement as an explanatory variable. Thus, if p_{ij} denotes the probability that patient i drops out at the jth time-point (so that the jth and all subsequent measurements are missing), then

$$\text{logit}(p_{ij}) = \phi_0 + \phi_1 y_{i,j-1}. \tag{13.8.2}$$

The parameter estimates for this simple dropout model are $\hat{\phi}_0 = -4.817$ and $\hat{\phi}_1 = 0.031$. In particular, the positive estimate of ϕ_1 confirms that high responders are progressively selected out by the dropout process. Within this assumed dropout model, the log-likelihood ratio statistic to test the sub-model with $\beta_1 = 0$ is $D = 103.3$ on 1 degree of freedom, which is overwhelmingly significant. We therefore reject completely random dropout in favour of random dropout. At this stage, the earlier results for the measurement process obtained by ignoring the dropout process remain valid, as they rely only on the dropout process being either completely random or random.

Within the random dropout framework, we now consider two possible extensions to the model: including a dependence on the previous measurement but one; and including a dependence on the treatment allocation. Thus, we replace (13.8.2) by

$$\text{logit}(p_{ij}) = \beta_{0k} + \beta_1 y_{i,j-1} + \beta_2 y_{i,j-2}, \tag{13.8.3}$$

where $k = k(i)$ denotes the treatment allocation for the ith subject. Both extensions yield a significant improvement in the log-likelihood, as indicated in the first three lines of Table 13.6.

Table 13.6. Maximized log-likelihoods under different dropout models.

$\text{logit}(p_{ij})$	Log-likelihood
$\beta_0 + \beta_1 y_{i,j-1}$	−20743.85
$\beta_0 + \beta_1 y_{i,j-1} + \beta_2 y_{i,j-2}$	−20728.51
$\beta_{0k} + \beta_1 y_{i,j-1} + \beta_2 y_{i,j-2}$	−20724.73
$\beta_{0k} + \gamma y_{ij} + \beta_1 y_{i,j-1} + \beta_2 y_{i,j-2}$	−20721.03

Finally, we test the random dropout assumption by embedding (13.8.3) within the informative dropout model

$$\text{logit}(p_{ij}) = \beta_{0k} + \gamma y_{ij} + \beta_1 y_{i,j-1} + \beta_2 y_{i,j-2}. \qquad (13.8.4)$$

From lines 3 and 4 of Table 13.6 we compute the log-likelihood ratio statistic to test the sub-model of (13.8.4) with $\gamma = 0$ as $D = 7.4$ on 1 degree of freedom This corresponds to a p-value of 0.007, leading us to reject the random dropout assumption in favour of informative dropout.

We emphasize at this point that rejection of random dropout is necessarily pre-conditioned by the particular modelling framework adopted, as a consequence of the Molenberghs *et al.* (1997) result. Nevertheless, the unequivocal rejection of random dropout within this modelling framework suggests that we should establish whether the conclusions regarding the measurement process are materially affected by whether or not we assume random dropout. Table 13.7 shows the estimates of the covariance parameters under the random and informative dropout models. Some of the numerical changes are substantial, but the values of the fitted variogram within the range of time-lags encompassed by the data are almost identical, as is demonstrated in Fig. 13.8.

Of more direct practical importance in this example is the inference concerning the mean response. Under the random dropout assumption, a linear hypothesis concerning the mean response profiles can be tested using either a generalized likelihood ratio statistic, comparing the maximized log-likelihoods for the two models in question, or a quadratic form based on the approximate multivariate normal sampling distribution of the estimated mean parameters in the full model. Under the informative dropout assumption, only the first of these methods is available, because the current methodology does not provide standard errors for the estimated treatment effects within the informative dropout model.

Under the random dropout model (13.8.3), the generalized likelihood ratio statistic to test the hypothesis of no difference between the three mean response profiles is $D = 42.32$ on 6 degrees of freedom, whereas under the

Table 13.7. Maximum likelihood estimates of covariance parameters under random dropout and informative dropout models.

	Parameter			
Dropout	σ^2	α_1	α_2	α_3
Random	170.091	0.560	0.951	0.056
Informative	137.400	0.755	1.277	0.070

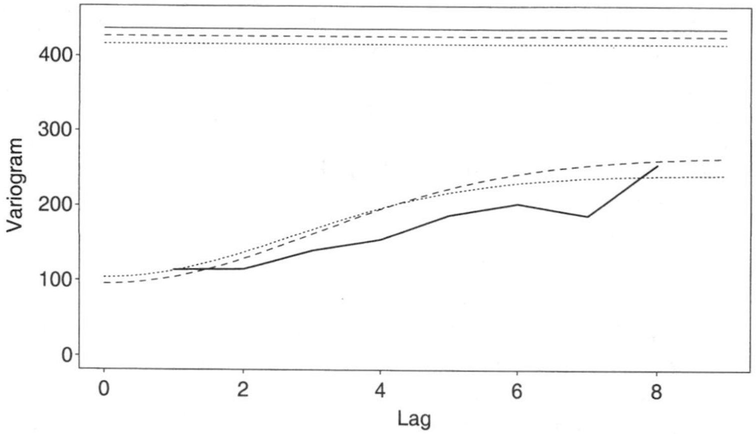

Fig. 13.8. The estimated variogram for the schizophrenia trial data (——), together with fitted parametric models assuming random dropouts (- - - - - -) and informative dropouts (……).

informative dropout model (13.8.4), the corresponding statistic is $D = 35.02$. The conclusion that the mean response profiles differ significantly between treatment groups is therefore unchanged. The estimated treatment effects also do not change substantially, relative to their estimated standard errors, when we move from the random dropout model to the informative dropout model. For each parameter, the absolute difference between the estimates under informative and under random dropout assumptions is less than the standard error of the estimate under the random dropout assumption.

Finally, to emphasize how the dependence between the measurement and dropout processes affects the interpretation of the observed mean response profiles, Fig. 13.9 compares the observed means in the three treatment groups with their simulated counterparts, calculated from a simulated realization of the fitted informative dropout model with 10 000 subjects in each treatment group. In contrast to Fig. 13.7, these fitted means *should* correspond to the observed means if the model fits the data well. The correspondence is reasonably close. The contrast between Figs. 13.7 and 13.9 encapsulates the important practical difference between an analysis which ignores the dropouts and one which takes account of them. By comparison, the distinction between the random dropout model (13.8.3) and the informative dropout model (13.8.4) is much less important.

In summary, our conclusions for the schizophrenia trial data are the following. Figure 13.9 demonstrates that all three treatment groups show a downward trend in the mean PANSS score conditional on not having

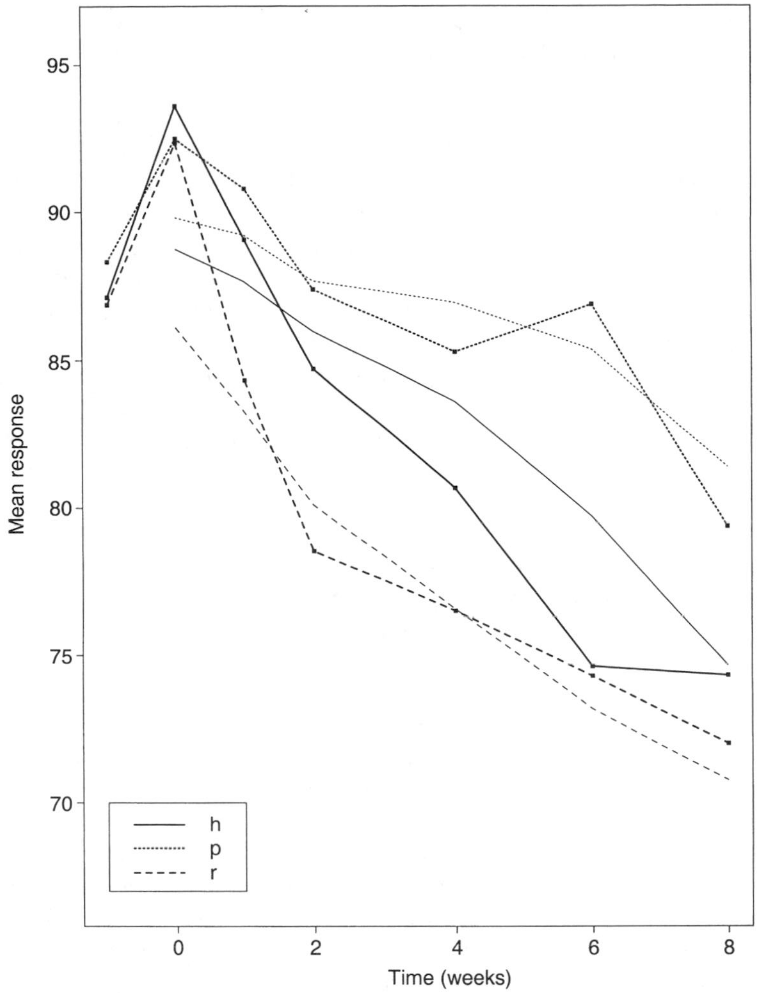

Fig. 13.9. Observed means in the placebo (**......**), haloperidol (——) and risperidone (**- - - - - -**) treatment groups, compared with simulated means conditional on not yet having dropped out (......, —— and - - - - - -, respectively), from an informative dropout model.

dropped out of the study; the reduction in the mean PANSS score between baseline and 8 weeks is from 86.1 to 70.8. If we want to adjust for the selection effect of the dropouts, the relevant fitted means are those shown in Fig. 13.7. In this case, the fitted mean PANSS score is almost constant in the placebo group but still shows a downward trend in each of the two active treatment groups. The 'on-average' change between baseline and 8 weeks in the risperidone group is now from 86.5 to 71.4. In view of the fact that the majority of dropouts are the result of an inadequate response, and that this artificially deflates the observed average PANSS score, we would argue that the fitted curves in Fig. 13.7 are more appropriate indicators of the biochemical effectiveness of the treatments than are those in Fig. 13.9. From either point of view, risperidone achieves a lower mean PANSS score than haloperidol throughout the trial, and the estimated mean reduction between baseline and 8 weeks comes close to the 20% criterion which is regarded as demonstrating a clinical improvement. With regard to the dropout process, there is significant variation in the dropout rates between the three treatment groups, with the highest rates in the placebo group and the lowest in the risperidone group. There is also significant evidence that, *within the selection modelling framework represented by equation (13.8.4)*, the dropout mechanism is informative. However, this does not materially affect the conclusions regarding the mean PANSS scores by comparison with the analysis under a random dropout assumption.

13.9 Discussion

There is fast-growing literature on dealing with dropouts in longitudinal studies, and the review in this chapter is necessarily incomplete. A useful introduction, from a somewhat different perspective to ours, is Little (1995).

An emerging consensus is that analysis of data with potentially informative dropouts necessarily involves assumptions which are difficult, or even impossible, to check from the observed data. Copas and Li (1997) reach a similar conclusion in their discussion of inference based on non-random samples. This suggests that it would be unwise to rely on the precise conclusions of an analysis based on a particular informative dropout model. This of course should not be taken as an excuse for avoiding the issue, but it may well be that the major practical value of informative dropout models is in sensitivity analysis, to provide some protection against the possibility that conclusions reached from a random dropout model are critically dependent on the validity of this stronger assumption. The discussion published alongside Scharfstein *et al.* (2000) contains a range of views on how such sensitivity analyses might be conducted.

One striking feature of longitudinal data with dropouts, which we first encountered with the simulated example in Section 13.3, is the frequent divergence of observed and fitted means when dropouts are ignored. This arises with likelihood-based methods of analysis when the dropout mechanism is not completely random and (as is almost universal in our experience) the data are correlated. In these circumstances, the likelihood implicitly recognizes the progressive selectivity of the non-dropout sub-population and adjusts its mean estimates accordingly. In fact, this represents a rather general counterexample to the commonly held view that ordinary least squares regression, which ignores the correlation structure of the data, usually gives acceptable estimates of the mean response function. As we have emphasized in the earlier sections of this chapter, the difficulty with ordinary least squares in this context lies not so much in the method itself (which is, of course, unbiased for the mean irrespective of the true correlation structure), but rather in a failure to specify precisely what is the required estimand.

Our discussion in this chapter has focused on linear, Gaussian measurement models, both for convenience of exposition and because it is the context in which most progress has been made with respect to the analysis of data with potentially informative dropouts. However, the ideas extend to discrete response models, as do the attendant complications of interpretation. Kenward *et al.* (1994) and Molenberghs *et al.* (1997) discuss selection models for discrete longitudinal data under random and informative dropout assumptions, respectively. Fitzmaurice *et al.* (1996) discuss both random and informative dropout mechanisms in conjunction with a binary response variable, with particular emphasis on the resulting problems of non-identifiability. Follman and Wu (1995) extend random effect models for dropout to discrete responses.

Generalized linear mixed models (Breslow and Clayton, 1993) provide an extension of linear Gaussian selection modelling ideas to discrete or categorical response as follows. Consider the linear model for a continuous response variable,

$$Y_{ij} = \mu_{ij} + d'_{ij}\boldsymbol{U}_i + W_i(t_{ij}) + Z_{ij},$$

in which $\mu_{ij} = \mathrm{E}[Y_{ij}]$, $\boldsymbol{U}_i$ is a vector of random effects for the ith subject with associated explanatory variables d_{ij}, $W_i(t)$ is a serially correlated random process for the ith subject and Z_{ij} is a set of mutually independent measurement errors. This can be trivially re-expressed as a set of conditional distributions for the Y_{ij} given the $\boldsymbol{U}_i$ and the $W_i(t)$ as

$$Y_{ij} \mid \boldsymbol{U}_i, W_i(t) \sim \mathrm{N}(\mu_{ij} + d'_{ij}\boldsymbol{U}_i + W_i(t_{ij}), \tau^2), \qquad (13.9.1)$$

where $\tau^2 = \mathrm{Var}(Z_{ij})$ and the Y_{ij} are mutually independent conditional on the $\boldsymbol{U}_i$ and the $W_i(t)$. To turn this into a generalized linear *mixed* model for a discrete or categorical response, we simply replace the Gaussian conditional in (13.9.1) by a more appropriate distribution, for example the Poisson for a count response, together with a suitable link function to transform the linear predictor, $\eta_{ij} = \mu_{ij} + d'_{ij}\boldsymbol{U}_i + W_i(t_{ij})$, onto the whole of the real line. To allow for informative dropout, we could then posit a model for the relationship between the η_{ij} and corresponding dropout probabilities. Models of this kind, in which the linear predictor η is a function of unobserved random variables, may be very useful for thinking about the kinds of mechanisms which could induce informative dropout behaviour. Modelling the probability of dropout conditional on η is a form of random effects modelling as defined in Section 13.7.3. Because η is a function of unobserved random variables $\boldsymbol{U}$ and $W(t)$, these models generally equate to informative dropout, and earlier remarks about the need to consider the sensitivity of conclusions to specific assumptions about the dropout mechanism continue to apply. More fundamentally, the example of Murray and Findlay (1988) reminds us that dropout can in some cases be directly related to observed measurements, whether or not these include a measurement error component.

Much of the above discussion is only indirectly relevant to the problems raised by intermittent missing values, which can be rather different in character from dropouts.

Intermittent missing values can arise through explicitly stated censoring rules. For example, values outside a stated range may be simply unreliable because of the limitations of the measuring techniques in use – this is a feature of many bioassay techniques. Methods for handling censored data are very well established in survival analysis (e.g. Cox and Oakes, 1984; Lawless, 1982), and have been developed more recently for the types of correlated data structures which arise with longitudinal data (Laird, 1988; Hughes, 1999).

When censoring is not an issue, it may be reasonable to assume that intermittent missing values are either completely random or random, in which case a likelihood-based analysis ignoring the missing values should give the relevant inferences. An exception would be in longitudinal clinical trials with voluntary compliance, where a patient may miss an appointment because they are feeling particularly unwell on the day. From a practical point of view, the fact that subjects with intermittent missing values remain in the study means that there should be more opportunity to ascertain the reasons for the missingness, and to take corrective action accordingly, than is often the case with dropouts who are lost to follow-up.

Perhaps the most important conclusion from this chapter is that if dropouts are *not* completely random we need to think carefully about what the relevant inferences are. Do we want to know about the dropout process; or about the conditional distribution of the measurements given that the unit has not dropped out; or about the distribution that the measurements would follow in the absence of dropouts? Diggle and Kenward (1994) used their model to investigate some of the consequences of informative dropouts. Using simulated data, they showed that wrongly treating informative dropouts as random dropouts introduces bias into parameter estimates, and that likelihood-based methods can be used to identify informative dropout processes from data sets of a realistic size. A much more difficult problem is to identify a unique model for any real dataset, where all aspects of the model are unknown *a priori* and, as we have suggested above, random or informative dropout processes may be partially confounded with time-trends in the mean response.

14
Additional topics

The field of longitudinal data analysis continues to develop. In this chapter, we give a short introduction to several topics, each of which can be pursued in greater detail through the literature cited.

14.1 Non-parametric modelling of the mean response

The case study on log-bodyweights of cows, discussed in Section 5.4, introduced the idea of describing the mean response profile non-parametrically. There, the approach was to use a separate value for the mean response at each time-point, with no attempt to link the mean responses at different times. This assumes firstly that the complete mean response curve is not of direct interest, and secondly that the times of measurement are common to all, or at least to a reasonable number, of the units, so as to give the required replication at each time. An instance in which neither of these assumptions holds is provided by the CD4+ data of Example 1.1. For these data, the CD4+ count as a function of time since seroconversion is of direct interest, and the sets of times of measurement are essentially unique to each person in the study. To handle this situation, we now consider how to fit *smooth* non-parametric models to the mean response profile as a function of time, whilst continuing to recognize the covariance structure within units.

In Section 3.3, we discussed the use of smooth, non-parametric curves as exploratory tools, drawing mainly on well-established methods for cross-sectional data. If we want to use these methods for confirmatory analyses, we need to consider more carefully how the correlation structure of longitudinal data impinges on considerations of how much to smooth the data, and how to make inferences.

To develop ideas, we assume that there are no experimental treatments or other explanatory variables. The data can be represented as $\{(y_{ij}, t_{ij}),\ j = 1, \ldots, n_i;\ i = 1, \ldots, m\}$, where n_i is the number of measurements on the ith of m units. We write $N = \sum_{i=1}^{m} n_i$ for the total number of measurements. Our model for the data takes the form

$$Y_{ij} = \mu(t_{ij}) + \epsilon_i(t_{ij}),$$

where $\{\epsilon_i(t),\ t \in R\}$ for $i = 1, \ldots, m$ are independent copies of a stationary random process, $\{\epsilon(t)\}$, with variance σ^2 and correlation function $\rho(u)$, and the mean response, $\mu(t)$, is a smooth function of t.

A simple, and intuitively appealing, non-parametric estimate of $\mu(t)$ is a weighted average of the data, with large weights given to measurements at times t_{ij} which are close to t. To implement this idea, we define a *kernel function*, $K(u)$, to be a symmetric, non-negative valued function taking large values close to $u = 0$ and small values when $|u|$ is large. For example, in what follows we use the Gaussian kernel,

$$K(u) = \exp(-u^2/2), \qquad (14.1.1)$$

as in Section 3.3. Now, choose a positive number, h, and define weights

$$w^*_{ij}(t) = h^{-1}K\{(t_{ij} - t)/h\}. \qquad (14.1.2)$$

Note that $w^*_{ij}(t)$ is large when t_{ij} is close to t and vice versa, and that the rate at which the $w^*_{ij}(t)$ decrease as $|t_{ij} - t|$ increases is governed by the value of h, a small value giving a rapid decrease. Define standardized weights,

$$w_{ij}(t) = w^*_{ij}(t)\left\{\sum_{i=1}^{m}\sum_{j=1}^{n_i} w^*_{ij}(t)\right\}^{-1},$$

so that $\sum_{i=1}^{m}\sum_{j=1}^{n_i} w_{ij}(t) = 1$ for any value of t. Then, a non-parametric estimate of $\mu(t)$ is

$$\hat{\mu}(t) = \sum_{i=1}^{m}\sum_{j=1}^{n_i} w_{ij}(t)y_{ij}. \qquad (14.1.3)$$

A useful refinement of (14.1.3) is an adaptive kernel estimator, in which we replace the constant, h, by a function of t such that $h(t)$ is small when there is a high density of data close to t, and vice versa. This is consistent with the view that for data which are highly replicated at a fixed set of times, the observed average at time t is a reasonable non-parametric estimate of $\mu(t)$ without any smoothing over a range of neighbouring times, that is, in effect setting $h = 0$. Also, using a function $h(t)$ with this qualitative behaviour can be shown more generally to improve the estimates of $\mu(t)$. See, for example, Silverman (1984) who demonstrates that a variable kernel estimate is approximately equivalent to a smoothing spline. In the remainder of this section, we consider in detail the case of a constant value of h. The essential ideas apply also to the case of adaptive kernel estimation where, typically, the function $h(t)$ is indexed by a scalar quantity, b say, which controls the overall degree of smoothing and takes on the role played by the constant h in non-adaptive kernel estimation.

While the choice of h has a direct and major impact on the resulting estimate $\hat{\mu}(t)$, the choice of kernel function is generally held to be of secondary importance. The Gaussian kernel (14.1.1) is intuitively sensible but not uniquely compelling.

Estimators of this kind were introduced by Priestley and Chao (1972) for independent data, and have been studied in the longitudinal data setting by Hart and Wehrly (1986), Müller (1988), Altman (1990), Rice and Silverman (1991), and Hart (1991). From our point of view, the most important question concerns the choice of h. In some applications, it will be sensible to choose h to have a particular substantive interpretation; for example, smoothing over a 'natural' time-window such as a day if we wish to eliminate ciradian variation. If we want to choose h automatically from the data, the main message from the above-cited work is that a good choice of h depends on the correlation structure of the data, and in particular that methods for choosing h based on a false assumption of independence between measurements can give very misleading results.

Rice and Silverman (1991) give an elegant, cross-validatory prescription for choosing h which makes no assumptions about the underlying correlation structure. Their detailed results are for smoothing spline estimates of $\mu(t)$, but the method is easily adaptable to kernel estimates. For a given h, let $\hat{\mu}^{(k)}(t)$ be the estimate of $\mu(t)$ obtained from (14.1.3) but omitting the kth subject, thus

$$\hat{\mu}^{(k)} = \sum_{i \neq k} \sum_{j=1}^{n_i} w_{ij}^{(k)}(t) y_{ij},$$

where $w_{ij}^{(k)}(t) = w_{ij}^*(t) / \left\{ \sum_{i \neq k} \sum_{j=1}^{n_i} w_{ij}^*(t) \right\}$. Then, the Rice and Silverman prescription chooses h to minimize the quantity

$$S(h) = \sum_{i=1}^{m} \sum_{j=1}^{n_i} \left\{ y_{ij} - \hat{\mu}^{(i)}(t_{ij}) \right\}^2 . \tag{14.1.4}$$

The rationale for minimizing (14.1.4) is that it is estimating the mean square error of $\hat{\mu}(t)$ for $\mu(t)$ averaged across the design points, t_{ij}, up to an additive constant which does not depend on h. To see this, write

$$\mathrm{E}\left[\{ y_{ij} - \hat{\mu}^{(i)}(t_{ij}) \}^2 \right] = \mathrm{E}\left[\left(\{ y_{ij} - \mu(t_{ij}) \} + \{ \mu(t_{ij}) - \hat{\mu}^{(i)}(t_{ij}) \} \right)^2 \right]$$

and expand the right-hand side into the following three terms:

$$\mathrm{E}\left[\{y_{ij}-\mu(t_{ij})\}^2\right]+2\mathrm{E}\left[\{y_{ij}-\mu(t_{ij})\}\{\mu(t_{ij})-\hat{\mu}^{(i)}(t_{ij})\}\right]$$
$$+\,\mathrm{E}\left[\{\mu(t_{ij})-\hat{\mu}^{(i)}\}^2\right].$$

Now, the first of the three terms in this expression is equal to $\mathrm{Var}(y_{ij})$ and does not depend on h, while the second is zero because $\mathrm{E}(y_{ij})=\mu(t_{ij})$ and y_{ij} is independent of $\hat{\mu}^{(i)}(t_{ij})$, by construction. Thus,

$$\mathrm{E}\left[\{y_{ij}-\hat{\mu}^{(i)}(t_{ij})\}^2\right]=\mathrm{Var}(y_{ij})+\mathrm{MSE}^{(i)}(t_{ij},h), \qquad (14.1.5)$$

where $\mathrm{MSE}^{(i)}(t,h)$ is the mean square error of $\hat{\mu}^{(i)}(t)$ for $\mu(t)$. Substitution of (14.1.5) into (14.1.4) gives the result.

One interesting thing about the Rice and Silverman prescription is that it does not explicitly involve the covariance structure of the data. However, this structure is accommodated implicitly by the device of leaving out all observations from a single subject in defining the criterion $S(h)$, whereas the standard method of cross-validation would leave out single observations to define a criterion

$$S_0(h)=\sum_{i=1}^{m}\sum_{j=1}^{n_i}\left\{y_{ij}-\hat{\mu}^{(ij)}(t_{ij})\right\}^2.$$

Direct computation of (14.1.4) would be very time-consuming with large numbers of subjects. An easier computation, again adapted from Rice and Silverman (1991), is the following. To simplify the notation, we temporarily suppress the dependence of $w_{ij}(t)$ on t, and write $w_i=\sum_{j=1}^{n_i}w_{ij}$, so that $\sum_{i=1}^{m}w_i=1$. Note that

$$\begin{aligned}
y_{ij}-\hat{\mu}^{(i)}(t_{ij}) &= y_{ij}-\left\{\hat{\mu}(t_{ij})-\sum_{j=1}^{n_i}w_{ij}y_{ij}\right\}\Big/(1-w_i)\\
&= y_{ij}-\left\{\hat{\mu}(t_{ij})-\sum_{j=1}^{n_i}w_{ij}y_{ij}\right\}\{1+w_i/(1-w_i)\}\\
&= \{y_{ij}-\hat{\mu}(t_{ij})\}+\{w_i/(1-w_i)\}\\
&\quad\times\left\{\sum_{j=1}^{n_i}w_{ij}y_{ij}/w_i-\hat{\mu}(t_{ij})\right\}.
\end{aligned} \qquad (14.1.6)$$

Using (14.1.6) to compute $S(h)$ avoids the need for explicit computation of the m leave-one-out estimates, $\hat{\mu}^{(i)}(t)$. Further, computational savings can be made by collecting the time-points, t_{ij}, into a reduced set, say t_r, $r = 1, \ldots, p$, and computing only the p estimates $\hat{\mu}(t_r)$ for each value of h.

To make inferences about $\hat{\mu}(t)$, we need to know the covariance structure of the data. Let V be the $N \times N$ block-diagonal covariance matrix of the data, where $N = \sum_{i=1}^{m} n_i$. For fixed h, the estimate $\hat{\mu}(t)$ defined by (14.1.3) is a linear combination of the data-vector $\boldsymbol{y}$, say $\hat{\mu}(t) = \boldsymbol{w}(t)'\boldsymbol{y}$. Now, for p values $t_r, r = 1, \ldots, p$, let $\hat{\boldsymbol{\mu}}$ be the vector with rth element $\hat{\mu}(t_r)$, and W the $p \times N$ matrix with rth row $\boldsymbol{w}(t_r)$. Then,

$$\hat{\boldsymbol{\mu}} = W\boldsymbol{y}, \tag{14.1.7}$$

and $\hat{\boldsymbol{\mu}}$ has an approximate multivariate Gaussian sampling distribution with

$$\mathrm{E}(\hat{\boldsymbol{\mu}}) = W\mathrm{E}(\boldsymbol{y})$$

and

$$\mathrm{Var}(\hat{\boldsymbol{\mu}}) = WVW'. \tag{14.1.8}$$

Note that in general, $\hat{\mu}(t)$ is a biased estimator for $\mu(t)$, but that the bias will be small if h is small so that the weights, w_{ij}, decay quickly to zero with increasing $|t_{ij} - t|$. Conversely, the variance of $\hat{\mu}(t)$ typically increases as h decreases. The need to balance bias against variance is characteristic of non-parametric smoothing problems, and explains the use of a mean-squared-error criterion for choosing h automatically from the data. In practice, a sensible choice of h is one which tends to zero as the number of subjects increases, in which case the bias becomes negligible, and we can use (14.1.8) to attach standard errors to the estimates $\hat{\mu}(t)$.

The covariance structure of the data can be estimated from the time-sequences of residuals, $r_{ij} = y_{ij} - \hat{\mu}(t_{ij})$. In particular, the empirical variogram of the r_{ij} can be used to formulate an appropriate model. Likelihood-based estimation of parameters in the assumed covariance structure is somewhat problematical. From a practical point of view, the computations will be extensive if the number of subjects is large and there is little replication of the observation times, t_{ij}, which is precisely the situation in which non-parametric smoothing is most likely required. Also, the absence of a parametric model for the mean puts the inference on a rather shaky foundation. Simple curve-fitting (moment) estimates of covariance parameters may be preferable.

A final point to note is that expressions (14.1.7) and (14.1.8) for the mean vector and variance matrix of $\hat{\boldsymbol{\mu}}$ assume that both V and the value of h are specified without reference to the data. The effect of estimating parameters in V will be small when the number of units is large, whilst the effect of calculating h from the data should also be small when $\mu(t)$ is a smooth function although the theoretical issues are less well understood here. The references cited above give detailed discussion of these and other issues.

We now consider how the analysis can be extended to incorporate experimental treatments. For a non-parametric analysis, we can simply apply the method separately to subjects from each treatment group. From an interpretive point of view, it is preferable to use a common value of the smoothing constant, h. When the data are from an experiment comparing several treatments, the mean-squared-error criterion (14.1.4) for choosing h consists of a sum of contributions from within each treatment group. Covariance structure is estimated from the empirical variogram of the residuals pooled across treatment groups, assuming a common covariance structure in all groups.

Another possibility is to model treatment contrasts parametrically using a linear model. This gives the following semi-parametric specification of a model for the complete set of data,

$$Y_{ij} = \boldsymbol{x}'_{ij}\boldsymbol{\beta} + \mu(t_{ij}) + \epsilon_i(t_{ij}), \tag{14.1.9}$$

where $\boldsymbol{x}_{ij}$ is a p-element vector of covariates. This formulation also covers situations in which explanatory variables other than indicators of treatment group are relevant, as will be the case in many observational studies. For the extended model (14.1.9), the kernel method for estimating $\mu(t)$ can be combined iteratively with a generalized least squares calculation for $\hat{\boldsymbol{\beta}}$, as follows:

1. Given the current estimate, $\hat{\boldsymbol{\beta}}$, calculate residuals, $r_{ij} = y_{ij} - \boldsymbol{x}'_{ij}\hat{\boldsymbol{\beta}}$, and use these in place of y_{ij} to calculate a kernel estimate, $\hat{\mu}(t)$.
2. Given $\hat{\mu}$, calculate residuals, $r_{ij} = y_{ij} - \hat{\mu}(t)$, and update the estimate $\hat{\boldsymbol{\beta}}$ using generalized least squares,

   $$\hat{\boldsymbol{\beta}} = (X'V^{-1}X)^{-1}X'V^{-1}\boldsymbol{r},$$

   where X is the $N \times p$ matrix with rows $\boldsymbol{x}'_{ij}, V$ is the assumed block-diagonal covariance matrix of the data and $\boldsymbol{r}$ is the vector of residuals, r_{ij}.
3. Repeat steps (1) and (2) to convergence.

This algorithm is an example of the back-fitting algorithm described by Hastie and Tibshirani (1990). Typically, few iterations are required unless there is a near-confounding between the linear and non-parametric parts of the model. This might well happen if, for example, we included a polynomial time-trend in the linear part. Further details of the algorithm, and a discussion of the asymptotic properties of the resulting estimators, are given in Zeger and Diggle (1994) and Moyeed and Diggle (1994).

Example 14.1. Estimation of the population mean CD4+ curve

For the CD4+ data, there are $N = 2376$ observations of CD4+ cell numbers on $m = 369$ men infected with the HIV virus. Recall that time is measured in years with the origin at the date of seroconversion, which is known approximately for each individual. As in our earlier, parametric analysis of these data, we include the following explanatory variables in the linear part of the model: smoking (packs per day); recreational drug use (yes/no); numbers of sexual partners; and depressive symptoms as measured by the CESD scale. For the non-parametric part of the model, we use a mildly adaptive kernel estimator, with $h(t) = b\{f(t)\}^{-0.25}$, where $f(t)$ is a crude estimate of the local density of observations times, t_{ij}, and b is chosen by cross-validation, as described above.

Figure 14.1 shows the data with the estimate $\hat{\mu}(t)$ and pointwise confidence limits calculated as plus and minus two standard errors. The standard errors were calculated from a parametric model for the covariance structure of the kind introduced in Section 5.2.3. We assume that the variance of each measurement is $\tau^2 + \sigma^2 + \nu^2$ and that the variogram within each unit is $\gamma(u) = \tau^2 + \sigma^2\{1 - \exp(-\alpha u)\}$. Figure 14.2 shows the empirical variogram and a parametric fit obtained by an *ad hoc* procedure, which gave estimates $\hat{\tau}^2 = 14.1$, $\hat{\sigma}^2 = 16.1$, $\hat{\nu}^2 = 6.9$, and $\hat{\alpha} = 0.22$.

Figure 14.1 suggests that the mean number of CD4+ cells is approximately constant at close to 1000 cells prior to seroconversion. Within the first six months after seroconversion, the mean drops to around 700. Subsequently, the rate of loss is much slower. For example, it takes nearly three years before the mean number reaches 500, the level at which, at the

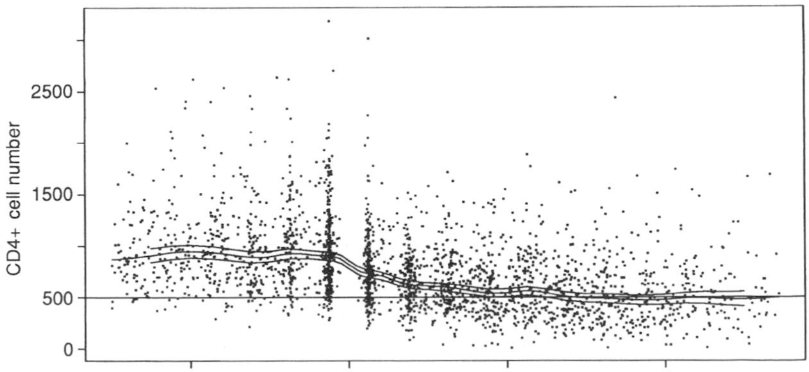

Fig. 14.1. CD4+ cell counts with kernel estimate and pointwise confidence limits for the mean response profile.

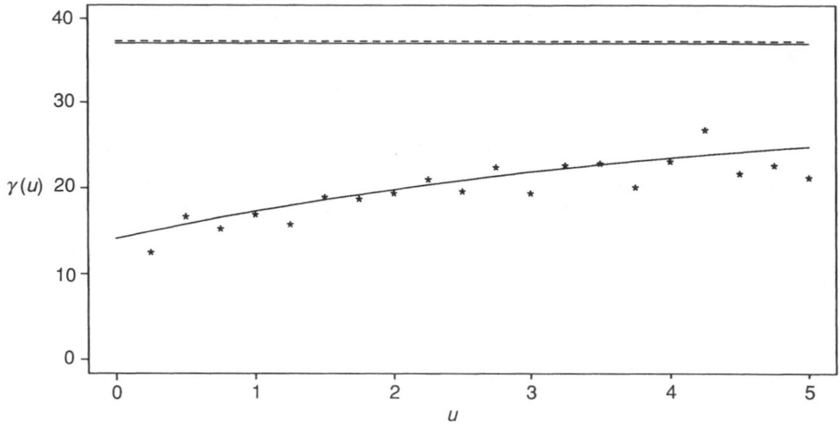

Fig. 14.2. CD4+ cell counts: observed and fitted variograms $\star$: sample variogram – – –: sample variance ——: fitted model.

time the data were collected, it was recommended that prophylactic AZT therapy should begin (Volberding *et al.*, 1990). As with Example 5.1 on the protein contents of milk samples, the interpretation of the fitted mean response is complicated by the possibility that subjects who become very ill may drop out of the study, and these subjects may also have unusually low CD4+ counts.

14.1.1 *Further reading*

Non- and semi-parametric methods for longitudinal data are areas of current research activity. See Brumback and Rice (1998), Wang (1998), and Zhang *et al.* (1998) for methods based on smoothing splines. Lin and Carroll (2000) develop methods based on local polynomial kernal regression, and Lin and Ying (2001) consider methods for irregularly spaced longitudinal data.

14.2 Non-linear regression modelling

In this section, we consider how to extend the framework of Chapter 5 to non-linear models for the mean response. Davidian and Giltinan (1995) give a much more detailed account of this topic. Another useful review, from a somewhat different perspective, is Glasbey (1988).

The cross-sectional form of the non-linear regression model is

$$Y_i = \mu(x_i; \beta) + Z_i \quad i = 1, \ldots, n, \tag{14.2.1}$$

where the Z_i are mutually independent deviations from the mean response and are assumed to be normally distributed with mean zero and common variance σ^2, whilst the mean response function, $\mu(\cdot)$, is a non-linear function of explanatory variables x_i measured on the ith subject and parameters β. For example, an exponential growth model with a single explanatory variable x would specify

$$\mu(x; \beta_1, \beta_2) = \beta_1 \exp(\beta_2 x).$$

Some non-linear models can be converted to a superficially linear form by transformation. For example, the simple exponential growth model above can be expressed as

$$\mu^*(x; \beta_1^*, \beta_2) = \beta_1^* + \beta_2 x,$$

where $\mu^*(\cdot) = \log \mu(\cdot)$ and $\beta_1^* = \log \beta_1$. However, it would not then be consistent with the original, non-linear formulation simply to add an assumed zero-mean, constant variance error term to define the linear regression model,

$$Y^* = \mu^*(x; \beta^*) + Z_i^* \quad i = 1, \ldots, n,$$

as this would be equivalent to assuming a multiplicative, rather than additive, error term on the unlogged scale. Moreover, there are many forms of non-linear regression model for which no transformation of $\mu(\cdot), \beta$ and/or x can yield an equivalent linear model.

Methods for fitting the model (14.2.1) to cross-sectional data are described in Bates and Watts (1988).

In the longitudinal setting, we make the notational extension to

$$Y_{ij} = \mu(x_{ij}; \beta) + Z_{ij} \quad j = 1, \ldots, n_i; \;\; i = 1, \ldots, n, \tag{14.2.2}$$

where, as usual, i indexes subjects and j occasions within subjects, and consider two generalizations of the cross-sectional model:

1. *Correlated error structures* – the sequence of deviations Z_{ij}: $j = 1, \ldots, n_i$ within the ith subject may be correlated;
2. *Non-linear random effects* – one or more of the regression parameters β may be modelled as subject-specific stochastic perturbations of a population average value, thus in (14.2.2) β is replaced by a random vector $\boldsymbol{B}_i$, realised independently for each subject from a distribution (usually assumed to be multivariate Gaussian) with mean β and variance matrix V_β.

Recall that in the linear case considered in Chapter 5, we could treat these two cases as one, because in that context the assumption of randomly varying subject-specific parameters leaves the population mean response unchanged and affects only the form of the covariance structure of the Y_{ij}.

For non-linear models, as for the generalized linear models dicussed in Chapter 7, the two cases have different implications, both for statistical analysis and for the interpretation of the model parameters.

14.2.1 *Correlated errors*

The model of interest is (14.2.2), with a parametric specification for the covariance structure of the Z_{ij}. Let $\boldsymbol{Z}_i = (Z_{i1}, \ldots, Z_{i,n_i})$ denote the vector of Z_{ij} associated with the ith subject, and $\boldsymbol{t}_i = (t_{i1}, \ldots, t_{i,n_i})$ the corresponding vector of measurement times. We assume that $\boldsymbol{Z}_i$ follows a multivariate Gaussian distribution with mean zero and variance matrix $V_i(\boldsymbol{t}_i; \alpha)$.

For exploratory analysis, we can use the general approach described in Chapter 3 to identify suitable parametric families for the mean function $\mu(\cdot)$ and the covariance matrices $V_i(\boldsymbol{t}_i; \alpha)$. However, often the reason for adopting a non-linear model will be that a particular form for $\mu(\cdot)$ is suggested by the scientific context in which the data arise. For example, in pharmaco-kinetic studies, $\mu(\cdot)$ is often obtained as the solution to a differential equation model of the underlying biochemical processes involved (Gibaldi and Perrier, 1982). The form of the covariance matrices $V_i(\boldsymbol{t}_i; \alpha)$ may also be derived from an explicit stochastic model but this appears to be rare in practice. More commonly, the correlation structure is chosen empirically to provide a reasonable fit to the data, its role being to ensure approximately valid inferences about $\mu(\cdot)$. If this is the case, it would be appropriate to develop the model for the $V_i(\cdot)$ from the variogram of the ordinary (nonlinear) least squares residuals after fitting the chosen parametric model for $\mu(\cdot)$.

Once parametric forms have been chosen for the mean and covariance structure, the log-likelihood function for the complete set of model parameters (β, α) follows as

$$L(\alpha, \beta) = \sum_{i=1}^{m} L_i(\alpha, \beta), \tag{14.2.3}$$

where

$$-2L_i(\alpha, \beta) = \log \mid V_i(\boldsymbol{t}_i; \alpha) \mid + (\boldsymbol{Y}_i - \mu_i)' V_i(\boldsymbol{t}_i; \alpha)^{-1} (\boldsymbol{Y}_i - \mu_i), \tag{14.2.4}$$

$\boldsymbol{Y}_i$ is the n_i-element vector with jth element Y_{ij} and μ_i is the n_i-element vector with jth element $\mu(x_{ij}; \beta)$.

Likelihood-based inference follows according to the same general principles as for the linear models discussed in Chapter 5 although, in the non-linear setting, there is not the same opportunity to exploit the existence of an explicit solution for $\hat{\beta}$ conditional on α.

14.2.2 *Non-linear random effects*

In this second generalization of the cross-sectional non-linear regression model, equation (14.2.2) is assumed to hold conditionally on the regression parameters β, which are then allowed to vary randomly between subjects. Thus, for the ith subject the parameter β is replaced by B_i, where the B_i for different subjects are mutually independent multivariate Gaussian random variables with common mean β and variance matrix V_β.

Let $\boldsymbol{b} = (b_1, \ldots, b_m)$ denote the set of realized values of $B_1, \ldots, B_m$. Then, the likelihood function for the model parameters α, β, and V_β is obtained by taking the expectation of the conditional likelihood given $\boldsymbol{b}$ with respect to the assumed multivariate Gaussian distribution of $\boldsymbol{b}$. Thus, if $\ell_i(\alpha, \boldsymbol{b}) = \exp L_i(\alpha, \boldsymbol{b})$, where $L_i(\cdot)$ is the contribution to the conditional log-likelihood from a single subject, as defined by (14.2.4), then the overall log-likelihood for the random effects model applied to data on m subjects is

$$L(\alpha, \beta, V_\beta) = \sum_{i=1}^{m} \log \int \ell_i(\alpha, \boldsymbol{b}) f(\boldsymbol{b}; \beta, V_\beta)\, \mathrm{d}\boldsymbol{b}, \tag{14.2.5}$$

where $f(\cdot)$ denotes the multivariate Gaussian density with mean β and variance matrix V_β.

Exact likelihood calculations for this model therefore require repeated numerical evaluation of an integral whose dimension is equal to p, the number of elements of β. While this task is computationally feasible for typical values of p it would require a specially written program for each particular class of non-linear models. Lindstrom and Bates (1990) therefore propose an approximate method of evaluation in which the contribution to the conditional likelihood, $\ell_i(\alpha, \boldsymbol{b})$, is replaced by a multivariate Gaussian density whose expectation is linear in $\boldsymbol{b}$. This allows explicit evaluation of the integral terms. The resulting algorithm provides a computationally fast, albeit approximate, method for a wide class of non-linear models and assumed covariance structures for the error terms Z_{ij}. The method is implemented in the Splus function `nlme()`.

14.3 Joint modelling of longitudinal measurements and recurrent events

Until now, we have worked mostly within a paradigm which either treats times of measurements as fixed by the study design or, in an observational setting, assumes that the measurement times are unrelated to the phenomenon of interest, and from a statistical modelling perspective can therefore be treated as if they had been fixed in advance. Thus, for example, in our earlier discussions of the Thall and Vail (1990) epilepsy data, the data were presented as counts of the numbers of events in fixed time-intervals prior to analysis. An alternative approach would have been to treat the actual times of the individual seizures as the response variable. Often, the aggregation of individual event-times into interval-counts will be a reasonable data-analytic strategy, but it represents a discarding of potential information. Indeed, a major branch of statistical methodology has developed in its own right to deal with such data, which are variously known as point process data, event history data or recurrent event data. See, for example, Andersen *et al.* (1993). Survival analysis, also a major area of statistical methodology in its own right, refers to the special case in which the outcome of interest is the time of occurrence of a single, terminating event.

In this section, we consider briefly how we might analyse data in which each subject in a longitudinal study provides both a sequence of measurements at a set of fixed times and a set of random times at which events of substantive interest occur. The resulting methods are potentially relevant to many kinds of investigation, including the following examples.

In AIDS research, many studies are concerned with using a longitudinally measured biomarker such as CD4 cell count or estimated viral load to predict the time to onset of clinical AIDS. In longitudinal clinical trials, inferences about mean response profiles may need to be adjusted to take account of informative dropout; in Chapter 13, we discussed this area under the implicit assumption that dropout occurs at one of a number of prespecified measurement times, but in some applications dropout will be a well-defined event occurring at a precisely recorded time. In psychiatric studies, it may be of interest to model jointly the times of onset of acute episodes and the longitudinal evolution of a general measure of psychiatric disturbance such as the Positive and Negative Syndrome Scale (PANSS) used in the case study of Section 13.8.

Models and methods for dealing with data of this kind have become widely studied in recent years. Hogan and Laird (1997*a*) give an excellent review. Other contributions include Pawitan and Self (1993), Tsiatis *et al.* (1995), Faucett and Thomas (1996), Lavalley and De Gruttola (1996), Hogan and Laird (1977*b*), Wulfsohn and Tsiatis (1997), Finkelstein and Schoenfeld (1999), Henderson *et al.* (2000) and Xu and Zeger (2001). Note that, according to the particular context, the focus for inference may be on modelling the distribution of the time to a terminal event conditional on a longitudinal measurement sequence, on adjusting inference about a longitudinal measurement sequence to allow for informative dropout, or on modelling the joint evolution of a measurement and an event-time process.

Much of the literature cited above is motivated by specific applications, and makes extensive use of random effects, or more generally underlying latent stochastic processes, to induce association between the measurement and event-time processes. Here, we give an outline of the general formulation given in Henderson *et al.* (2000) and note some unresolved issues concerning inference for the resulting class of models.

We assume that the data-format for a single subject is a measurement sequence Y_j: $j = 1, \ldots, n$ at times t_j: $j = 1, \ldots, n$ and a counting process $\{N(u): 0 \leq u \leq d\}$ which identifies event-times within the interval $(0, d)$. Events which occur after time d are therefore censored.

One aim is to provide a bivariate modelling framework which includes the standard methods of choice for separate, univariate analyses of the measurement and event processes. For the measurement process, we therefore assume that

$$Y_j = \mu(t_j) + W_1(t_j) + Z_j \quad j = 1, \ldots, n, \tag{14.3.1}$$

where the mean response $\mu(t)$ is described by a linear model, Z_j is a measurement error, normally distributed with mean zero and variance τ^2, and $W_1(t)$ is a Gaussian stochastic process which can be decomposed into a random effect term and a stationary term, say

$$W_1(t) = d_1(t)'U_1 + V_1(t),$$

as discussed in Chapter 5.

For the event process, we adopt a semi-parametric proportional hazards formulation as in the seminal work of Cox (1972), with a second latent stochastic process providing a time-dependent frailty term. Thus, we model the intensity of events as

$$\lambda(t) = \lambda_0(t) \exp\{\alpha(t) + W_2(t)\}, \tag{14.3.2}$$

where $\lambda_0(t)$ is a non-parametric baseline intensity, $\alpha(t)$ is a linear model which describes the proportional effects of explanatory variables measured at time t, and the Gaussian process $W_2(t)$ has a decomposition comparable to that of $W_1(t)$, namely

$$W_2(t) = d_2(t)'U_2 + V_2(t).$$

Association between the measurement and event-time processes is induced by postulating a joint multivariate Gaussian distribution for the two random effect vectors U_1 and U_2, and a non-zero cross-covariance structure, $\gamma_{12}(u) = \text{Cov}\{W_1(t), W_2(t-u)\}$, for the bivariate process $W(t)$.

Inference in this model is not entirely straightforward. Using Y and N to denote the measurement and event data respectively, and $\mathcal{W}$ to denote the complete path of $W_1(t)$ for $0 \leq t \leq d$, we can express the likelihood contribution from a single subject in the form

$$\ell(\theta) = \ell_1(\theta; Y) \text{E}_{\mathcal{W} \mid Y}[\ell_2(\theta; N \mid \mathcal{W}_2].\tag{14.3.3}$$

In (14.3.3), the term $\ell_1(\theta; Y)$ is of the standard form corresponding to the multivariate Gaussian distribution of Y, as discussed in Chapters 4 and 5.

The second term is generally more complicated. It reduces to the standard form for a proportional hazards model with frailty if the component latent processes $W_1(\cdot)$ and $W_2(\cdot)$ are independent, although this case is of limited interest here.

A simple method of estimation is to use standard methods to analyse the measurement data, including evaluation of the minimum mean square predictor for $W_2(\cdot)$, then to analyse the event-time data using predicted values of $W_2(t)$ in place of the true, unknown values.

It will usually be preferable to base inference on the full likelihood function (14.3.3). Faucett and Thomas (1996) and Xu and Zeger (2001) use Bayesian methods, implemented via Markov chain Monte Carlo. Wulfsohn and Tsiatis (1997) obtain maximum likelihood estimators using an EM algorithm, in the special case when $W_2(t) = \gamma W_1(t)$ and $W_1(t) = d_1(t)'U_1$. Henderson *et al.* (2000) extend the method of Wulfsohn and Tsiatis to a wider class of models and note the identifiability problems which can arise when $W_2(t)$ is allowed to be time-varying in conjunction with a non-parametric specification of the baseline intensity $\lambda_0(t)$.

Some authors have questioned the wisdom of relying on the assumption of Gaussian random effect or latent process models, on the grounds that the resulting inferences can be sensitive to assumptions which cannot easily be checked from the available data. This echos the concerns expressed in Chapter 13 about reliance on specific informative dropout models to adjust inferences about the mean response in incomplete longitudinal measurement data. These issues are raised, for example, in the discussion of Scharfstein *et al.* (1999).

14.4 Multivariate longitudinal data

There is a trend in biomedical and public health research toward outcome measures of increasing complexity. This book primarily considers complexities that arise with repeated measures of a scalar outcome. But it is also common to observe multivariate outcomes repeatedly. For example, we measure the severity of schizophrenic symptoms with the PANSS which comprises 30 different symptom reports, producing a 30×1 response vector at each time. In neuroimaging, we record repeated images on an individual, each of which is a high-dimensional vector of voxel intensities. A final example is time series studies of gene expression arrays where the outcome is a 10 000-dimensional vector of estimates of mRNA levels. In this section, we briefly discuss extensions of longitudinal data analysis methods appropriate for multivariate responses. We focus on the PANSS example with a 30-dimensional outcome. We also only consider linear models; non-linear models are set up similarly. Early work on this topic was by O'Brien (1984) and Pocock *et al.* (1987) who focused on statistical tests. Dupuis *et al.* (1996) and Gray and Brookmeyer (1998, 2000) have more recently developed latent variable models and generalized estimating equations for regression analysis with multivariate responses.

We illustrate the approach to multivariate longitudinal data by considering a simple pre-post design in which a vector response is observed at baseline and then again after a period of treatment for two groups, one receiving a placebo, the other a new treatment. The basic model takes the form

$$Y_{ijk} = \beta_{0k} + \beta_{1k}\text{Post}_j + \gamma_k \text{Post}_j * \text{Trt}_i + \epsilon_{ijk}, \tag{14.4.1}$$

where Y_{ijk} is the response for item k at time t_{ij} for person i, Post_j is the indicator of the post-treatment time and Trt_i indicates the treatment group to which the ith person belongs (0-placebo; 1-active treatment). If we let $Y_{ij} = (Y_{ij1}, Y_{ij2}, \ldots, Y_{ij30})$ be the 30-dimensional vector response, then the model can be written as

$$Y_{ij} = \beta_0 + \beta_1 \cdot \text{Post}_j + \gamma \cdot \text{Post}_j * \text{Trt}_i + \epsilon_{ij},$$

where $\beta_0 = (\beta_{01}, \ldots, \beta_{030})$ is the vector of expected responses at baseline for each of the 30 items, $\beta_1 = (\beta_{11}, \ldots, \beta_{130})$ is the vector of changes from baseline for the placebo group and $\gamma = (\gamma_1, \gamma_2, \ldots, \gamma_{30})$ comprise the 30 item-specific differences γ_k in the average change from baseline for the treatment and placebo groups. Here, γ is the parameter vector of interest. In the classic linear model, we would further assume that $\epsilon_i = (\epsilon'_{i1}, \epsilon'_{i2})'$ is a 60×1 vector of near zero residuals with 60×60 covariance matrix:

$$\text{Var}(\epsilon_i) = V = \begin{pmatrix} V_{11} & V_{12} \\ V_{21} & V_{22} \end{pmatrix},$$

where $V_{11} = \text{Var}(\epsilon_{i1}), V_{22} = \text{Var}(\epsilon_{12})$, and $V_{12} = \text{Cov}(\epsilon_{i1}, \epsilon_{i2})$. The goal of statistical inference is to estimate the regression coefficients as efficiently as possible.

Suppose, we observe $Y_i = (Y'_{i1}, Y'_{i2})'$ for each of m persons and let X_i be the three (predictors) by two (times) design matrix for each item:

$$X_i^* = \overset{\quad\text{Int}\ \text{Post}_j\ \text{Trt}_i}{\begin{pmatrix} 1 & 0 & 0 \\ 1 & 1 & \text{Trt}_i \end{pmatrix}}.$$

Let $X_i = X_i^* \otimes I_{30}$ be the Kronecker product with X_i^* on the diagonal and 0 elsewhere. Finally, collect the regression coefficients into $\beta = \{(\beta_{0k}, \beta_{1k}, \gamma_k), k = 1, \ldots, 30\}$. Then, we can write the model for a single person as

$$\underset{60\times 1}{Y_i} = \underset{60\times 90}{X_i}\ \underset{90\times 1}{\beta} + \underset{60\times 1}{\epsilon_i}, \qquad \epsilon_i \sim N(0, V).$$

Suppose V is known. Then, by the Guass–Markov theorem, the minimum varianced unbiased estiamte of β (and the MLE under the Gaussian assumption) is given by

$$\hat{\beta} = \left(\sum_{i=1}^{m} X_i' V^{-1} X_i\right)^{-1} \left(\sum_{i=1}^{m} X_i' V^{-1} Y_i\right),$$

and we have then $\hat{\beta} \sim N\left(\beta, \left(\sum_{i=1}^{m} X_i' V^{-1} X_i\right)^{-1}\right)$.

Figure 14.3(a) shows estimates of γ_k for the 30 items along with approximate 95% confidence intervals for a data set of PANSS scores for $m = 174$ schizophrenic patients who participated in a clinical trial comparing risperidol (6 mg) to placebo.

We can see that for every item, the estimate of γ_k is negative indicating less severe symptoms for patients receiving risperidone. To obtain these estimates, we used the REML estimate of V as discussed in Section 4.5.

The challenge in the analysis of multivariate longitudinal data, particularly with a high-dimensional response, is to choose a sensible approximations to V. Note, even in this simple pre-post design, V is 60×60 and has $\binom{60}{2} = 1770$ parameters. We are likely to lose any gains in efficiency that are available from joint longitudinal modelling of the 30 items by weighting the data with $\widehat{V}^{-1}$ if V is poorly estimated.

One simple approach is to weight the data by $W_i = \text{diag}\left(\hat{\sigma}_1^2, \ldots, \hat{\sigma}_{30}^2\right)^{-1}$, where $\hat{\sigma}^2$ is an estimate of $\text{Var}(Y_{ijk})$. The resulting estimator

$$\hat{\beta}_W = \left(\sum_{i=1}^{m} X_i' W X_i^*\right)^{-1} \sum_{i=1}^{m} X_i' W Y_i = I_0^{-1} \sum_{i=1}^{m} X_i' W Y_i,$$

is approximately normal with mean β and variance which can be estimated by the empirical variance formula

$$\widehat{\text{Var}}(\hat{\beta}_W) = I_0^{-1} \left[\sum_{i=1}^{m} X_i' W (Y_i - X_i\hat{\beta})(Y_i - X_i\hat{\beta})' W X_i\right] I_0^{-1}.$$

Here, we are accounting for the possibly different variances of the items but ignoring correlations among items at the same or different times.

A better strategy might be to consider an hierarchical random effects model with random effects for individuals but also for items. Returning to the basic model, we might assume for the first level, that

$$Y_{ijk} = X_{jk}^* \beta_{ik} + \epsilon_{ijk},$$

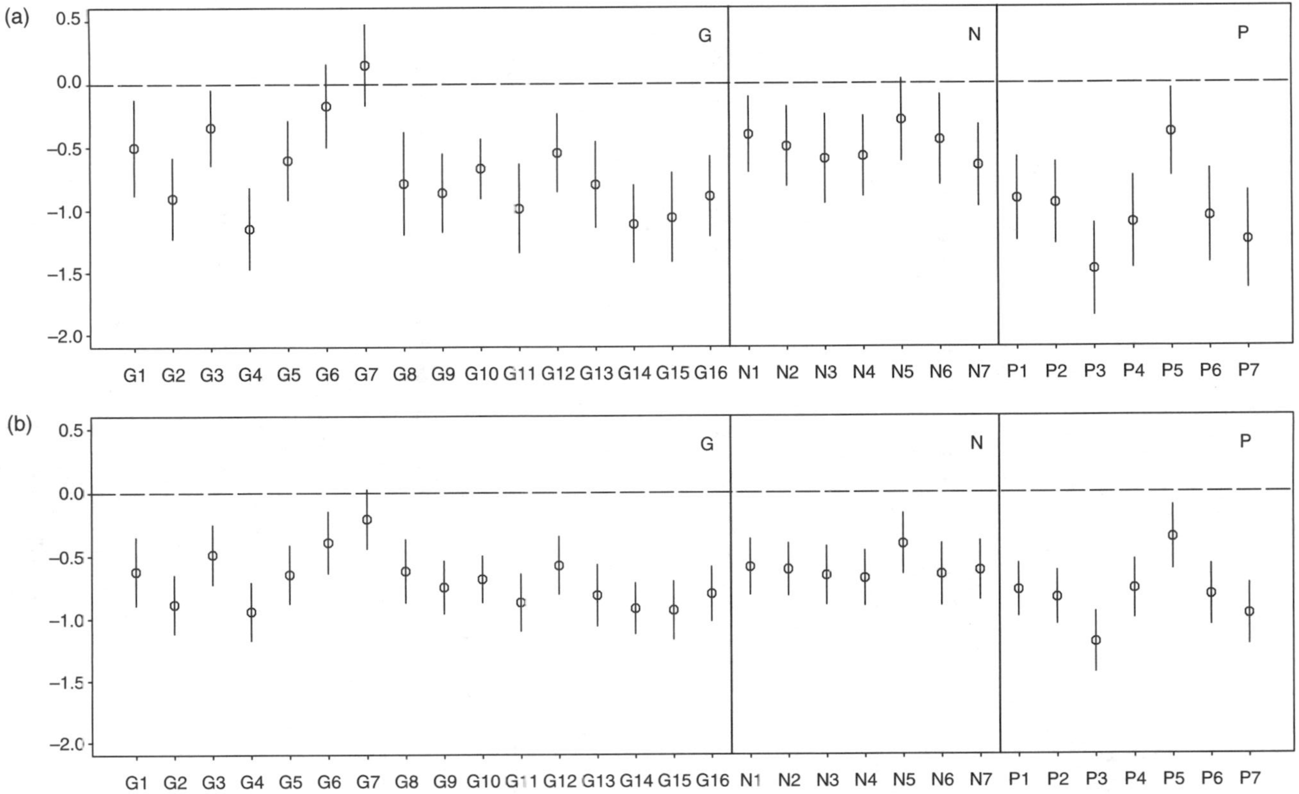

Fig. 14.3. Estimated treatment effects for each of the 30 items in the PANSS instrument for measuring symptoms of schizophrenia. Negative values indicate the treatment is better than the control. The items are classified as general (G), positive (P) for symptoms which are added to the personality, and negative (N) for symptoms which represent a loss of personality traits. (a) Maximum likelihood estimates using unstructured covariance matrix; (b) approximate empirical Bayes' estimates which shrink each item coefficient toward the across-item mean value.

where $\beta_{ik} = (\beta_{0_{ik}}, \beta_{1_{ik}}, \gamma_{ik})$. In a second level, we assume, for example, that

$$\underset{3\times 1}{\beta_{ik}} = \underset{3\times 1}{\bar{\beta}} + \underset{3\times 1}{\delta_k} + \underset{3\times 1,}{b_i}$$

where $\bar{\beta}$ is the population and item average regression coefficients, δ_k is the deviation of the coefficients for item k from $\bar{\beta}$ and b_i is the deviation of subject i's coefficients from $\bar{\beta}$. Note, this particular second level model assumes there are no interactions of item and subject; the subject deviation is the same for all items. To complete the specification, we can assume δ_k and b_i are independent, mean zero Gaussian variables with variances D_δ and D_b, respectively. In some applications, we might allow only a subset of the coefficients to have random effects so that D_δ or D_b might be degenerate.

This multilevel formulation provides a lower-dimensional parameterization of the variance matrix $\text{Var}(Y) = V$. To see the specifics, we write

$$\underset{60\times 1}{Y_i} = \underset{60\times 90}{X_i} \underset{(90\times 1}{(\bar{\beta}\otimes 1_{30}} + \underset{90\times 1}{\delta} + \underset{90\times 1)}{b_i \otimes 1_{30})} + \underset{60\times 1,}{\epsilon_i}$$

where 1_{30} is a 30×1 vector of ones and $\delta = (\delta_1', \delta_2', \ldots, \delta_{30}')'$. Then, we have

$$Y_i = X_i\bar{\beta}\otimes 1_{30} + \epsilon_i^* \;\;,\; \epsilon_i^* = X_i^*(\delta + b_i \otimes 1_{30}) + \epsilon_i,$$

where $\text{Var}(\epsilon_i^*) = X_i(D_\delta \otimes I_{30} + D_b \otimes 1_{30}1_{30}')X_i' + V$ and $V = \text{Var}(\epsilon_i)$. If we assume $V = \text{diag}\left(\sigma_1^2, \ldots, \sigma_{30}^2, \sigma_1^2, \ldots, \sigma_{30}^2\right)$, then the only correlation among items at the same or different times derives from shared random effects. This model reduces the parameters necessary to specify V from $\binom{60}{2} = 1770$ down to $\binom{3}{2} + \binom{3}{2} + 30 = 36$.

We can estimate the fixed effects of $\bar{\beta}$ and the covariance parameters by restricted maximum likelihood. Also of interest are the empirical Bayes' estimates of $\bar{\beta} + \delta_k$, the population average coefficients for item $k, k = 1, \ldots, 30$. These can be estimated by a simpler approximate method as follows. First, obtain the maximum likelihood estimates $\hat{\beta}_k$ and $\hat{V}_k = \text{Var}(\hat{\beta}_k \mid \beta_k), k = 1, \ldots, 30$. If we assume the β_ks are independent with mean $\bar{\beta}$ and variance D_δ, then $\hat{\beta}_k \sim N(\bar{\beta}, D_\delta + \hat{V}_k)$ and the empirical Bayes' estimate is given by

$$\tilde{\beta}_k = (\hat{D}_\delta + \hat{V}_K)^{-1}[\hat{D}_\delta\hat{\beta}_i + \hat{V}_k\hat{\bar{\beta}}].$$

Figure 14.3(b) shows these estimates for the treatment effect for the 30 PANSS items. Comparing these results to those from Fig. 14.3(a), one can see the value of borrowing strength across items.

Appendix
Statistical background

A.1 Introduction

This appendix provides a brief review of some basic statistical concepts used throughout the book. Readers should find sections A.2 and A.3 useful for the material that is presented in Chapters 4, 5, 6 and 13 which deal with methods for analysing data with a continuous response variable. These four chapters also make extensive use of the method of maximum likelihood, which is the subject of section A.4. Sections A.5 and A.6 outline the basic concepts of generalised linear models, which provide a unified methodology for the analysis of data with continuous or discrete responses. This material is most relevant for Chapters 7–11.

A.2 The linear model and the method of least squares

In many scientific studies, the main goal is to predict or describe an *outcome* or *response* variable, in terms of other variables which we will refer to as *predictors, covariates* or *explanatory variables.* The explanatory variables can either be fixed in advance, such as the treatment assignment in an experiment, or uncontrolled, such as smoking status in an observational study. Regression analysis has been used since the early nineteenth century to describe the relationship between the expectation of a response variable, Y, and a set of explanatory variables, x_j: $j = 1, \ldots, p$. The *linear regression model* assumes that the response variable and the explanatory variables are related through

$$Y_i = \beta_1 x_{i1} + \beta_2 x_{i2} + \cdots + \beta_p x_{ip} + \epsilon_i = \boldsymbol{x}_i' \boldsymbol{\beta} + \epsilon_i, \quad i = 1, \ldots, m,$$

where Y_i is the response for the ith of m subjects and x_{ij} is the value of the jth explanatory variable for the ith subject. Usually, $x_{i1} = 1$ for every subject, so that β_1 is the *intercept* of this regression model. The ϵ_i are random variables which are assumed to be uncorrelated with each other, and to have $\mathrm{E}(\epsilon_i) = 0$ and $\mathrm{Var}(\epsilon_i) = \sigma^2$. This implies that the first two moments of Y_i are $\mathrm{E}(Y_i) = \boldsymbol{x}_i' \boldsymbol{\beta}$ and $\mathrm{Var}(Y_i) = \sigma^2$, where $\boldsymbol{x}_i$ and $\boldsymbol{\beta}$ are p-element vectors. Note that these statements involve no distributional assumption about Y_i, although a common assumption is that the joint distribution of $Y_1, \ldots, Y_m$ is multivariate Gaussian. Models of this kind have been widely used in both experimental and observational studies. In fact, linear models include as special cases

(1) the analysis of variance, in which the x_j are dummy variables, used to indicate the allocation of experimental units to treatments,

(2) multiple regression, in which the x_j are quantitative variables,

(3) the analysis of covariance, in which the x_j are a mixture of continuous and dummy variables.

Each regression coefficient, β_j, describes the change in the expected value of the response variable, Y, per unit change of its corresponding explanatory variable, x_j, all other variables held fixed.

The method of *least squares* (Legendre, 1805; Gauss, 1809) is a long-standing method for estimating the vector of regression coefficients, $\boldsymbol{\beta}$. The idea is to find an estimate, $\hat{\boldsymbol{\beta}}$ say, which minimizes the sum of squares

$$\mathrm{RSS} = \sum_{i=1}^{m} (Y_i - \boldsymbol{x}_i'\boldsymbol{\beta})^2.$$

This procedure is formally equivalent to solving

$$\frac{\partial \mathrm{RSS}}{\partial \boldsymbol{\beta}} = -2\sum_{i=1}^{m} \boldsymbol{x}_i(Y_i - \boldsymbol{x}_i'\boldsymbol{\beta}) = 0,$$

which gives rise to

$$\hat{\boldsymbol{\beta}} = \left(\sum_{i=1}^{m} \boldsymbol{x}_i\boldsymbol{x}_i'\right)^{-1} \sum_{i=1}^{m} \boldsymbol{x}_i Y_i.$$

An alternative, and more familiar, form of the least-squares estimate $\hat{\boldsymbol{\beta}}$ is obtained by defining an m-element vector $\boldsymbol{Y} = (Y_1, \ldots, Y_m)$ and an m by p matrix X with ijth element x_{ij}. Then,

$$\hat{\boldsymbol{\beta}} = (X'X)^{-1}X'\boldsymbol{Y}.$$

The least-squares estimate, $\hat{\boldsymbol{\beta}}$, enjoys many desirable statistical properties. Firstly, it is an unbiased estimator of $\boldsymbol{\beta}$, that is, $\mathrm{E}(\hat{\boldsymbol{\beta}}) = \boldsymbol{\beta}$. Its variance matrix is

$$\mathrm{Var}(\hat{\boldsymbol{\beta}}) = \sigma^2(X'X)^{-1}.$$

Secondly, for any vector $\boldsymbol{a}$ of known coefficients, if we let $\phi = \boldsymbol{a}'\boldsymbol{\beta}$ then $\hat{\phi} = \boldsymbol{a}'\hat{\boldsymbol{\beta}}$ has the smallest possible variance amongst all unbiased estimators for ϕ which are linear combinations of the Y_i. This optimality property of least-squares estimation is known as the Gauss–Markov Theorem.

The constant variance, σ^2, of the ϵ_i is usually unknown but can be estimated by

$$\hat{\sigma}^2 = \sum_{i=1}^{m}(Y_i - \boldsymbol{x}_i'\hat{\boldsymbol{\beta}})^2/(m-p).$$

Many books, including Seber (1977) and Draper and Smith (1981), give more detailed discussions of least-squares estimation.

A.3 Multivariate Gaussian theory

This section reviews some of the important results for multivariate Gaussian observations. For more detailed treatment of multivariate Gaussian theory see, for example, Graybill (1976) or Rao (1973).

A random vector $\boldsymbol{Y} = (Y_1, \ldots, Y_n)$ is said to follow a multivariate Gaussian distribution if its probability density is of the form

$$f(\boldsymbol{y}; \boldsymbol{\mu}, V) = (2\pi)^{-n/2} \,|\, V \,|^{-1/2} \exp\{-(\boldsymbol{y} - \boldsymbol{\mu})'V^{-1}(\boldsymbol{y} - \boldsymbol{\mu})/2\},$$

where $-\infty < y_j < \infty, \quad j = 1, \ldots, n$. As in the univariate case, this distribution is fully specified by its first two moments, $\boldsymbol{\mu} = \mathrm{E}(\boldsymbol{Y})$ and $V = \mathrm{Var}(\boldsymbol{Y})$. A convenient shorthand notation is $\boldsymbol{Y} \sim MVN(\boldsymbol{\mu}, V)$.

The following properties of the multivariate Gaussian distribution are used extensively in the book:

1. Each Y_j has a univariate Gaussian distribution.
2. More generally, if $\boldsymbol{Z}_1 = (Y_1, \ldots, Y_{n_1})$ with $n_1 < n$, then $\boldsymbol{Z}_1$ also follows a multivariate Gaussian distribution with mean $\boldsymbol{\mu}_1 = (\mu_1, \ldots, \mu_{n_1})$ and covariance matrix V_1 which is the upper left n_1 by n_1 submatrix of V.
3. If, additionally, $\boldsymbol{Z}_2 = (Y_{n_1+1}, \ldots, Y_n)$, then the conditional distribution of $\boldsymbol{Z}_1$ given $\boldsymbol{Z}_2 = \boldsymbol{z}_2$ is multivariate Gaussian. Its conditional mean vector is

$$\boldsymbol{\mu}_1 + V_{12}{V_{22}}^{-1}(\boldsymbol{z_2} - \boldsymbol{\mu}_2),$$

   and its conditional variance matrix is

$$V_{11} - V_{12}{V_{22}}^{-1}V_{12}',$$

   where $\boldsymbol{\mu}_2 = (\mu_{n_1+1}, \ldots, \mu_n)$ and V is partitioned as

$$V = \begin{pmatrix} V_{11} & V_{12} \\ V_{12}' & V_{22} \end{pmatrix}.$$

4. If B is an $m \times n$ matrix of rank $m \leq n$, then $B\boldsymbol{Y}$ is also distributed as a multivariate Gaussian, with mean vector $B\boldsymbol{\mu}$ and variance matrix BVB'.
5. The random variable $U = (\boldsymbol{Y} - \boldsymbol{\mu})'V^{-1}(\boldsymbol{Y} - \boldsymbol{\mu})$ has a *chi-squared distribution* with n degrees of freedom, which we write as $U \sim \chi^2_n$.

A.4 Likelihood inference

Likelihood inference is based on a specification of the probability or probability density for the observed data, $\boldsymbol{y}$. This expression, $f(\boldsymbol{y};\boldsymbol{\theta})$, is indexed by a vector of unknown parameters, $\boldsymbol{\theta}$. Once the data are observed, the only quantities in $f(\cdot)$ that are unknown to the investigators are $\boldsymbol{\theta}$. Then, the *likelihood function* for $\boldsymbol{\theta}$ is the function

$$L(\boldsymbol{\theta} \,|\, \boldsymbol{y}) = f(\boldsymbol{y};\boldsymbol{\theta}).$$

Note that the likelihood is interpreted as a function of $\boldsymbol{\theta}$, with $\boldsymbol{y}$ held fixed at its observed value.

The *maximum likelihood estimate* of $\boldsymbol{\theta}$ is the value, $\hat{\boldsymbol{\theta}}$, which maximizes the likelihood function or, equivalently, its logarithm. That is, for any value of $\boldsymbol{\theta}$,

$$L(\boldsymbol{\theta} \,|\, \boldsymbol{y}) \leq L(\hat{\boldsymbol{\theta}} \,|\, \boldsymbol{y}).$$

According to the likelihood principle, $\hat{\boldsymbol{\theta}}$ is then regarded as the value of $\boldsymbol{\theta}$ which is most strongly supported by the observed data. In practice, $\hat{\boldsymbol{\theta}}$ is obtained either by direct maximisation of $\log L$, or by solving the set of equations

$$\boldsymbol{S}(\boldsymbol{\theta}) = \partial \log L / \partial \boldsymbol{\theta} = 0. \tag{A.4.1}$$

The function $\boldsymbol{S}(\boldsymbol{\theta})$ is known as the *score function* for $\boldsymbol{\theta}$. Very often, numerical methods are required to evaluate the maximum likelihood estimate. Popular methods include the Nelder and Mead (1965) simplex algorithm for direct maximisation of $\log L$, or Newton–Raphson iteration for solution of the score equations (A.4.1).

The maximum likelihood estimate is known to enjoy many optimality properties in large samples. In particular, under mild regularity conditions, $\hat{\boldsymbol{\theta}}$ is asymptotically unbiased, and asymptotically efficient in the sense that the elements of $\boldsymbol{\theta}$ are estimated with the smallest possible asymptotic variances of any asymptotically unbiased estimators. The asymptotic variance matrix of $\hat{\boldsymbol{\theta}}$ is given by the expression

$$V = \{-\mathrm{E}(\partial^2 \log L / \partial \boldsymbol{\theta}^2)\}^{-1}.$$

The matrix V^{-1} is also known as the *Fisher information matrix* for $\boldsymbol{\theta}$.

Example A.1. Consider Y_1 and Y_2 to be two independent binomial observations with sample sizes and probabilities (n_1, p_1) and (n_2, p_2), respectively. A typical example for which this setting is appropriate is a clinical trial where two treatments are being compared. Here, Y_i denotes the number of patients responding negatively to the treatment i, to which n_i subjects were assigned, and p_i is the corresponding probability of negative response for $i = 1, 2$. It is convenient to transform the parameters (p_1, p_2) to (θ_1, θ_2), where

$$\theta_1 = \log\left(\frac{p_1(1-p_2)}{p_2(1-p_1)}\right), \quad \theta_2 = \log\left(\frac{p_2}{1-p_2}\right).$$

This leads to a likelihood function for $\boldsymbol{\theta} = (\theta_1, \theta_2)$ of the form

$$\begin{aligned} L(\boldsymbol{\theta} \mid y_1, y_2) &\propto p_1^{y_1}(1-p_1)^{n_1-y_1} p_2^{y_2}(1-p_2)^{n_2-y_2} \\ &= \left(\frac{p_1}{1-p_1}\right)^{y_1}\left(\frac{p_2}{1-p_2}\right)^{y_2}(1-p_1)^{n_1}(1-p_2)^{n_2} \\ &= \exp\{\theta_1 + \theta_2 y_1 + \theta_2 y_2 - n_1 \log\left(1+\mathrm{e}^{\theta_1+\theta_2}\right) - n_2 \log\left(1+\mathrm{e}^{\theta_2}\right)\}. \end{aligned}$$

The parameter θ_1 is called the *log-odds ratio*. A zero value for θ_1 denotes equality of p_1 and p_2. The maximum likelihood estimate, $\hat{\boldsymbol{\theta}}$, can be derived as the solution of the pair of equations,

$$y_1 - \frac{n_1 \exp(\theta_1+\theta_2)}{1+\exp(\theta_1+\theta_2)} = y_1 - n_1 p_1 = 0,$$

and

$$y_1 + y_2 - \frac{n_1 \exp(\theta_1+\theta_2)}{1+\exp(\theta_1+\theta_2)} - \frac{n_2 \exp(\theta_2)}{1+\exp(\theta_2)} = y_1 + y_2 - n_1 p_1 - n_2 p_2 = 0.$$

This gives

$$\hat{\theta}_1 = \log\left(\frac{y_1(n_2-y_2)}{y_2(n_1-y_1)}\right), \quad \hat{\theta}_2 = \log\left(\frac{y_2}{n_2-y_2}\right).$$

Fisher's information matrix for θ can be obtained by straightforward algebra, and is

$$V^{-1} = \begin{pmatrix} \dfrac{n_1 \exp(\theta_1+\theta_2)}{\{1+\exp(\theta_1+\theta_2)\}^2} & \dfrac{n_1 \exp(\theta_1+\theta_2)}{\{1+\exp(\theta_1+\theta_2)\}^2} \\ \dfrac{n_1 \exp(\theta_1+\theta_2)}{\{1+\exp(\theta_1+\theta_2)\}^2} & \dfrac{n_1 \exp(\theta_1+\theta_2)}{\{1+\exp(\theta_1+\theta_2)\}^2} + \dfrac{n_2 \exp(\theta_2)}{\{1+\exp(\theta_2)\}^2} \end{pmatrix}.$$

The asymptotic variance of $\hat{\theta}_1$ is the upper left entry of V, namely

$$[n_1 \exp(\theta_1+\theta_2)/\{1+\exp(\theta_1+\theta_2)\}^2]^{-1} + [n_2 \exp(\theta_2)/\{1+\exp(\theta_2)\}^2]^{-1},$$

which can be estimated consistently by

$$\frac{1}{y_1} + \frac{1}{n_1 - y_1} + \frac{1}{y_2} + \frac{1}{n_2 - y_2}.$$

The word 'asymptotic' in this example means that both n_1 and n_2 are large.

Likelihood inference proceeds by fitting a series of sub-models which are *nested*. This means that each sub-model in the sequence is contained within the previous one. In Example A.1, an interesting hypothesis, or sub-model, to test is that $\theta_1 = 0$, corresponding to equality of p_1 and p_2. The difference between this sub-model and the full model with no restriction on θ_1 can be examined by calculating the *likelihood ratio test statistic*, which is defined as

$$G = 2\{\log L(\hat{\boldsymbol{\theta}} \mid y) - \log L(\hat{\boldsymbol{\theta}}_0 \mid y)\},$$

where $\hat{\boldsymbol{\theta}}_0$ and $\hat{\boldsymbol{\theta}}$ are the maximum likelihood estimates of $\boldsymbol{\theta}$ under the null hypothesis or sub-model, and the unrestricted model, respectively. Assuming that the sub-model is correct, the sampling distribution of G is approximately chi-squared, with number of degrees of freedom equal to the difference between the numbers of parameters specified under the sub-model and the unrestricted model.

An alternative testing procedure is to examine the *score statistic*, $\boldsymbol{S(\theta)}$, as in (A.4.1). The score test statistic is

$$\boldsymbol{S}(\hat{\boldsymbol{\theta}}_0)V(\hat{\boldsymbol{\theta}}_0)\boldsymbol{S}'(\hat{\boldsymbol{\theta}}_0),$$

whose null sampling distribution is also chi-squared, with the same degrees of freedom as for the likelihood ratio test statistic. In either case, the sub-model is rejected in favour of the unrestricted model if the test statistic is too large.

Example A.2. (continued)

Suppose that we want to test whether the probabilities, p_1 and p_2, from two treatments are identical. This is equivalent to testing the sub-model with $\theta_1 = 0$. Note that the value of θ_2 is unspecified by the null hypothesis and therefore has to be estimated. The algebraic form of the likelihood ratio test statistic G is complicated, and we do not give it here, although in applications it can easily be evaluated numerically. The score statistic has the simple form

$$\frac{(y_1 - E_1)^2}{E_1} + \frac{(y_2 - E_2)^2}{E_2}$$

where $E_i = n_i(y_1 + y_2)/(n_1 + n_2)$ is the expected value for Y_i under the null model that the two groups are the same. This statistic is also known as the Pearson's chi-squared test statistic. The number of degrees of freedom in this example is one, because the sub-model has one parameter, whereas the unrestricted model has two.

A.5 Generalized linear models

Regression models for independent, discrete and continuous responses have been unified under the class of *generalized linear models*, or GLMs (McCullagh and Nelder, 1989), thus providing a common body of statistical methodology for different types of response. Here, we review the salient features of this class of models.

We begin by considering two particular GLMs, logistic and Poisson regression models, and then discuss the general class. Because GLMs apply to independent responses, we focus on the cross-sectional situation, as in section A.2, with a single response Y_i and a vector $\boldsymbol{x_i}$ of p explanatory variables associated with each of m experimental units. The objective is to describe the dependence of the mean response, $\mu_i = \mathrm{E}(Y_i)$, on the explanatory variables.

A.5.1 *Logistic regression*

This model has been used extensively for dichotomous response variables such as the presence or absence of a disease. The logistic model assumes that the logarithm of the odds of a positive response is a linear function of explanatory variables, so that

$$\log \frac{\Pr(Y_i = 1)}{\Pr(Y_i = 0)} = \log \frac{\mu_i}{1 - \mu_i} = \boldsymbol{x}_i' \boldsymbol{\beta}.$$

Figure A.1 shows plots of $\Pr(Y = 1)$ against a single explanatory variable x, for several values of β. A major distinction between the logistic regression model and the linear model in Section A.2 is that the linearity applies to a transformation of the expectation of Y_i, in this case the log odds transformation, rather than to the expectation itself. Thus, the regression coefficients, $\boldsymbol{\beta}$, represent the change of the log odds of the response variable per unit change of x. Another feature of the dichotomous response variable is that the variance of Y_i is completely determined by its mean, μ_i. Specifically,

$$\mathrm{Var}(Y_i) = \mathrm{E}(Y_i)\{1 - \mathrm{E}(Y_i)\} = \exp(\boldsymbol{x}_i'\boldsymbol{\beta})/\{1 + \exp(\boldsymbol{x}_i'\boldsymbol{\beta})\}^2.$$

This is to be contrasted with the linear model, where $\mathrm{Var}(Y_i)$ is usually assumed to be a constant, σ^2, which is independent of the mean.

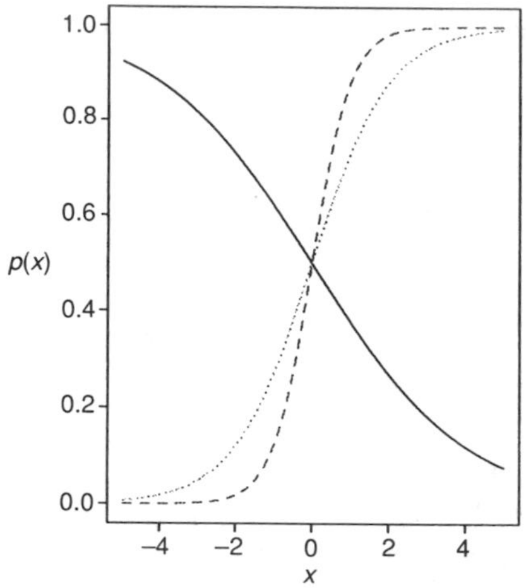

Fig. A.1. The logistic model, $p(x) = \exp(\beta x)/\{1 + \exp(\beta x)\}$; ——: $\beta = -0.5$; ....: $\beta = 1$; – – –: $\beta = 2$.

A.5.2 *Poisson regression*

Poisson regression, or *log-linear*, models are applicable to problems in which the response variable represents the number of events occurring in a fixed period of time. One instance is the number of seizures in a given time-interval, as in Example 1.6. Because of the discrete and non-negative nature of count data, a reasonable assumption is that the *logarithm* of the expected count is a linear function of explanatory variables, so that

$$\log \mathrm{E}(Y_i) = \boldsymbol{x}_i'\boldsymbol{\beta}.$$

Here, the regression coefficient for a particular explanatory variable can be interpreted as the logarithm of the ratio of expected counts before and after a one unit increase in that explanatory variable, with all other explanatory variables held constant. The term 'Poisson' refers to the distribution for counts derived by Poisson (1837),

$$p(y) = \exp(-\mu)\mu^y/y!, \quad y = 0, 1, \ldots.$$

As in logistic regression, the assumption that Y_i follows a Poisson distribution implies that the variance of Y_i is determined by its mean. In this case, the mean and variance are the same,

$$\mathrm{Var}(Y_i) = \mathrm{E}(Y_i) = \exp(\boldsymbol{x}_i'\boldsymbol{\beta}).$$

A.5.3 *The general class*

Linear, logistic and Poisson regression models are all special cases of generalized linear models, which share the following features.

First, the mean response, $\mu_i = \mathrm{E}(Y_i)$, is assumed to be related to a vector of covariates, $\boldsymbol{x}$, through

$$h(\mu_i) = \boldsymbol{x}_i'\boldsymbol{\beta}.$$

For logistic regression, $h(\mu_i) = \log\{\mu_i/(1-\mu_i)\}$; in Poisson regression, $h(\mu_i) = \log(\mu_i)$. The function $h(\cdot)$ is called the *link function.*

Second, the variance of Y_i is a specified function of its mean, μ_i, namely

$$\mathrm{Var}(Y_i) = v_i = \phi v(\mu_i).$$

In this expression, the known function $v(\cdot)$ is referred to as the *variance function*; the scaling factor, ϕ, is a known constant for some members of the GLM family, whereas in others it is an additional parameter to be estimated.

Third, each class of GLMs corresponds to a member of the exponential family of distributions, with a likelihood function of the form

$$f(y_i) = \exp[\{y_i\theta_i - \psi(\theta_i)\}/\phi + c(y_i, \phi)]. \tag{A.5.1}$$

The parameter θ_i is known as the *natural parameter*, and is related to μ_i through $\mu_i = \partial\psi(\theta_i)/\partial\theta_i$. For example, the Poisson distribution is a special case of the exponential family, with

$$\theta_i = \log\mu_i,\ \ \psi(\theta_i) = \exp(\theta_i),\ \ c(y_i,\phi) = -\log(y_i!),\ \ \phi = 1.$$

Other distributions within this family include the Gaussian or Normal distribution, the binomial distribution and the two-parameter gamma distribution.

In any GLM the regression coefficients, $\boldsymbol{\beta}$, can be estimated by solving the same estimating equation,

$$\boldsymbol{S}(\boldsymbol{\beta}) = \sum_{i=1}^{m}\left(\frac{\partial\mu_i}{\partial\boldsymbol{\beta}}\right)' v_i^{-1}\{Y_i - \mu_i(\boldsymbol{\beta})\} = 0, \tag{A.5.2}$$

where $v_i = \mathrm{Var}(Y_i)$. Note that $\boldsymbol{S}(\boldsymbol{\beta})$ is the derivative of the logarithm of the likelihood function. The solution $\hat{\boldsymbol{\beta}}$, which is the maximum likelihood estimate, can be obtained by iteratively reweighted least squares; see McCullagh and Nelder (1989) for a detailed discussion. Finally, in large samples $\hat{\boldsymbol{\beta}}$ follows a Gaussian distribution with mean $\boldsymbol{\beta}$ and variance

$$V = \left(\sum_{i=1}^{m} \left(\frac{\partial \mu_i}{\partial \boldsymbol{\beta}} \right)' v_i^{-1} \frac{\partial \mu_i}{\partial \boldsymbol{\beta}} \right)^{-1}. \qquad \text{(A.5.3)}$$

This variance can be estimated by $\hat{V}$ which is obtained by replacing $\boldsymbol{\beta}$ with $\hat{\boldsymbol{\beta}}$ in the expression (A.5.3).

A.6 Quasi-likelihood

One important property of the GLM family is that the score function, $\boldsymbol{S}(\boldsymbol{\beta})$, depends only on the mean and the variance of the Y_i. Wedderburn (1974) was the first to point out that the estimating equation (A.5.2) can therefore be used to estimate the regression coefficients for any choices of link and variance functions, whether or not they correspond to a particular member of the exponential family. The name *quasi-score function* was coined for $\boldsymbol{S}(\boldsymbol{\beta})$ in (A.5.2), since its integral with respect to $\boldsymbol{\beta}$ can be thought of as a 'quasi-likelihood' even if it does not constitute a proper likelihood function. This suggests an approach to statistical modelling in which we make assumptions about the link and variance functions without attempting to specify the entire distribution of Y_i. This is desirable, since we often do not understand the precise details of the probabilistic mechanisms by which data were generated. McCullagh (1983) showed that the solution, $\hat{\boldsymbol{\beta}}$, of the quasi-score function has a sampling distribution which, in large samples, is approximately Gaussian with mean $\boldsymbol{\beta}$ and variance given by equation (A.5.3).

Example A.2. Let $Y_1, \ldots, Y_m$ be independent counts whose expectations are modelled as

$$\log \mathrm{E}(Y_i) = \boldsymbol{x}_i' \boldsymbol{\beta}, \quad i = 1, \ldots, m.$$

In biomedical studies, frequently the variance of Y_i is greater than $\mathrm{E}(Y_i)$, the variance expression induced by the Poisson assumption. This phenomenon is known as *over-dispersion*. One way to account for this is to assume that $\mathrm{Var}(Y_i) = \phi \mathrm{E}(Y_i)$ where ϕ is a non-negative scalar parameter. Note that for the Poisson distribution, $\phi = 1$; if we allow $\phi > 1$, we no longer have a distribution from the exponential family. However, if we define $\hat{\boldsymbol{\beta}}$ as the solution to

$$\sum_{i=1}^{m} \boldsymbol{x}_i \{Y_i - \exp(\boldsymbol{x}_i' \boldsymbol{\beta})\} = 0,$$

then a simple calculation gives the asymptotic variance matrix of $\hat{\boldsymbol{\beta}}$ as

$$\phi \left(\sum_{i=1}^{m} \boldsymbol{x}_i \exp(x_i'\boldsymbol{\beta})\boldsymbol{x}_i' \right)^{-1}.$$

Thus, by comparison with (A.5.3) the variance of $\hat{\boldsymbol{\beta}}$ is inflated by a factor of ϕ. Clearly, ignoring over-dispersion in the analysis would lead to under-estimation of standard errors, and consequent over-statement of significance in hypothesis testing.

In the above example, $\phi \mathrm{E}(Y_i)$ is but one of many possible choices for the variance formula which would take account of over-dispersion in count data. Fortunately, the solution, $\hat{\boldsymbol{\beta}}$, is a consistent estimate of $\boldsymbol{\beta}$ as long as $h(\mu_i) = \boldsymbol{x}_i'\boldsymbol{\beta}$, whether or not the variance function is correctly specified. This robustness property holds because the expectation of $\boldsymbol{S}(\boldsymbol{\beta})$ remains zero so long as $\mathrm{E}(Y_i) = \mu_i(\boldsymbol{\beta})$. However, the asymptotic variance matrix of $\hat{\boldsymbol{\beta}}$ has the form

$$V_2 = V \left(\sum_{i=1}^{m} \left(\frac{\partial \mu_i}{\partial \boldsymbol{\beta}} \right)' v_i^{-1} \mathrm{Var}(Y_i) v_i^{-1} \frac{\partial \mu_i}{\partial \boldsymbol{\beta}} \right) V.$$

Note that V_2 is identical to V in (A.5.3) only if $\mathrm{Var}(Y_i) = v_i$. When this assumption is in doubt, confidence limits for $\boldsymbol{\beta}$ can be based on the estimated variance matrix

$$\hat{V}_2 = \hat{V} \left(\sum_{i=1}^{m} \left(\frac{\partial \mu_i}{\partial \boldsymbol{\beta}} \right)' v_i^{-1} \{Y_i - \mu_i(\boldsymbol{\beta})\}^2 v_i^{-1} \frac{\partial \mu_i}{\partial \boldsymbol{\beta}} \right) \hat{V}, \tag{A.6.1}$$

evaluated at $\hat{\boldsymbol{\beta}}$. We call $\hat{V}$ a *model-based* variance estimate of $\hat{\boldsymbol{\beta}}$ and $\hat{V}_2$ a *robust* variance estimate in that $\hat{V}_2$ is consistent regardless of whether the specification of $\mathrm{Var}(Y_i)$ is correct.

Example A.2. (continued)
An alternative to the variance function

$$v_i = \phi \mu_i,$$

is the form induced by the Poisson-gamma distribution (Breslow, 1984),

$$v_i = \mu_i(1 + \mu_i \phi).$$

With a limited amount of data available, it is difficult to choose empirically between these two variance functions (Liang and McCullagh, 1993). The availability of the robust variance estimate, $\hat{V}_2$, helps to alleviate the concern regarding the choice of variance formula in larger samples.

It is interesting to note that in the special case where $\mu_i = \mu$ and hence $\log \mu_i = \beta_0$, the estimate $\hat{V}_2$ reduces to

$$\sum_{i=1}^{m} (Y_i - \bar{Y})^2 / m^2,$$

the sampling variance of $\hat{\beta}_0 = \log \bar{Y}$ (Royall, 1986).

Bibliography

Aerts, M. and Claeskens, G. (1997). Local polynomial estimation in multi-parameter likelihood models. *Journal of the American Statistical Association*, **92**, 1536–45.

Afsarinejad, K. (1983). Balanced repeated measurements designs. *Biometrika*, **70**, 199–204.

Agresti, A. (1990). *Categorical data analysis.* John Wiley, New York.

Agresti, A. and Lang, J. (1993). A proportional odds model with subject-specific effects for repeated ordered categorical responses. *Biometrika*, **80**, 527–34.

Agresti, A. (1999). Modelling ordered categorical data: recent advances and future challenges. *Statistics in Medicine*, **18**, 2191–207.

Aitkin, M., Anderson, D., Francis, B., and Hinde, J. (1989). *Statistical modelling in GLIM.* Oxford University Press, Oxford.

Albert, J.H. and Chib, S. (1993). Bayesian analysis of binary and polytomous data. *Journal of the American Statistical Association*, **88**, 669–79.

Alexander, C.S. and Markowitz, R. (1986). Maternal employment and use of pediatric clinic services. *Medical Care*, **24**(2), 134–47.

Almon, S. (1965). The distributed lag between capital appropriations and expenditures. *Econometrica*, **33**, 178–96.

Altman, N.S. (1990). Kernel smoothing of data with correlated errors. *Journal of the American Statistical Association*, **85**, 749–59.

Amemiya, T. (1985). *Advanced econometrics.* Harvard University Press, Cambridge Massachusetts.

Amemiya, T. and Morimune, K. (1974). Selecting the optimal order of polynomial in the Almon distributed lag. *The Review of Economics and Statistics*, **56**, 378–86.

Andersen, P.K., Borgan, Ø., Gill, R.D., and Keiding, N. (1993). *Statistical models based on counting processes.* Springer-Verlag, New York.

Anderson, J.A. (1984). Regression and ordered categorical variables (with Discussion). *Journal of the Royal Statistical Society*, **B**, **46**, 1–30.

Anderson, D.A. and Aitkin, M. (1985). Variance component models with binary response: interviewer variability. *Journal of the Royal Statistical Society*, **B**, **47**, 203–10.

Atkinson, A.C. (1985). *Plots, transformations and regression. An introduction to graphical methods of diagnostic regression analysis.* Oxford University Press, Oxford.

Azzzalini, A. (1994). Logistic regression for autocorrelated data with application to repeated measures. *Biometrika*, **81**, 767–75.

Bahadur, R.R. (1961). A representation of the joint distribution of responses to n dichotomous items. In *Studies on item analysis and prediction* (ed. H. Solomon), pp. 158–68. Stanford Mathematical Studies in the Social Sciences VI, Stanford University Press, Stanford, California.

Barnard, G.A. (1963). Contributions to the discussion of Professor Bartlett's paper. *Journal of the Royal Statistical Society*, **B**, **25**, 294.

Bartholomew, D.J. (1987). *Latent variable models and factor analysis.* Oxford University Press, New York.

Bates, D.M. and Watts, D.G. (1988). *Nonlinear regression analysis and its Applications.* Wiley, New York.

Becker, R.A., Chambers, J.M., and Wilks, A.R. (1988). *The new S language.* Wadsworth and Brooks-Cole, Pacific Grove.

Besag, J. (1974). Spatial interaction and the statistical analysis of lattice systems. *Journal of the Royal Statistical Society*, **B**, **36**, 192–236.

Billingsley, P. (1961). *Statistical inference for Markov processes.* University of Chicago Press, Chicago, Illinois.

Bishop, S.H. and Jones, B. (1984). A review of higher-order cross-over designs. *Journal of Applied Statistics*, **11**, 29–50.

Bishop,Y.M.M., Fienberg, S.E., and Holland, P.W. (1975). *Discrete multivariate analysis: theory and practice.* MIT Press, Cambridge, Massachussetts.

Bloomfield, P. and Watson, G.S. (1975). The inefficiency of least squares. *Biometrika*, **62**, 121–28.

Booth, J.G. and Hobert, J.P. (1999). Maximizing generalized linear mixed model likelihoods with an automated Monte Carlo EM algorithm. *Journal of the Royal Statistical Society*, **B**, **61**, 265–85.

Box, G.P. and Jenkins, G.M. (1970). *Time series analysis – forecasting and control* (revised edn). Holden-Day, San Francisco, California.

Breslow, N.E. (1984). Extra-Poisson variation in log linear models. *Applied Statistics*, **33**, 38–44.

Breslow, N.E. and Clayton, D.G. (1993). Approximate inference in generalized linear mixed models. *Journal of the American Statistical Association*, **88**, 125–34.

Breslow, N.E. and Day, N.E. (1980). *Statistical methods in cancer research, Volume I.* IARC Scientific Publications No. 32. Lyon.

Breslow, N.E. and Lin, X. (1995). Bias correction in generalized linear mixed models with a single component of dispersion. *Biometrika*, **82**, 81–91.

Brumback, B.A. and Rice, J.A. (1998). Smoothing spline models for the analysis of nested and crossed samples of curves (C/R: p976–994). *Journal of the American Statistical Association*, **93**, 961–76.

Carey, V.C. (1992). Regression analysis for large binary clusters. Unpublished PhD thesis, Department of Biostatistics, The Johns Hopkins University, Baltimore, Maryland.

Carey, V.C., Zeger, S.L., and Diggle, P.J. (1993). Modelling multivariate binary data with alternating logistic regressions. *Biometrika*, **80**, 517–26.

Carlin, B.P. and Louis, T.A. (1996), *Bayes and empirical Bayes methods for data analysis*, Chapman and Hall, London.

Chambers, J.M. and Hastie, T.J. (1992). *Statistical models in* S. Wadsworth and Brooks-Cole, Pacific Grove.

Chambers, J.M., Cleveland, W.S., Kleiner, B., and Tukey, P.A. (1983). *Graphical methods for data analysis.* Wadsworth, Belmont, California.

Chib, S. and Carlin, B. (1999). On MCMC sampling in hierarchical longitudinal models. *Statistics and Computing*, **9**, 17–26.

Chib, S. and Greenberg, E. (1998). Analysis of multivariate probit models. *Biometrika*, **85**, 347–61.

Clayton, D.G. (1974). Some odds ratio statistics for the analysis of ordered categorical data. *Biometrika*, **61**, 525–31.

Clayton, D.G. (1992). Repeated ordinal measurements: a generalised estimating equation approach. *Medical Research Council Biostatistics Unit Technical Reports*, Cambridge, England.

Cleveland, W.S. (1979). Robust locally weighted regression and smoothing scatterplots. *Journal of the American Statistical Association*, **74**, 829–36.

Cochran, W.G. (1977). *Sampling techniques.* John Wiley, New York.

Conaway, M.R. (1990). A random effects model for binary data. *Biometrics*, **46**, 317–28.

Cook, D. and Weisberg, S. (1982). *Residuals and influence in regression.* Chapman and Hall, London.

Copas, J.B. and Li, H.G. (1997). Inference for non-random samples (with Discussion). *Journal of the Royal Statistical Society*, **B**, **59**, 55–95.

Courcier. Reissued with a supplement, 1806. Second supplement published 1820. A portion of the appendix was translated, 1929, pp. 576–9 in *A source book in mathematics*, D.E. Smith, ed., trans. by H.A. Ruger and H.M. Walker, McGraw Hill, New York; reprinted 1959 in 2 volumes, Dover, New York.

Cox, D.R. (1970). *Analysis of binary data.* Chapman and Hall, London.

Cox, D.R. (1972). Regression models and life tables (with discussion). *Journal of the Royal Statistical Society*, **B**, **74**, 187–200.

Cox, D.R. (1990). Role of models in statistical analysis. *Statistical science*, **5**, 169–74.

Cox, D.R. and Miller, H.D. (1965). *The theory of stochastic processes.* John Wiley, New York.

Cox, D.R. and Oakes, D. (1984). *Analysis of survival data.* Chapman and Hall, London.

Cox, D.R. and Snell, E.J. (1989). *Analysis of binary data.* Chapman and Hall, London.

Cressie, N.A.C. (1993). *Statistics for spatial data.* Wiley, New York.

Crouch, A.C. and Spiegelman, E. (1990). The evaluation of integrals of the form $\int f(t)\exp(-t^2)\,dt$: application to logistic-normal models. *Journal of the American Statistical Association*, **85**, 464–69.

Cullis, B.R. (1994). Contribution to the Discussion of the paper by Diggle and Kenward. *Applied Statistics*, **43**, 79–80.

Cullis, B.R. and McGilchrist, C.A. (1990). A model for the analysis of growth data from designed experiments. *Biometrics*, **46**, 131–42.

Davidian, M. and Gallant, A.R. (1992). The nonlinear mixed effects model with a smooth random effects density. *Department of Statistics Technical Report, North Carolina State University*, Campus Box 8203, Raleigh, North Carolina 27695.

Davidian, M. and Giltinan, D.M. (1995). *Nonlinear mixed effects models for repeated measurement data.* Chapman and Hall, London.

Deming, W.E. and Stephan, F.F. (1940). On a least squares adjustment of a sampled frequency table when the expected marginal totals are known. *Annals of Mathematical Statistics*, **11**, 427–44.

Dempster, A.P., Laird, N.M., and Rubin, D.B. (1977). Maximum likelihood from incomplete data via the EM algorithm. *Journal of the Royal Statistical Society*, **B**, **39**, 1–38.

Dhrymes, P.J. (1971). *Distributed lags: problems of estimation and formulation.* Holden-Day, San Francisco.

Diggle, P.J. (1988). An approach to the analysis of repeated measures. *Biometrics*, **44**, 959–71.

Diggle, P.J. (1989). Testing for random dropouts in repeated measurement data. *Biometrics*, **45**, 1255–58.

Diggle, P.J. (1990). *Time series: a biostatistical introduction.* Oxford University Press, Oxford.

Diggle, P.J. and Kenward, M.G. (1994). Informative dropout in longitudinal data analysis (with discussion). *Applied Statistics*, **43**, 49–73.

Diggle, P.J. (1998). Dealing with missing values in longitudinal studies. In *Advances in the statistical analysis of medical data* (ed. B.S. Everitt and G. Dunn), pp. 203–28. Edward Arnold, London.

Diggle, P.J. and Verbyla, A. (1998). Nonparametric estimation of covariance structure in longitudinal data. *Biometrics*, **54**, 401–15.

Draper, N. and Smith, H. (1981). *Applied regression analysis (2nd edn).* Wiley, New York.

Drum, M.L. and McCullagh, P. (1993). REML estimation with exact covariance in the logistic mixed model. *Biometrics*, **49**, 677–89.

Dupuis Sammel, M. and Ryan, L.M. (1996). Latent variable models with fixed effects. *Biometrics*, **52**, 650–63.

Emond, M.J., Ritz, J., and Oakes, D. (1997). Bias in GEE estimates from misspecified models for longitudinal data. *Communications in Statistics*, **26**, 15–32.

Engle, R.F., Hendry, D.F., and Richard, J.-F. (1983). Exogeneity. *Econometrica*, **51**, 277–304.

Evans, J.L. and Roberts, E.A. (1979). Analysis of sequential observations with applications to experiments on grazing animals and perennial plants. *Biometrics*, **35**, 687–93.

Evans, M. and Swartz, T. (1995). Methods for approximating integrals in statistics with special emphasis on Bayesian integration problems. *Statistical Science*, **10**, 254–72.

Faucett, C.L. and Thomas, D.C. (1996). Simultaneously modelling censored survival data and repeatedly measured covariates: a Gibbs sampling approach. *Statistics in Medicine*, **15**, 1663–86.

Fearn, T. (1977). A two-stage model for growth curves which leads to Rao's covariance-adjusted estimates. *Biometrika*, **64**, 141–43.

Feller, W. (1968). *An introduction to probability theory and its applications* (3rd edn). John Wiley, New York.

Finkelstein, D.M. and Schoenfeld, D.A. (1999). Combining mortality and longitudinal measures in clinical trials. *Statistics in Medicine*, **18**, 1341–54.

Fitzmaurice, G.M. (1995). A caveat concerning independence estimating equations with multivariate binary data. *Biometrics*, **51**, 309–17.

Fitzmaurice, G.M., Heath, A.F., and Clifford, P. (1996). Logistic regression models for binary panel data with attrition. *Journal of the Royal Statistical Society*, **A**, **159**, 249–63.

Fitzmaurice, G.M. and Laird, N.M. (1993). A likelihood-based method for analysing longitudinal binary responses. *Biometrika*, **80**, 141–51.

Fitzmaurice, G.M., Laird, N.M., and Rotnitzky, A.G. (1993). Regression models for discrete longitudinal responses. *Statistical Science*, **8**, 284–99.

Follman, D. and Wu, M. (1995). An approximate generalized linear model with random effects for informative missing data. *Biometrics*, **51**, 151–68.

Frison, L.J. and Pocock, S.J. (1992). Repeated measures in clinical trials: analysis using mean summary statistics and its implication for design. *Statistics in Medicine*, **11**, 1685–1704.

Frison, L.J. and Pocock, S.J. (1997). Linearly divergent treatment effects in clinical trials with repeated measures: efficient analysis using summary statistics. *Statistics in Medicine*, **16**, 2855–72.

Gabriel, K.R. (1962). Ante dependence analysis of an ordered set of variables. *Annals of Mathematical Statistics*, **33**, 201–12.

Gauss, C.F. (1809). *Theoria motus corporum celestium.* Hamburg: Perthes et Besser. Translated, 1857, as *Theory of motion of the heavenly bodies moving about the sun in conic sections*, trans. C. H. Davis. Little, Brown, Boston. Reprinted, 1963; Dover, New York. French translation of the portion on least squares, pp. 11–134 in Gauss, 1855.

Gelfand, A.E. and Smith, A.F.M. (1990). Sampling-based approaches to calculating margina densities. *Journal of the American Statistical Association*, **85**, 398–409.

Gelfand, A.E., Hills, S.E., Racine-Poon, A., and Smith, A.F.M. (1990). Illustration of Bayesian inference in normal data models using Gibbs sampling. *Journal of the American Statistical Association*, **85**, 972–85.

Gelman, A., Carlin, J.B, Stern, H.S. and Rubin, D.B. (1995). *Bayesian data analysis.* Chapman and Hall, London.

Gibaldi, M. and Perrier, D. (1982). *Pharmacokinetics.* Marcel Dekker, New York.

Gilks, W., Richardson, S., and Speigelhalter, D. (1996). *Markov chain Monte Carlo in practice.* Chapman and Hall, London.

Gilmour, A.R., Anderson, R.D., and Rae, A.L. (1985). The analysis of binomial data by a generalized linear mixed model, *Biometrika*, **72**, 593–99.

Glasbey, C.A. (1988). Examples of regression with serially correlated errors. *The Statistician*, **37**, 277–92.

Glonek, G.F.V. and McCullagh, P. (1995). Multivariate logistic models. *Journal of the Royal Statistical Society*, **B**, **57**, 533–46.

Godambe, V.P. (1960). An optimum property of regular maximum likelihood estimation. *Annals of Mathematical Statistics*, **31**, 1208–12.

Godfrey, L.G. and Poskitt, D.S. (1975). Testing the restrictions of the Almon lag technique. *Journal of the American Statistical Association*, **70**, 105–8.

Goldfarb, N. (1960). *An introduction to longitudinal statistical analysis: the method of repeated observations from a fixed sample.* Free Press of Glencoe, Illinois.

Goldstein, H. (1979). *The design and analysis of longitudinal studies: their role in the measurement of change.* Academic Press, London.

Goldstein, H. (1986). Multilevel mixed linear model analysis using iterative generalised least squares. *Biometrika*, **73**, 43–56.

Goldstein, H. (1995). *Multilevel statistical models* (2nd edn). Edward Arnold, London.

Goldstein, H. and Rasbash, J. (1996). Improved approximations for multilevel models with binary responses. *Journal of the Royal Statistical Society*, **A**, **159**, 505–13.

Gourieroux, C., Monfort, A., and Trognon, A. (1984). Psuedo-maximum likelihood methods: theory. *Econometrica*, **52**, 681–700.

Graubard, B.I. and Korn, E.L. (1994). Regression analysis with clustered data. *Statistics in Medicine*, **13**, 509–22.

Gray, S.M. and Brookmeyer, R. (1998). Estimating a treatment effect from multidimensional longitudinal data. *Biometrics*, **54**, 976–88.

Gray, S. and Brookmeyer, R. (2000). Multidimensional longitudinal data: estimating a treatment effect from continuous, discrete or time to event response variables. *Journal of American Statistical Association*, **95**, 396–406.

Graybill, F. (1976). *Theory and application of the linear model.* Wadsworth, California.

Greenwood, M. and Yule, G.U. (1920). An enquiry into the nature of frequency distributions to the occurrence of multiple attacks of disease or of repeated accidents. *Journal of the Royal Statistical Socieity, Series A*, **83**, 255–79.

Grieve, A.P. (1994). Contribution to the Discussion of the paper by Diggle and Kenward. *Applied Statistics*, **43**, 74–6.

Griffiths, D.A. (1973). Maximum likelihood estimation for the beta-binomial distribution and an application to the household distribution of the total number of cases of a disease. *Biometrics*, **29**, 637–48.

Grömping, U. (1996). A note on fitting a marginal model to mixed effects loglinear regression data via GEE. *Biometrics*, **52**, 280–5.

Guo, S.W. and Lin, D.Y. (1994). Regression analysis of multivariate grouped survival data. *Biometrics*, **50**, 632–39.

Hall, D.B. and Severini, T.A. (1998). Extended generalized estimating equations for clustered data, *Journal of the American Statistical Association*, **93**, 1365–75.

Härdle, W. (1990). *Applied nonparametric regression.* Cambridge University Press, New York.

Harrell, F.E., Lee, K.L., Califf, R.M., Pryor, D.B., and Rosati, R.A. (1984). Regression modelling strategies for improved prognostic prediction. *Statistics in Medicine*, **3**, 143–52.

Hart, J.D. (1991). Kernel regression estimation with time series errors. *Journal of the Royal Statistical Society*, **B**, **53**, 173–87.

Hart, J.D. and Wehrly, T.E. (1986). Kernel regression estimation using repeated measurements data. *Journal of the American Statistical Association*, **81**, 1080–88.

Harville, D. (1974). Bayesian inference for variance components using only error contrasts. *Biometrika*, **61**, 383–85.

Harville, D. (1977). Maximum likelihood estimation of variance components and related problems. *Journal of the American Statistical Association*, **72**, 320–40.

Hastie, T.J. and Tibshirani, R.J. (1990). *Generalized additive models.* Chapman and Hall, New York.

Hausman, J.A. (1978). Specification tests in econometrics. *Econometrica*, **46**, 1251–72.

Heagerty, P.J. (1999). Marginally specified logistic-normal models for longitudinal binary data. *Biometrics*, **55**, 247–57.

Heagerty, P.J. (2002). Marginalized transition models and likelihood inference for longitudinal categorical data. *Biometrics* **58** (to appear).

Heagerty P.J. and Kurland, B.F. (2001). Misspecified maximum likelihood estimates and generalized linear mixed models. *Biometrika*, **88**, 973–85.

Heagerty, P.J. and Zeger, S.L. (1996). Marginal regression models for clustered ordinal measurements. *Journal of the American Statistical Association*, **91**, 1024–36.

Heagerty, P.J. and Zeger, S.L. (1998). Lorelogram: a regression approach to exploring dependence in longitudinal categorical responses. *Journal of the American Statistical Association*, **93**, 150–62.

Heagerty, P.J. and Zeger, S.L. (2000). Marginalized multilevel models and likelihood inference. *Statistical Science*, **15**, 1–26.

Heagerty, P.J. and Zeger, S.L. (2000). Multivariate continuation ratio models: connections and caveats. *Biometrics*, **56**, 719–32.

Heckman, J.J. (1976). The common structure of statistical models of truncation, sample selection and limited dependent variables, and a simple estimation method for such models. *Annals of Economic and Social Measurement*, **5**, 475–92.

Heckman, J.J. and Singer, B. (1985). *Longitudinal analysis of labour market data.* Cambridge University Press, Cambridge.

Hedayat, A. and Afsarinejad, K. (1975). Repeated measures designs, I. In *A survey of statistical design and linear models* (Ed. J.N. Srivastava). North-Holland, Amsterdam.

Hedayat, A. and Afsarinejad, K. (1978). Repeated measures designs, II. *Annals of Statistics*, **6**, 619–28.

Hedeker, D. and Gibbons, R. (1994). A random-effects ordinal regression model for multilevel analysis. *Biometrics*, **50**, 933–44.

Henderson, R., Diggle, P., and Dobson, A. (2000). Joint modelling of longitudinal measurements and recurrent events. *Biostatistics*, **1**, 465–80.

Hernán, M.A., Brumback, B., and Robins, J.M. (2001). Marginal structural models to estimate the joint causal effect of nonrandomized treatments. *Journal of the American Statistical Association*, **96**, 440–8.

Heyting, A., Tolboom, J.T.B.M., and Essers, J.G.A. (1992). Statistical handling of dropouts in longitudinal clinical trials. *Statistics in Medicine*, **11**, 2043–62.

Hogan, J.W. and Laird, N.M. (1977a). Model-based approaches to analysing incomplete longitudinal and failuretime data. *Statistics in Medicine*, **16**, 259–72.

Hogan, J.W. and Laird, N.M. (1977b). Mixture models for the joint distribution of repeated measures and event times. *Statistics in Medicine*, **16**, 239–57.

Holland, P. (1986). Statistics and causal inference. *Journal of the American Statistical Association*, **81**, 945–61.

Huber, P.J. (1967). The behaviour of maximum likelihood estimators under nonstandard conditions. *Proceedings of the Fifth Berkeley Symposium on Mathematical Statistics and Probability*, **1**, LeCam, L.M. and Neyman, J. editors, University of California Press, pp. 221–33.

Hughes, J.P. (1999). Mixed effects models with censored data with application to HIV RNA levels. *Biometrics*, **55**, 625–9.

Jones, B. and Kenward, M.G. (1987). Modelling binary data from a three-point cross-over trial. *Statistics in Medicine*, **6**, 555–64.

Jones, B. and Kenward, M.G. (1989). *Design and analysis of cross-over trials.* Chapman and Hall, London.

Jones, M.C. and Rice, J.A. (1992). Displaying the important features of large collections of similar curves. *The American Statistician*, **46**, 140–45.

Jones, R.M. (1993). *Longitudinal data with serial correlation: a state-space approach.* Chapman and Hall, London.

Jones, R.H. and Ackerson, L.M. (1990). Serial correlation in unequally spaced longitudinal data. *Biometrika*, **77**, 721–31.

Jones, R.H. and Boadi-Boteng, F. (1991). Unequally spaced longitudinal data with serial correlation. *Biometrics*, **47**, 161–75.

Journel, A.G. and Huijbregts, C.J. (1978). *Mining geostatistics.* Academic Press, New York.

Jowett, G.H. (1952). The accuracy of systematic sampling from conveyor belts. *Applied Statistics*, **1**, 50–9.

Kalbfleisch, J.D. and Prentice, R.L. (1980). *The statistical analysis of failure time data.* John Wiley, New York.

Kalman, R.E. (1960). A new approach to linear filtering and prediction problems. *Journal of Basic Engineering*, **82**, 34–45.

Karim, M.R. (1991). Generalized linear models with random effects: a Gibbs sampling approach. Unpublished PhD thesis from the Johns Hopkins University Department of Biostatistics, Baltimore, Maryland.

Kaslow, R.A., Ostrow, D.G., Detels, R. *et al.* (1987). The Multicenter AIDS Cohort Study: rationale, organization and selected characteristics of the participants. *American Journal of Epidemiology*, **126**, 310–18.

Kaufmann, H. (1987). Regression models for nonstationary categorical time series: asymptotic estimation theory. *Annals of Statistics*, **15**, 863–71.

Kenward, M.G. (1987). A method for comparing profiles of repeated measurements. *Applied Statistics*, **36**, 296–308.

Kenward, M.G., Lesaffre, E., and Molenberghs, G. (1994). An application of maximum likelihood and estimating equations to the analysis of ordinal data from a longitudinal study with cases missing at random. *Biometrics*, **50**, 945–53.

Korn, E.L. and Whittemore, A.S. (1979). Methods for analyzing panel studies of acute health effects of air pollution. *Biometrics*, **35**, 795–802.

Laird, N.M. (1988). Missing data in longitudinal studies. *Statistics in Medicine*, **7**, 305–15.

Laird, N.M. and Wang, F. (1990). Estimating rates of change in randomized clinical trials. *Controlled Clinical Trials*, **11**, 405–19.

Laird, N.M. and Ware, J.H. (1982). Random-effects models for longitudinal data. *Biometrics*, **38**, 963–74.

Lang, J.B. and Agresti, A. (1994). Simultaneously modeling joint and marginal distributions of multivariate categorical responses. *Journal of the American Statistical Association*, **89**, 625–32.

Lang, J.B., McDonald, J.W., and Smith, P.W.F. (1999). Association-marginal modeling of multivariate categorical responses: a maximum likelihood approach. *Journal of the American Statistical Association*, **94**, 1161–71.

Lange, N. and Ryan, L. (1989). Assessing normality in random effects models. *Annals of Statistics*, **17**, 624–42.

Lauritzen, S.L. (2000). Causal inference from graphical models. Research Report R-99-2021, Department of Mathematical Sciences, Aalborg University.

Lavalley, M.P. and De Gruttola, V. (1996). Models for empirical Bayes estimators of longitudinal CD4 counts. *Statistics in Medicine*, **15**, 2289–305.

Lawless, J.F. (1982). *Statistical models and methods for lifetime data*. John Wiley, New York.

Lee, Y. and Nelder, J.A. (1996). Hierarchical generalized linear models (with discussion). *Journal of the Royal Statistical Society, Series B*, **58**, 619–78.

Lee, Y. and Nelder, J.A. (2001). Hierarchical generalised linear models, a synthesis of generalised linear models, random-effects models and structured dispersions. *Biometrika* **88**, 987–1006.

Legendre, A.M. (1805). *Nouvelles Méthodes pour la detérmination des orbites des comètes*. John Wiley, New York.

Lepper, A.W.D. (1989). Effects of altered dietary iron intake in *Mycobacterium paratuberculosis*-infected dairy cattle: sequential observations on growth, iron and copper metabolism and development of paratuberculosis. *Res. Vet. Sci.*, **46**, 289–96.

Liang, K.-Y. and McCullagh, P. (1993). Case studies in binary dispersion. *Biometrics*, **49**, 623–30.

Liang, K.-Y. and Zeger, S.L. (1986). Longitudinal data analysis using generalized linear models. *Biometrika*, **73**, 13–22.

Liang, K.-Y. and Zeger, S.L. (2000). Longitudinal data analysis of continuous and discrete responses for pre-post designs. *Sankya*, **B**, **62**, 134–48.

Liang, K.-Y., Zeger, S.L., and Qaqish, B. (1992). Multivariate regression analyses for categorical data (with Discussion). *Journal of the Royal Statistical Society*, **B**, **54**, 3–40.

Lin, D.Y. and Ying, Z. (2001). Semiparametric and nonparametric regression analysis of longitudinal data. *Journal of the American Statistical Association*, **96**, 103–26.

Lin, X. and Breslow, N.E. (1996). Bias correction in generalized linear mixed models with multiple components of dispersion. *Journal of the American Statistical Association*, **91**, 1007–16.

Lin, X. and Carroll, R.J. (2000). Nonparametric function estimation for clustered data when the predictor is measured without/with error. *Journal of the American Statistical Association*, **95**, 520–34.

Lindstrom, M.J. and Bates, D.M. (1990). Nonlinear mixed effects models for repeated measures data. *Biometrics*, **46**, 673–87.

Lipsitz, S. (1989). Generalized estimating equations for correlated binary data: using the odds ratio as a measure of association. Technical report, Department of Biostatistics, Harvard School of Public Health.

Lipsitz, S., Laird, N., and Harrington, D. (1991). Generalized estimating equations for correlated binary data: using odds ratios as a measure of association. *Biometrika*, **78**, 153–60.

Little, R.J.A. (1993). Pattern-mixture models for multivariate incomplete data. *Journal of the American Statistical Association*, **88**, 125–34.

Little, R.J.A. (1995). Modelling the drop-out mechanism in repeated-measures studies. *Journal of the American Statistical Association*, **90**, 1112–21.

Little, R.J.A. and Rubin, D.B. (1987). *Statistical analysis with missing data.* John Wiley, New York.

Little, R.J. and Rubin, D.B. (2000). Causal effects in clinical and epidemiological studies via potential outcomes: concepts and analytical approaches. *Annual Review in Public Health*, **21**, 121–45.

Liu, G. and Liang, K.-Y. (1997). Sample size calculations for studies with correlated observations. *Biometrics*, **53**, 937–47.

Liu, Q. and Pierce, D.A. (1994). A note on Gauss–Hermite quadrature. *Biometrika*, **81**, 624–9.

Lindsey, J.K. (2000). Obtaining marginal estimates from conditional categorical repeated measurements models with missing data. *Statistics in Medicine*, **19**, 801–9.

Lunn, D.J., Wakefield, J., and Racine-Poon, A. (2001). Cumulative logit models for ordinal data, a case study involving allergic rhinitis severity scores. *Statistics in Medicine*, **20**, 2261–85.

Mason, W.B. and Fienberg, S.E. (eds) (1985). *Cohort analysis in social research: beyond the identification problem.* Springer-Verlag, New York.

McCullagh, P. (1980). Regression models for ordinal data (with discussion). *Journal of the Royal Statistical Society*, **B**, **42**, 109–42.

McCullagh, P. (1983). Quasi-likelihood functions. *Annals of Statistics*, **11**, 59–67.

McCullagh, P. and Nelder, J.A. (1989). *Generalized linear models.* Chapman and Hall, New York.

McCulloch, C.E. (1997). Maximum likelihood algorithms for generalized linear mixed models. *Journal of the American Statistical Association*, **92**, 162–70.

Mead, R. and Curnow, R.N. (1983). *Statistical methods in agriculture and experimental biology.* Chapman and Hall, London.

Molenberghs, G., Kenward, M.G., and Lesaffre, E. (1997). The analysis of longitudinal ordinal data with informativedvi dropout. *Biometrika*, **84**, 33–44.

Molenberghs, G. and Lesaffre, E. (1994). Marginal modeling of correlated ordinal data using a multivariate Plackett distribution. *Journal of the American Statistical Association*, **89**, 633–44.

Molenberghs, G. and Lesaffre, E. (1999). Marginal modeling of multivariate categorical data. *Statistics in Medicine*, **18**, 2237–55.

Molenberghs, G., Michiels, B., Kenward, M.G., and Diggle, P.J. (1997). Missing data mechanisms and pattern-mixture models. *Statistica Neerlandica*, **52**, 153–61.

Monahan, J.F. and Stefanski, L.A. (1992). Normal scale mixture approximations to $F^*(x)$ and computation of the logistic-normal integral. In *Handbook of the logistic distribution* (ed. N. Balakrishnan), pp. 529–40. Marcel Dekker, New York.

Morton, R. (1987). A generalized linear model with nested strat of extra-Poisson variation. *Biometrika*, **74**, 247–57.

Mosteller, F. and Tukey, J.W. (1977). *Data analysis and regression: a second course in statistics.* Addison-Wesley, Reading, Massachusetts.

Moyeed, R.A. and Diggle, P.J. (1994). Rates of convergence in semi-parametric modelling of longitudinal data. *Australian Journal of Statistics*, **36**, 75–93.

Müller, M.G. (1988). *Nonparametric regression analysis of longitudinal data.* Lecture Notes in Statistics, **41**. Springer-Verlag, Berlin.

Munoz, A., Carey, V., Schouten, J.P., Segal, M., and Rosner, B. (1992). A parametric family of correlation structures for the analysis of longitudinal data. *Biometrics*, **48**, 733–42.

Murray, G.D. and Findlay, J.G. (1988). Correcting for the bias caused by dropouts in hypertension trials. *Statistics in Medicine*, **7**, 941–46.

Nelder, J.A. and Mead, R. (1965). A simplex method for function minimisation. *Computational Journal*, **7**, 303–13.

Neuhaus, J.M., Hauck, W.W., and Kalbfleisch, J.D. (1992). The effects of mixture distribution misspecification when fitting mixed-effects logistic models. *Biometrika*, **79**, 755–62.

Neuhaus, J.M. and Jewell, N.P. (1990). Some comments on Rosner's multiple logistic model for clustered data. *Biometrics*, **46**, 523–34.

Neuhaus, J.M. and Kalbfleisch, J.D. (1998). Between- and within-cluster covariate effects in the analysis of clustered data. *Biometrics*, **54**, 638–45.

Neuhaus, J.M., Kalbfleisch, J.D., and Hauck, W.W. (1991). A comparison of cluster-specific and population averaged approaches for analyzing correlated binary data. *International Statistical Review*, **59**, 25–36.

Neyman, J. (1923). On the application of probability theory to agricultural experiments: essay on principles, section 9, translated in *Statistical Science*, 1990, **5**, 65–80.

Neyman, J. and Scott, E.L. (1948). Consistent estimates based on partially consistent observations. *Econometrica*, **16**, 1–32.

O'Brien, P.C. (1984). Procedures for comparing samples with multiple endpoints. *Biometrics*, **40**, 1079–87.

Paik, M.C. (1992). Parametric variance function estimation for non-normal repeated measurement data. *Biometrics*, **48**, 18–30.

Palta, M., Lin, C-Y., and Chao, W.-H. (1997). Effect of confounding and other misspecification in models for longitudinal data. In *Modelling longitudinal and spatially correlated data: methods, applications, and future directions (Springer Lecture Notes in Statistics, Volume 122)*, 77–87.

Pan, W., Louis, T.A., and Connett, J.E. (2000). A note on marginal linear regression with correlated response data. *American Statistician*, **54**, 191–5.

Pantula, S.G. and Pollock, K.H. (1985). Nested analysis of variance with autocorrelated errors. *Biometrics*, **41**, 909–20.

Patterson, H.D. (1951). Change-over trials. *Journal of the Royal Statistical Society*, **B**, **13**, 256–71.

Patterson, H.D. and Thompson, R. (1971). Recovery of inter-block information when block sizes are unequal. *Biometrika*, **58**, 545–54.

Pawitan, Y. and Self, S. (1993). Modelling disease marker processes in AIDS. *Journal of the American Statistical Association*, **88**, 719–26.

Pearl, J. (2000). Causal inference in the health sciences: a conceptual introduction. Contributions to Health Services and Outcomes Research Methodology, Technical report R-282, Department of Computer Science, University of California, Los Angeles.

Pepe, M.S. and Anderson, G.A. (1994). A cautionary note on inference for marginal regression models with longitudinal data and general correlated response data. *Communication in Statistics – Simulation*, **23**(4), 939–51.

Pepe, M.S. and Couper, D. (1997). Modeling partly conditional means with longitudinal data. *Journal of the American Statistical Association*, **92**, 991–8.

Pepe, M.S., Heagerty, P.J., and Whitaker, R. (1999). Prediction using partly conditional time-varying coefficients regression models. *Biometrics*, **55**, 944–50.

Pierce, D.A. and Sands, B.R. (1975). Extra-Bernoulli variation in binary data. Technical Report 46, Department of Statistics, Oregon State University.

Pinheiro, J.C. and Bates, D.M. (1995). Approximations to the log-likelihood function in the non-linear mixed-effects model. *Journal of Computational and Graphical Statistics*, **4**, 12–35.

Plewis, I. (1985). *Analysing change: measurement and explanation using longitudinal data.* John Wiley, New York.

Pocock, S.J., Geller, N.L., and Tsiatis, A.A. (1987). The analysis of multiple endpoints in clinical trials. *Biometrics*, **43**, 487–98.

Poisson, S.D. (1837). Recherches sur la Probabilite des Jugements en Matiere Criminelle et en Matiere Civile, Precedees des Regles Generales du Calcul des Probabilities. Bachelier, Imprimeur-Libraire pour les Mathematiques, la Physique, etc., Paris.

Pourahmadi, M. (1999). Joint mean-covariance models with application to longitudinal data: unconstrained parameterisation. *Biometrika*, **86**, 677–90.

Prentice, R.L. (1986). Binary regression using an extended beta-binomial distribution, with discussion of correlation induced by covariate measurement errors. *Journal of the American Statistical Association*, **81**, 321–27.

Prentice, R.L. (1988). Correlated binary regression with covariates specific to each binary observation. *Biometrics*, **44**, 1033–48.

Prentice, R.L. and Zhao, L.P. (1991). Estimating equations for parameters in means and covariances of multivariate discrete and continuous responses. *Biometrics*, **47**, 825–39.

Priestley, M.B. and Chao, M.T. (1972). Non-parametric function fitting. *Journal of the Royal Statistical Society*, **B**, **34**, 384–92.

Rao, C.R. (1965). The theory of least squares when the parameters are stochastic and its application to the analysis of growth curves. *Biometrika*, **52**, 447–58.

Rao, C.R. (1973). *Linear statistical inference and its applications* (2nd edn). John Wiley, New York.

Ratkowsky, D.A. (1983). *Non-linear regression modelling.* Marcel Dekker, New York.

Rice, J.A. and Silverman, B.W. (1991). Estimating the mean and covariance structure nonparametrically when the data are curves. *Journal of the Royal Statistical Society*, **B**, **53**, 233–43.

Ridout, M. (1991). Testing for random dropouts in repeated measurement data. *Biometrics*, **47**, 1617–21.

Robins, J.M. (1986). A new approach to causal inference in mortality studies with sustained exposure periods – application to control of the healthy worker survivor effect. *Mathematical Modelling*, **7**, 1393–512.

Robins, J.M. (1987). Addendum to 'A new approach to causal inference in mortality studies with sustained exposure periods – application to control of the healthy worker survivor effect.' *Computers and Mathematics with Applications*, **14**, 923–45.

Robins, J.M. (1998). Correction for non-compliance in equivalent trials. *Statistics in Medicine*, **17**, 269–302.

Robins, J.M. (1999). Marginal structural models versus structural nested models as tools for causal inference. In *Statistical models in epidemiology: the environment and clinical trials*. (ed. M.E. Halloran and D. Berry), pp. 95–134, *IMA Volume 116*, Springer-Verlag New York.

Robins, J.M., Greenland, S., and Hu, F.-C. (1999). Estimation of the causal effect of a time-varying exposure on the marginal mean of a repeated binary outcome (with Discussion). *Journal of the American Statistical Association*, **94**, 687–712.

Robins, J.M., Rotnitzky, A., and Zhao, L.P. (1995). Analysis of semiparametric regression models for repeated outcomes in the presence of missing data. *Journal of the American Statistical Association*, **90**, 106–21.

Rosner, B. (1984). Multivariate methods in ophthalmology with application to other paired-data situations. *Biometrics*, **40**, 1025–35.

Rosner, B. (1989). Multivariate methods for clustered binary data with more than one level of nesting. *Journal of the American Statistical Association*, **84**, 373–80.

Rothman, K.J. and Greenland, S. (1998). *Modern epidemiology*. Lippincott-Raven.

Rowell, J.G. and Walters, D.E. (1976). Analysing data with repeated observations on each experimental unit. *Journal of Agricultural Science*, **87**, 423–32.

Royall, R.M. (1986). Model robust inference using maximum likelihood estimators. *International Statistical Review*, **54**, 221–26.

Rubin, D.B. (1974). Estimating causal effects of treatment in randomized and non-randomized studies. *Journal of Educational Psychology*, **66**, 688–701.

Rubin, D.B. (1976). Inference and missing data. *Biometrika*, **63**, 581–92.

Rubin, D.B. (1978). Bayesian inference for causal effects: the role of randomization. *Annals of Statistics*, **6**, 34–58.

Samet, J.M., Dominici, F., Curriero, F.C., Coursac, I., and Zeger, S.L. (2000). Fine particulate air pollution and mortality in 20 US cities, 1987–1994. *New England Journal of Medicine*, **343**(24), 1798–9.

Sandland, R.L. and McGilchrist, C.A. (1979). Stochastic growth curve analysis. *Biometrics*, **35**, 255–71.

Schall, R. (1991). Estimation in generalized linear models with random effects. *Biometrika*, **78**, 719–27.

Scharfstein, D.O., Rotnitzky, A., and Robins, J.M. (1999). Adjusting for non-ignorable dropout using semiparametric non-response models (with Discussion). *Journal of the American Statistical Association*, **94**, 1096–1120.

Seber, G.A.F. (1977). *Linear regression analysis*. John Wiley, New York.

Self, S. and Mauritsen, R. (1988). Power/sample size calculations for generalized linear models. *Biometrics*, **44**, 79–86.

Senn, S.J. (1992). *Crossover trials in clinical research.* John Wiley, Chichester.

Sheiner, L.B., Beal, S.L., and Dunne, A. (1997). Analysis of nonrandomly censored ordered categorical longitudinal data from analgesic trials (with Discussion). *Journal of the American Statistical Association*, **92**, 1235–55.

Shih, J. (1998). Modeling multivaraite discrete failure time data. *Biometrics*, **54**, 1115–28.

Silverman, B.W. (1984). Spline smoothing: the equivalent variable kernel method. *Annals of Statistics*, **12**, 898–916.

Silverman, B.W. (1985). Some aspects of the spline smoothing approach to non-parametric regression curve fitting (with Discussion). *Journal of the Royal Statistical Society*, **B**, **47**, 1–52.

Skellam, J.G. (1948). A probability distribution derived from the binomial distribution by regarding the probability of success as variable between the sets of trials. *Journal of the Royal Statistical Society*, **B**, **10**, 257–61.

Snedecor, G.W. and Cochran, W.G. (1989). *Statistical methods* (8th edn). Iowa State University Press, Ames, Iowa.

Snell, E.J. (1964). A scaling procedure for ordered categorical data. *Biometrics*, **40**, 592–607.

Solomon, P.J. and Cox, D.R. (1992). Nonlinear components of variance models. *Biometrika*, **79**, 1–11.

Sommer, A. (1982). *Nutritional blindness.* Oxford University Press, New York.

Sommer, A., Katz, J., and Tarwotjo, I. (1984). Increased risk of respiratory infection and diarrhea in children with pre-existing mild vitamin A deficiency. *American Journal of Clinical Nutrition*, **40**, 1090–95.

Spall, J. C. (1988). *Bayesian analysis of time series and Dynamic models.* Marcel Dekker, New York.

Stanek, E.J. (1988). Choosing a pre-test-post test analysis. *American Statistician*, **42**, 178–83.

Stefanski, L.A. and Carroll, R.J. (1985). Covariate measurement error in logistic regression. *Annals of Statistics*, **13**, 1335–51.

Stern, R.D. and Coe, R. (1984). A model fitting analysis of daily rainfall data. *Journal of the Royal Statistical Society*, **A**, **147**, 1–34.

Stiratelli, R., Laird, N., and Ware, J.H. (1984). Random effects models for serial observations with binary responses. *Biometrics*, **40**, 961–71.

Stram, D.O., Wei, L.J., and Ware, J.H. (1988). Analysis of repeated ordered categorical outcomes with possibly missing observations and time-dependent covariates. *Journal of the American Statistical Association*, **83**, 631–37.

Sun, D., Speckman, P.L., and Tsutakawa, R.K. (2000). Random effects in generalized linear mixed models (GLMMs). In *Generalized linear models, a Bayesian perspective* (ed. D. Dey, S. Ghosh, and B. Mallick), pp. 23–39, Marcel-Dekker, New York.

TenHave, T.R., Kunselman, A.R., and Tran, L. (1999). A comparison of mixed effects logistic regression model for binary response data with two nested levels of clustering. *Statistics in Medicine*, **18**, 947–60.

TenHave, T.R. and Uttal, D.H. (1994). Subject-specific and population-averaged contination ratio logit models for multiple discrete survival profiles. *Applied Statistics*, **43**, 371–84.

Thall, P.F. and Vail, S.C. (1990). Some covariance models for longitudinal count data with overdispersion. *Biometrics*, **46**, 657–71.

Thara, R., Henrietta, M., Joseph, A., Rajkumar, S., and Eaton, W. (1994). Ten year course of schizophrenia – the Madras Longitudinal study. *Acta Psychiatrica Scandinavica*, **90**, 329–36.

Tsay, R. (1984). Regression models with time series errors. *Journal of the American Statistical Association*, **79**, 118–24.

Tsiatis, A.A., De Gruttola, V., and Wulfsohn, M.S. (1995). Modelling the relationship of survival to longitudinal data measured with error. Applications to survival and CD4 counts in patients with AIDS. *Journal of the American Statistical Association*, **90**, 27–37.

Tufte, E.R. (1983). *The visual display of quantitative information.* Graphics Press, Cheshire, Connecticut.

Tufte, E.R. (1990). *Envisioning information.* Graphics Press, Cheshire, Connecticut.

Tukey, J.W. (1977). *Exploratory data analysis.* Addison-Wesley, Reading, Massachusetts.

Tunnicliffe-Wilson, G. (1989). On the use of marginal likelihood in time series model estimation. *Journal of the Royal Statistical Society*, **B**, **51**, 15–27.

Velleman, P.F. and Hoaglin, D.C. (1981). *Applications, basics, and computing of exploratory data analysis.* Duxbury Press, Boston, Massachusetts.

Verbeke, G. and Molenberghs, G. (2000). *Linear Mixed Models for Longitudinal Data.* Springer, New York.

Verbyla, A.P. (1986). Conditioning in the growth curve model. *Biometrika*, **73**, 475–83.

Verbyla, A.P. and Cullis, B.R. (1990). Modelling in repeated measures experiments. *Applied Statistics*, **39**, 341–56.

Verbyla, A.P. and Venables, W.N. (1988). An extension of the growth curve model. *Biometrika*, **75**, 129–38.

Volberding, P.A., Lagakos, S.W., Koch, M.A. *et al.* (1990). Zidovudine in asymptomatic human immunodeficiency virus infection. *The New England Journal of Medicine*, **322**, 941–9.

Waclawiw, M.A. and Liang, K.-Y. (1993). Prediction of random effects in the generalized linear model. *Journal of the American Statistical Association*, **88**, 171–78.

Wakefield, J. (1996). The Bayesian analysis of population pharmacokinetic models. *Journal of the American Statistical Association*, **91**, 62–75.

Wang, Y. (1998). Smoothing spline models with correlated random errors. *Journal of the American Statistical Association*, **93**, 341–48.

Ware, J.H. (1985). Linear models for the analysis of longitudinal studies. *The American Statistician*, **39**, 95–101.

Ware, J.H., Lipsitz, S., and Speizer, F.E. (1988). Issues in the analysis of repeated categorical outcomes. *Statistics in Medicine*, **7**, 95–107.

Ware, J.H., Dockery, D., Louis, T.A. *et al.* (1990). Longitudinal and cross-sectional estimates of pulmonary function decline in never-smoking adults. *American Journal of Epidemiology*, **32**, 685–700.

Wedderburn, R.W.M. (1974). Quasi-likelihood functions, generalized linear models and the Gaussian method. *Biometrika*, **61**, 439–47.

West, M., Harrison, P.J., and Migon, H.S. (1985). Dynamic generalized linear models and Bayesian forecasting (with Discussion). *Journal of the American Statistical Association*, **80**, 73–97.

White, H. (1982). Maximum likelihood estimation of misspecified models. *Econometrics*, **50**, 1–25.

Whittaker, J.C. (1990). *Graphical models in applied multivariate statistics*. John Wiley, New York.

Williams, E.J. (1949). Experimental designs balanced for the estimation of residual effects of treatments. *Australian Journal of Scientific Research*, **2**, 149–68.

Williams, D.A. (1975). The analysis of binary responses from toxicological experiments involving reproduction and teratogenicity. *Biometrics*, **31**, 949–52.

Williams, D.A. (1982). Extra-binomial variation in logistic linear models. *Applied Statistics*, **31**, 144–48.

Winer, B.J. (1977). *Statistical principles in experimental design* (2nd edn). McGraw-Hill, New York.

Wishart, J. (1938). Growth-rate determinations in nutrition studies with the bacon pig, and their analysis. *Biometrika*, **30**, 16–28.

Wong, W.H. (1986). Theory of partial likelihood. *Annals of Statistics*, **14**, 88–123.

Wu, M.C. and Bailey, K.R. (1989). Estimation and comparison of changes in the presence of informative right censoring: conditional linear model. *Biometrics*, **45**, 939–55.

Wu, M.C. and Carroll, R.J. (1988). Estimation and comparison of changes in the presence of right censoring by modeling the censoring process. *Biometrics*, **44**, 175–88.

Wulfsohn, M.S. and Tsiatis, A.A. (1997). A joint model for survival and longitudinal data measured with error. *Biometrics*, **53**, 330–39.

Xu, J. and Zeger, S.L. (2001). Joint analysis of longitudinal data comprising repeated measures and times to events. *Applied Statistics*, **50**, 375–87.

Yu, O., Sheppard, L., Lumley, T., Koenig, J.Q., and Shapiro, G. (2000). Effects of ambient carbon monoxide and atmospheric particles on asthma symptoms, results from the CAMP air pollution ancillary study. *Environmental Health Perspectives*, **12**, 1–10.

Yule, G.U. (1927). On a method of investigating periodicities in disturbed series with special reference to Wolfer's sunspot numbers. *Philosophical Transactions of the Royal Society of London*, **A**, **226**, 267–98.

Zeger, S.L. and Diggle, P.J. (1994). Semi-parametric models for longitudinal data with application to CD4 cell numbers in HIV seroconverters. *Biometrics*, **50**, 689–99.

Zeger, S.L. and Karim, M.R. (1991). Generalized linear models with random effects: a Gibbs sampling approach. *Journal of the American Statistical Association*, **86**, 79–86.

Zeger, S.L. and Liang, K.-Y. (1986). Longitudinal data analysis for discrete and continuous outcomes. *Biometrics*, **42**, 121–30.

Zeger, S.L. and Liang, K.Y. (1991). Feedback models for discrete and continuous time series. *Statistica Sinica*, **1**, 51–64.

Zeger, S.L. and Liang, K.-Y. (1992). An overview of methods for the analysis of longitudinal data. *Statistics in Medicine*, **11**, 1825–39.

Zeger, S.L., Liang, K.-Y., and Albert, P.S. (1988). Models for longitudinal data: a generalized estimating equation approach. *Biometrics*, **44**, 1049–60.

Zeger, S.L., Liang, K.-Y., and Self, S.G. (1985). The analysis of binary longitudinal data with time-indpendent covariates. *Biometrika*, **72**, 31–8.

Zeger, S.L. and Qaqish, B. (1988). Markov regression models for time series: a quasi-likelihood approach. *Biometrics*, **44**, 1019–31.

Zhang, D., Lin, X., Raz, J., and Sowers, M.F. (1998). Semiparametric stochastic mixed models for longitudinal data. *Journal of the American Statistical Association*, **93**, 710–19.

Zhao, L.P. and Prentice, R.L. (1990). Correlated binary regression using a generalized quadratic model. *Biometrika*, **77**, 642–48.

Index

Note: Figures and Tables are indicated by *italic page numbers.*

adaptive quadrature technique 212–13
  examples of use *232*, *238*
age effect 1, 157
  in example 157–9, *159*
AIDS research 3, 330
  see also CD4+ cell numbers data
alternating logistic regressions (ALRs) 147
  see also generalized estimating equations
analysis of variance (ANOVA) methods 114–25
  advantages 125
  limitations 114
  split-plot ANOVA 56, 123–5
    example of use 124–5
  time-by-time ANOVA 115–16, 125
    example of use 116, *118*
    limitations 115, 125
ante-dependence models 87–9, 115
approximate maximum likelihood methods 175, 210
  advantage 212
autocorrelated/autoregressive random effects model 210, *211*
  in example 239
autocorrelation function 46, 48
  for CD4+ data *48*, *49*
  for exponential model *57*, 84
autoregressive models 56–7, 87–8, 134
available case missing value restrictions 300

back-fitting algorithm 324
Bahadur representation 144
bandwidth, curve-fitting 45
Bayesian methods
  for generalized linear mixed models 214–16
    examples of use *232*, *238*
beta-binomial distribution 178–9
  uses 179
bias 22–4
bibliography 349–68
binary data, simulation under generalized linear mixed models 210, *211*
binary responses
  logistic regression models 175–84
    conditional likelihood approach 175–8
    with Gaussian random effects 180–4
    random effects models 178–80
  log-linear models 142–3
  marginal models 143–6
    examples 148–60
  sample size calculations 30–1
boxcar window 43
boxplots 10, *12*
BUGS software 216

calf intestinal parasites experiment
  data *117*
  time-by-time ANOVA applied 116, *118*
canonical parameters, in log-linear models 143, 153
carry-over effect
  experimental assessment of 7, 151–3
  ignored 149
categorical data
  generalized linear mixed models for 209–16
    examples 231, *232*, 237–40

categorical data (*cont.*)
likelihood-based methods for 208–44
marginalized models for 216–31
examples 231–3, 240–3
ordered, transition models for 201–4
transition models for 194–204
examples 197–201
categorical responses, association among 52–3
causal estimation methods 273–4
causal models 271
causal targets of inference 269–73
CD4+ cell numbers data 3–4
correlation in 46–8
and depressive symptoms score 39–41
estimation of population mean curve 325–6
graphical representation *3*, 35–9
marginal analysis 18
parametric modelling 108–10
prediction of individual trajectories 110, 112–13
random effects models 18, 130
time-dependent covariates 247
variograms 50, *51*, *326*
cerebrovascular deficiency treatment trial 148
conditional likelihood estimation 177
data *148*
marginal model used 148–50, *181*
maximum likelihood estimation 180–1
random effects model used *181*
chi-squared distributions 342
chi-squared test statistic, in cow-weight study 107
c-index 264
clinical trials
dropouts in *13*, 285
as prospective studies 2
see also epileptic seizure ...; schizophrenia clinical trial
cohort effects 1
complete case analysis 288
complete case missing variable restrictions 300
complete data score functions 173
completely random dropouts
testing for 288–90
in examples 290–3
completely random missing values 283, 284
conditional generalized linear regression model 209
conditional likelihood
advantages of approach 177–8
for generalized linear mixed models 171–2
maximization in transition model 138, 193
for random intercept logistic regression model 175–8
random intercept log-linear model for count data 184–6
see also maximum likelihood
conditional maximum likelihood estimation
random effects model
for count data 184–6
generalized linear mixed model 171–2
for transition models 138, 192–3, 203
conditional means 13, 191, 209
full covariate conditional mean 253
likelihood-based estimates *232*, *238*
partly conditional mean 253
conditional models 153, 190
conditional modes 174
conditional odds ratios 144, 146–7
confirmatory analysis 33
confounders
meaning of term 265
time-dependent 265–80
connected-line graphs 35, *35*, *36*, *37*
alternative plots 37–8
continuous responses, sample size calculations 28–30
correlated errors
general linear model with 55–9
non-linear models with 327, 328
correlation
among repeated observations 28
in longitudinal data 46–52
consequences of ignoring 19
correlation matrix 24–5, 46
for CD4+ data 46, *48*
correlation models
exponential 56–7
uniform 55–6
count data
examples 160–1
generalized estimating equations for 162–3
log-linear transition models for 204–6

marginal model for 137, 160–5
over-dispersed 161, 186
parametric modelling for 160–2
random effects model for 137, 186–8
counted responses
marginal model used 160–5
random effects model used 184–9
counterfactual outcomes 269
regression model for 276–7
covariance structure
modelling of 81–113, 323, 324
reasons for 79–80
covariate endogeneity 245, 246
covariates 337
external 246
internal 246
lagged 259–65
stochastic 253–8
time-dependent 245–81
cow weight data 103–4
parametric modelling 104–8
crossover trials 148
examples 7, 9, *10*, 148–53, 176–7
further reading recommended 31–2, 168
GLMMs compared with marginalized models 231–3
marginal models applied 148–53
random effects models applied 176–7
relative efficiency of OLS estimation 63
time-dependent covariates in 247
see also cerebrovascular deficiency treatment trial; dysmenorrhoeal pain treatment trial
cross-sectional analysis, example 257–8
cross-sectional association in data 251, 254
cross-sectional data, fitting of non-linear regression model to 327
cross-sectional models
correlated error structures 327, 328
estimation issues for 254–5, 256
non-linear random effects 327, 329
cross-sectional studies
bias in 22–4
compared with longitudinal studies 1, 16–17, 22–31, *41*, 159–60
cross-validation 45
crowding effect 205
cubic smoothing spline 44
curve-fitting methods 41–5

data score functions 173
derived variables 17, 116–23
examples of use 119–23
design considerations 22–32
bias 22–4
efficiency 24–6
further reading recommended 31–2
sample size calculations 25–31
diagnostics, for models 98
Diggle–Kenward model 295
fitted to milk protein data 298–9
informative dropouts investigated by 298, 318
distributed lag models 260–1
in examples 262, *263*
dropout process
modelling of 295–8
in examples 298–9, 301
graphical representation of various models 303–5
pattern mixture models 299–301, 304
random effects models 301–3, 304, 305
selection models 295–8, 304–5
dropouts 284–7
in clinical trials *13*, 285
completely random, testing for 288–90
divergence of fitted and observed means when ignored *311*, 316
in milk protein study 285
random 285
reasons for 12, 285, 299
ways of dealing with 287–8
complete case analysis 288
last-observation-carried-forward method 287–8
dysmenorrhoeal pain treatment trial 7, 9
data *10*, *151*
GLMMs compared with marginalized models 231–3
marginal model used 150–3
random intercept model fitted 177

efficiency, longitudinal compared with cross-sectional studies 24–6
EM algorithm 173–4, 284, 332
empirical Bayes estimates 112
endogeneity, in example 268–9
endogenous variables 246, 253
epileptic seizure clinical trial 10
boxplots of data *12*

epileptic seizure clinical trial (*cont.*)
  data *11*
    summary statistics *163*
  marginal model 163–5
  Poisson model used 161–2
  random effects model 185–6, 188, *189*
estimation stage of model-fitting process 95–7
event history data 330
exogeneity 245, 246–7
exogenous variables 246
explanatory variables 337
exploratory data analysis (EDA) 33–53, 198–9, 328
exponential correlation model 56–7, 84, 89
  compared with Gaussian correlation model 87
  efficiency of OLS estimator in 61–2
  variograms for *85*
external covariates 246
extra-binomial variation 178

feedback, covariate–response 253, 258, 266–8
first-order autoregressive models 56–7, 87–8
first-order marginalized transition model/MTM(1) 226–7, 230, 241
  in example 241, *242*
Fisher's information matrix 340
  in example 341
fixed quadrature technique 212
  examples of use *232*
formulation of parametric model 94–5
F-statistic 115, 120, 122–3, 123–4, 125
full covariate conditional mean 253
full covariate conditional mean (FCCM) assumption 255
  further reading recommended 258
  simulation illustration 256–7

Gauss–Hermite quadrature 212, 213
Gaussian adaptive quadrature 212–13
Gaussian assumptions
  further reading recommended 189
  general linear model 55
  maximum likelihood estimation under 64–5, 180, 181
Gaussian correlation model 86
  compared with exponential correlation model 87
  variograms for *86*
Gaussian kernel 43, 320, 321
Gaussian linear model, marginalized models using 218–20
Gaussian random effects
  logistic models with 180–4
  Poisson regression with 188
Gauss–Markov Theorem 334, 339
g-computation, estimation of causal effects by 273–4
  advantages 276
  in example 275–6
generalized estimating equations (GEEs) 138–40, 146–7
  advantages 293–4
  for count data 162–3
    example 163–5
  and dropouts 293–5
  further reading recommended 167, 168
  for logistic regression models 146–7, 203, 240, *241*
    in examples 149, *150*, 154
  for random missingness mechanism 293–5
  and stochastic covariates 257, 258, *258*
  and time-dependent covariates 249–50, *251*
generalized linear mixed models (GLMMs) 209–16
  Bayesian methods 214–16
  and conditional likelihood 171–2
  and dropouts 317
  examples of use 231, *232*, 237–40
  maximum likelihood estimation for 172–5, 212–14
generalized linear models (GLMs) 343–6
  contrasting approaches 131–7
  extensions 126–40
    marginal models 126–8, 141–68
    random effects models 128–30, 169–89
    transition models 130–1, 190–207
  generic features 345–6
  inferences 137–40
general linear model (GLM) 54–80
  with correlated errors 55–9
    exponential correlation model 56–7
    uniform correlation model 55–6
geostatistics 49
Gibbs sampling 174, 180, 214

Granger non-causality 246
graphical representation of longitudinal data 6–7, *12*, 34–41
  further reading recommended 53
  guidelines 33
growth curve model 92

Hammersly–Clifford Theorem 21
hat notation 60
hierarchical random effects model 334, 336
holly leaves, effect of pH on drying rate 120–3
human immune deficiency virus (HIV) 3
  see also CD4+ cell numbers data

ignorable missing values 284
independence estimating equations (IEEs) 257
individual trajectories
  prediction of 110–13
    example using CD4+ data 112–13
Indonesian Children's Health Study (ICHS) 4, *5*
  marginal model used 17–18, 127, 132, 135–6, 141, 156–60
  random effects model used 18, 129, 130, 132–3, 182–4
  time-dependent covariates 247
  transition model used 18, 130–1, 133, 197–201
inference(s)
  about generalized linear models 137–40
  about model parameters 94, 97–8
informative dropout mechanisms 295, 316
  in example 313–16
  representation by pattern mixture models 299–301
informative dropouts
  consequences 318
  investigation of 298, 318, 330
informative missing values 80, 283
intercept
  of linear regression model 337
  random intercept models 90–1, 170, 210, *211*
intermediate variable, meaning of term 265
intermittent missing values 284, 287, 318
internal covariates 246
inverse probability of treatment weights (IPTW)
  estimation of causal effects using 277–9
    in example 279–80
iterative proportional fitting 221

joint modelling, of longitudinal measurements and recurrent events 329–32
joint probability density functions 88–9

kernel estimation 42–3
  compared with other curve-fitting techniques *42*, *45*
  in examples *42*, *43*, *325*
kernel function 320
Kolmogorov–Smirnov statistic 290, 291

lag 46
lagged covariates 259–65
  example 261–5
  multiple lagged covariates 260–1
  single lagged covariate 259–60
last observation carried forward 287–8
latent variable models 129
  marginalized models 222–5
least-squares estimation 338–9
  further reading recommended 339
  optimality property 338–9
least-squares estimator 338
  bias in 23–4
  variance of 63
  weighted 59–64, 70
likelihood-based methods
  for categorical data 208–44
  for generalized linear mixed models 209–16
  for marginalized models 216–31
  for non-linear models 328
likelihood functions 138, 171, 173, 340
likelihood inference 340–3
  examples 341–3
likelihood ratio testing 98, 342
likelihood ratio test statistic 342
linear links 191
linear models 337–8
  and least-squares estimation method 338–9
  marginal modelling approach 132
  random effects model 132–3
  transition model 133–4
linear regression model 337

link functions 191–2, 345
logistic regression models 343, *344*
  and dropouts 292
  generalized estimating equations for 146–7
    example *251*
  and lagged covariates 261–5
  marginal-modelling approach 127, 135–6, 146–7
  and Markov chain 191
  random effects modelling approach 134–5, 175–80
    examples 176–7, 180–4
logit links 191
log likelihood ratio (test) statistic 98, 309
log-linear models 142–3, 344
  canonical parameters in 143, 153
  marginalized models 220–1
  marginal-modelling approach 137, 143–6, 162, 164–5
  random effects modelling approach 137
log-linear transition models, for count data 204–6
log-links 191
log odds ratios 52, 129, 147, 341
  in examples 200, 235, *236*
  standard error (in example) 148–9
longitudinal data
  association among categorical responses 52–3
  collection of 1–2
  correlation structure 46–52
    consequences of ignoring 19
  curve smoothing for 41–5
  defining feature 2
  example data sets 3–15
    calf intestinal parasites experiment *117*
    CD4+ cell numbers data 3–4
    cow weight data *103*
    dysmenorrhoeal pain treatment trial 7, 9, *10*
    epileptic seizure clinical trial 10, *11*, *12*
    Indonesian children's health study 4, 5
    milk protein data 5–7, *8*, *9*
    pig weight data *34*
    schizophrenia clinical trial 10–13, *14*
    Sitka spruce growth data 4–5, *6*, *7*
  general linear models for 54–80
  graphical representation 6–7, *12*, 34–41
    further reading recommended 53
    guidelines 33
  missing values in 282–318
longitudinal data analysis
  approaches 17–20
    marginal analysis 17–18
    random effects model 18
    transition model 18
    two-stage/derived variable analysis 17
  classification of problems 20
  confirmatory analysis 33
  exploratory data analysis 33–53
longitudinal studies 1–3
  advantages 1, 16–17, 22, 245
  compared with cross-sectional studies 1, 16–17, 22–31
  efficiency 24–6
lorelogram 34, 52–3
  further reading recommended 53
lowess smoothing 41, 44
  compared with other curve-fitting methods *42*, *45*
  examples *3*, *36*, *40*

Madras Longitudinal Schizophrenia Study 234–7
  analysis using marginalized models 240–3
marginal analysis 18
marginal generalized linear regression model 209
marginalized latent variable models 222–5, 232
  maximum likelihood estimation for 225
marginalized log-linear models 220–1, 233
marginalized models
  for categorical data 216–31
  examples of use 231–3, 240–3
  example using Gaussian linear model 218–20
marginalized random effects models 222, *223*, 225
marginalized transition models 225–31
  advantages 230–1
  in examples 233, 241–3
  first-order/MTM(1) 226–7, 230, 241
    in example 241, *242*
  second-order/MTM(2) 228
    in example *242*

marginal mean response 17
marginal means
  definition 209
  likelihood-based estimates *232*, *242*
  log-linear model for 143–6
marginal models 17–18, 126–8, 141–68
  advantages of direct approach 216–17
  assumptions 126–7
  examples of use 17–18, 127, 132, 135–6, 148–60
  further reading recommended 167–8
  and likelihood 138
marginal odds ratios 145, 147
marginal quasi-likelihood (MQL) methods 232
marginal structural models (MSMs) 276
  advantage(s) 280
  estimation using IPTW 277–9
    in example 279–80
Markov Chain Monte Carlo (MCMC) methods 214–16, 332
  in examples *232*, *238*
Markov chains 131, 190
Markov models 87, 190–206
  further reading recommended 206–7
  see also transition models
Markov–Poisson time series model 204–5
  realization of *206*
maximum likelihood algorithms 212
maximum likelihood estimation 64–5
  compared with REML estimation 69, 95
  for generalized linear mixed models 212–14
  in parametric modelling 98
  for random effects models 137–8, 172–5
  restricted 66–9
  for transition models 138, 192–3
  see also conditional likelihood; generalized estimating equations
maximum likelihood estimator 60, 64, 340
  variance 60
MCEM method *see* Monte Carlo Expectation-Maximization method
MCMC methods *see* Markov Chain Monte Carlo methods
MCNR method *see* Monte Carlo Newton–Raphson method
mean response
  non-parametric modelling of 319–26
  parametric modelling of 105–7
mean response profile(s)
  for calf intestinal parasites experiment *118*
  for cow weight data *106*
  defined in ANOVA 114
  for milk protein data 99, *100*, *102*, *302*
  for schizophrenia trial data *14*, *307*, 309, *311*, *315*
measurement error
  and random effects 91–3
  and serial correlation 89–90
and random intercept 90–1
  as source of random variation 83
measurement variation 28
micro/macro data-representation strategy 37
milk protein data 5–7, *8*, *9*
  dropouts in 290–1
    reasons for 285
    testing for completely random dropouts 291–3
  mean response profiles 99, *100*, *102*, *302*
  parametric model fitted 99–103
  pattern mixture analysis of 301, *302*
  variogram 50, 52, 99
missing value mechanisms
  classification of 283–4
  completely random 283, 284
  random 283, 284
missing values 282–318
  effects 282
  ignorable 284
  informative 80, 283
  intermittent 284, 287, 318
  and parametric modelling 80
model-based variance 347
model-fitting 93–8
  diagnostic stage 98
  estimation stage 95–7
  formulation stage 94–5
  inference stage 97–8
moments of response 138
Monte Carlo Expectation-Maximization (MCEM) method 214
Monte Carlo maximum likelihood algorithms 214
Monte Carlo Newton–Raphson (MCNR) method 214
Monte Carlo test(s), for completely random dropouts 290, 291

Mothers' Stress and Children's Morbidity (MSCM) Study 247–53
cross-sectional analysis 257–8
and endogeneity 268–9
g-computation 275–6
and lagged covariates 261–5
marginal structural models using IPTW 279–80
sample of data *252*
Multicenter AIDS Cohort Study (MACS) 3
CESD (depressive symptoms) scores 39–40, *41*
objective(s) 3–4
see also CD4+ cell numbers data
multiple lagged covariates 260–1
multivariate Gaussian theory 339–40
multivariate longitudinal data 332–6
examples 332

natural parameter 345
negative-binomial distribution 161, 186–7
Nelder–Mead simplex algorithm 340
nested sub-models 342
Newton–Raphson iteration 340
non-linear random effects, in cross-sectional models 327, 329
non-linear regression model 326–7
fitting to cross-sectional data 327
non-linear regression modelling 326–9
non-parametric curve-fitting techniques 41–5
see also kernel estimation; lowess; smoothing spline
non-parametric modelling of mean response 319–26
notation 15–16
causal models 271
conditional generalized linear model 209
dropout models 295
marginal generalized linear model 209
maximum likelihood estimator 60
multivariate Gaussian distribution 339–40
non-linear regression model 326–7
parametric models 83–4
time-dependent covariates 245
no-unmeasured-confounders assumption 270–1, 273
numerical integration methods 212–14

odds ratio, in marginal model 127, 128
ordered categorical data 201–4
proportional odd modelling of 201–3
ordering statistic, data representation using 38
ordinary least squares (OLS) estimation
and ignoring correlation in data 19
naive use 63
errors arising 63–4
in nonlinear regression modelling 119
relative efficiency
in crossover example *63*
in exponential correlation model 61–2
in linear regression example *62*
in uniform correlation model 60–1
in robust estimation of standard errors 70, 75, *76*
and sample variogram 50, 52
outliers, and curve fitting 44–5
over-dispersed count data, models for 161, 186–7
over-dispersion 162, 178, 346
ozone pollution
effect on tree growth 4–5
see also Sitka spruce growth data

panel studies 2
parametric modelling 81–113
for count data 160–2
example applications 99–110
CD4+ data 108–10
cow weight data 103–8
milk protein data 99–103
fitting model to data 93–8
further reading recommended 113
notation 83–4
pure serial correlation model 84–9
random effects + measurement error model 91–3
random intercept + serial correlation + measurement error model 90–1
serial correlation + measurement error model 89–90
and sources of random variation 82–3
partly conditional mean 253
partly conditional models 259–60
pattern mixture dropout models 299–301
graphical representation *303*, 304
Pearson chi-squared statistic 186
Pearson's chi-squared test statistic 343

penalized quasi-likelihood (PQL) methods 175, 210, 232
example of use *232*
period 1
pig weight data *34*
graphical representation 34–5, *35*, *36*
robust estimation of standard errors for 76–9
point process data 330
Poisson distribution 161, 186, 344
Poisson-gamma distribution 347
Poisson–Gaussian random effects models 188–9
Poisson regression models 344
population growth 205
Positive And Negative Syndrome Scale (PANSS) measure 11, 153, 330, 332
subset of placebo data *305*
treatment effects 334, *335*
potential outcomes 269–70
power of statistical test 28
predictive squared error (PSE) 45
predictors 337
principal components analysis, in data representation 38
probability density functions 88–9
proportional odds model 201–2
application to Markov chain 202–3
prospective collection of longitudinal data 1, 2

quadratic form (test) statistic 97, 309
quadrature methods 212–14
limitations 214
quasi-likelihood methods 232, 346–8
in example 347–8
see also marginal quasi-likelihood (MQL) methods; penalized quasi-likelihood (PQL) methods
quasi-score function 346

random dropout mechanism 285
random effects + measurement error models 91–3
random effects dropout models 301–3
in example 312–14
graphical representation *303*, 304, 305
random effects models 18, 82, 128–30, 169–89
assumptions 170–1
basic premise 129, 169
examples of use 18, 129, 130, 132–3
fitting using maximum likelihood method 137–8
further reading recommended 189
hierarchical 334, 336
marginalized 222, *223*, 225
multi-level 93
and two-stage least-squares estimation 57–9
random intercept models 90–1, 170, 210, *211*
in example 239
random intercept + random slope (random line) models 210, *211*, 238
in example 238–9
random intercept + serial correlation + measurement error model 90–1
random missingness mechanism 283
generalized estimating equations under 293–5
random missing values 283, 284
random variation
separation from systematic variation 217, 218
sources 82–3
two-level models 93
reading ability/age example 1, 2, 16
recurrent event data 330
recurrent events, joint modelling with longitudinal measurements 329–32
regression analysis 337
regression models
notation 15
see also linear ...; non-linear regression model
relative growth rate (RGR) 92
repeated measures ANOVA 123–5
see also split-plot ANOVA approach
repeated observations
correlation among 28
number per person 28
respiratory disease/infection, in Indonesian children 4, 131–6, 156–60, 182–4
restricted maximum likelihood (REML) estimation 66–9
compared with maximum likelihood estimation 69, 95
in parametric modelling 96, 99, *100*

restricted maximum likelihood (REML) estimation (*cont.*)
in robust estimation of standard errors 70–1, 73–4, 79
retrospective collection of longitudinal data 1–2
Rice–Silverman prescription 321, 322
robust estimation of standard errors 70–80
examples 73–9
robust variance 194, 347
roughness penalty 44

sample size calculations 25–31
binary responses 30–1
continuous responses 28–30
for marginal models 165–7
parameters required 25–8
sample variogram(s) 49
examples *51*, *90*, *102*, *105*, *107*
SAS software 180, 214
saturated models 50, 65
graphical representation *303*
limitations 65
robust estimation of standard errors in 70–1, 73
scatterplots 33, 40
and correlation structure 46, *47*
examples *36*, *38–43*, *45*, *47*
schizophrenia clinical trial 10–13
dropouts in 12, *13*, 306–16
marginal model used 153–6
mean response profiles *14*, *307*, *311*, *315*
multivariate data 332, 334, *335*
PANSS measure 11, 153, 330, 332
subset of placebo data *305*
treatment effects 334, *335*
random effects model used 181–2
variograms *308*, *314*
schizophrenia study (Madras Longitudinal Study) 234–7
analysis of data 237–43
score equations 173–4, 340
score function 340
score test statistic(s) 241, 242, 342
second-order marginalized transition model/MTM(2) 228
in example *242*
selection dropout models 295–8
in example 312–16
graphical representation *303*, 304–5
semi-parametric modelling 324
sensitivity analysis, and informative dropout models 316
serial correlation 82
plus measurement error 89–90
and random intercept 90–1
pure 84–9
as source of random variation 82
Simulated Maximum Likelihood (SML) method 214
single lagged covariate 259–60
Sitka spruce growth data 4–5, *6*, *7*
derived variables used 119–20
robust estimation of standard errors for 73–6, *77*
split-plot ANOVA applied 124–5
size-dependent branching process 204–5
smallest meaningful difference 27
smoothing spline 44, 320
compared with other curve-fitting techniques *42*
smoothing techniques 33–4, 41–5, 319
further reading recommended 41, 53
spline 44
see also smoothing spline
split-plot ANOVA approach 56, 123–5
example of use 124–5
split-plot model 92, 123, 124
stabilized weights 277
in example *278*
standard errors
robust estimation of 70–80
examples 73–9
standardized residuals, in graphical representation 35, *36*
STATA software 214
stochastic covariates 253–8
strong exogeneity 246–7
structural nested models, further reading recommended 281
survival analysis 2
systematic variation, separation from random variation 217, 218

time-by-time ANOVA 115–16, 125
example of use 116, *118*
time-dependent confounders 265–80
time-dependent covariates 245–81
time series analysis 2
time-by-time ANOVA, limitations 115–16
tracking 35

trajectories *see* individual trajectories
transition matrix 194, 195
transition models 18, 130–1, 190–207
  for categorical data 194–204
    examples 197–201
  for count data 204–6
  examples of use 18, 130–1, 133, 197–201
  fitting of 138, 192–4
  marginalized 225–31
  for ordered categorical data 201–4
  see also Markov models
transition ordinal regression model 203
tree growth data *see* Sitka spruce growth data
Tufte's micro/macro data-representation strategy 37
two-level models of random variation 93
two-stage analysis 17
two-stage least-squares estimation 57–9
type I error rate 26–7

unbalanced data 282
uniform correlation model 55–6, 285

variance functions 345
variograms 34, 48–50
  autocorrelation function estimated from 50
  in examples *51*, *52*, *308*, *314*, *326*
  for exponential correlation model *85*
  further reading recommended 53
  for Gaussian correlation model *86*
  for parametric models *102*, *105*, *107*
  for random intercepts + serial correlation + measurement error model *91*
  for serial correlation models 84–7
  for stochastic process 48, 82
  see also sample variogram
vitamin A deficiency
  causes and effects 4, 197
  see also Indonesian Children's Health Study

Wald statistic 233, 241
weighted average 320
weighted least-squares estimation 59–64
working variance matrix 70
  choice not critical 76
  in examples 76, 78

xerophthalmia 4, 197
  see also Indonesian Children's Health Study